While the Music Lasts

on Music and Dementia

ISBN: 978-90-5972-846-2

Research Group Lifelong Learning in Music

Prince Claus Conservatoire / Hanze Research 'Art and Society'

Hanze University of Applied Sciences, Groningen

Veemarktstraat 76

9724 GA Groningen, The Netherlands

www.lifelonglearninginmusic.nl

Eburon Academic Publishers

Oude Delft 224

2611 HJ Delft

tel.: 015-2131484

info@eburon.nl / www.eburon.nl

Cover design and production: digiTAAL, duurzaam communiceren, Groningen, www.dt.nl

Design content: Studio Frank & Lisa, Groningen

DTP content: Peter van Munster

Scores: Kate Page / Syberen van Munster

Graphics: Karoline Dausien

Photo cover: Linda Rose

With gratitude to Hanze University of Applied Sciences, Groningen

While the Music Lasts

on Music and Dementia

Rineke Smilde, Kate Page and Peter Alheit

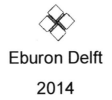

Eburon Delft

2014

For most of us, there is only the unattended
Moment, the moment in and out of time,
The distraction fit, lost in a shaft of sunlight,
The wild thyme unseen, or the winter lightning
Or the waterfall, or music heard so deeply
That it is not heard at all, but you are the music
While the music lasts.

T.S. Eliot (from: The Dry Salvages, 1941)

For Sieb Smilde

TABLE OF CONTENTS

Chapter

Preface

This book has been written for musicians who want to engage with audiences beyond the concert hall and other traditional venues. The study is equally worthwhile for conservatoires and music academies aiming to change the increasingly unrealistic goal of training young musicians solely for the stage.

When taking the changing music profession and its market opportunities seriously, higher music education institutions can become aware of creative opportunities for establishing professional music practices in areas in society that are remote from concert halls and big festivals, from public media and stardom, and instead look for settings which reach out to various kinds of audiences. This does not mean, of course, that the results presented here wish to diminish the wonderful gift of being an accomplished soloist or chamber musician, but they would like to show that the role of music can be exhaustive, where artistic connection can bring about strong communication between people. Music can make a difference and be deeply influential, especially in social fields of illness and suffering, weakness and depression.

'Music and dementia' is the challenging topic of this book. It is not about educational suggestions to care staff to sing well-known children's songs in care homes for residents with dementia, just to lift the mood. Through engaging in music as a participatory process, its goal is to make *the person behind the dementia* visible again. The project presented in this study not only shows that this idea can be realised for people with dementia and their caregivers, but it has also opened up learning processes for the musicians involved which nobody would have expected before, nurturing their professional lives and development. The project has changed their understanding of the place of music in people's lives; it has touched their personality and stimulated deep reflections about their identity. This positive effect should benefit young musicians in their music education.

However, musicians are not the only target group. The discoveries of the study are also helpful and inspiring for caregivers of people with dementia and for families of a loved one living with dementia.

The book explores the interaction between music and dementia through the stories of people who have been working closely together: three musicians, eight women living with dementia, five caregivers, a staff development practitioner, a project coordinator and three scientific observers. The result is a book in which all of them have participated in their own way. It consists of field observations, reflective journals, conversations, interviews and careful scientific analyses. If it can be read by many people at a profit, the project has worked. There will be, in the words of Clifford Geertz,[1] a 'thick description' of a new friendship between music and dementia, a story about a fascinating practice that will stimulate and bolster committed people.

---

[1] Geertz 1973.

The authors would like to thank first of all Linda Rose, founder of the project 'Music for Life' and in addition Wigmore Hall and Dementia UK as well as the organisation Jewish Care in London, in particular Padraic Garrett, for their trust and cooperation. We would also like to thank Peter Renshaw for his invaluable reflective contribution to this book.

First and for all however, we are deeply grateful to the protagonists of the story, who were willing to share their learning path and experiences. We will meet and get to know them in the next chapters where we will unfold our fascinating journey.

Rineke Smilde, Groningen (The Netherlands)

Kate Page, Perth (Australia)

Peter Alheit, Berlin (Germany)

1

If music be the food of love, play on…

Introduction

If music be the food of love, play on…

William Shakespeare[2]

1   Introduction

During approximately the last fifteen years we have seen an increase in the creative work of musicians and other artists engaging with new audiences in the wider community beyond the concert hall and other traditional venues. This happened first and foremost in the United Kingdom, gradually spreading throughout Europe. A decade ago, Peter Renshaw already argued that, "It is imperative that musicians and the whole arts community begin to engage in both a local and global debate about who we are and what we can achieve together."[3] He felt that a fundamental challenge to the arts was to ensure that performers, composers, teachers and artistic leaders "create live, shared experiences which have something to say and make sense to audiences in different contexts."[4]

Active participation in cultural activities, as for instance in participatory music-making, can be seen at the heart of building up individual and collective identity. This goes for all audiences, be it a classroom with children or a group of people living with dementia. The aim of the research into 'Music and Dementia' as described in this book was to explore the practice of music workshops created for elderly people with dementia and their care staff as they take place within the project 'Music for Life' in the United Kingdom. Music for Life was founded by music educator Linda Rose[5] since 1993 and has been developed in association with the organisation Jewish Care[6] and a growing team of musicians. Since 2009 the project has been managed by the well known concert venue Wigmore Hall, London in partnership with Dementia UK.[7]

The practice

The project comprises a series of interactive creative music workshops in care homes and day care centres for people with dementia. During a period of eight weeks three musicians work with a group of eight residents and five

---

[2] From Twelfth Night, 1601.
[3] Renshaw 2001.
[4] Ibid.
[5] See for more information Appendix III.
[6] Jewish Care is described in Appendix I.
[7] Wigmore Hall and Dementia UK are described in Appendix I.

members of the care staff, using musical improvisation as a catalyst to bring about communication in the widest sense at various levels. The objectives of the project are to strengthen the relationships between people with dementia and those with their caregivers. Musicians and care staff work as a team within the sessions.[8]

The musicians use a wide range of verbal and non-verbal ways in order to reach the individual residents and the residents and care staff as a *group*. Both the pleasure in music-making and the reflection of the care staff on the impact of the sessions are important. The insights and motivation which the care staff may gain can result in positive long-term effects on their work with the residents.[9] This is why, during a project, a professional development trajectory for the care staff takes place, led by a staff development practitioner of Jewish Care or Dementia UK. It is important: "Staff (...) come away from the project knowing each individual better. The knowledge is not based on facts about that person's life, even though it often sparks further interest into the person's history; it is based on having seen that person express their personality."[10]

One project takes eight successive weeks. Three musicians, one of which serves as the workshopleader, work together with the care staff development practitioner and care staff. During each weekly session, which lasts an hour, residents and members of the care staff are seated in a circle together with the musicians. In the middle of the circle a number of easy-to-play instruments are displayed in an attractive way. At the beginning of the session the musicians play a short piece that they composed especially for the group. This 'framing piece' serves as a framework for improvisation, "it marks the cornerstone of each workshop, providing a secure and predictable start and end to each session, but also with the opportunity to be shaped in response to the mood of individuals or to the group as a whole."[11] The opening piece is always followed by the 'welcome song', where the names of the participants within the circle are sung, serving as a recurring tool for recognition in the sessions. From there, through active sensitive and applied improvisation, an hour of shorter and longer music pieces follows, in which the residents and care staff are activated to participate, or sometimes even to make their own piece, together with one of the musicians.[12]

The musicians try to reach the residents by having their antennae on full alert. The smallest verbal and non-verbal signals of the residents can be picked up by the musicians, and the care staff gradually join in the process. Once musical communication is established, for example when one of the

---

[8] Smilde 2011.
[9] Rose and Schlingensiepen 2001.
[10] Rose and De Martino 2008: 23.
[11] Linda Rose in Renshaw 2010: 223.
[12] Smilde 2011.

residents holds a baton and the musicians respond to the person's movements, however minute, often a very special kind of interaction can be observed: "The workshop space becomes a place for all kinds of exploration, experiences ranging from the most joyful and celebratory to the gently amusing and teasing to the saddest sharing."[13]

In the workshops musicians need a '360 degrees radar' to keep everyone in the group safe enough to cope with unpredictability, risk, and trying something new. They need to be prepared to be out of their comfort zone whilst at the same time inspiring confidence in the group.[14] The musicians' sensitivity toward the people with dementia is of key importance. Often people with dementia have lost their language skills. The musicians do not perceive this as a problem; one of them interviewed in the preparatory phase of the research addressed this as "listening to something that is not tied to the words they use."

After each workshop there is a debriefing session between the musicians and members of the care staff, with the aim of providing an opportunity for reflection, discussion and learning. Members learn to articulate emerging issues, and the growing trust in the team enables staff, trainers and musicians to share dilemmas, pose questions, explore insights and express vulnerabilities, creating further opportunities for lasting change.[15]

Research shows that being engaged in musical communication can be beneficial for people living with dementia.[16] The Music for Life projects also show significant relevance for the interaction between the residents and the care staff, often deepened at a tacit and non-verbal level. The projects therefore are especially concerned with identity in its broadest sense, with finding, or rather 're-finding' the person behind the dementia.[17]

Focus of the research and the questions

With the key question being what learning and development takes place in each project, the focus of the research in this book was to explore the practice specifically from the musicians' perspective in order to inform future musician development. The research also aimed at building a clearer understanding of the dementia care context in which the musicians work in this project in order to inform their wider needs for professional development. The underpinning research questions were therefore:

[13] Linda Rose in Renshaw 2010: 221.
[14] Ibid: 224.
[15] Rose and De Martino 2008: 21.
[16] See e.g. Sacks 2008.
[17] Kitwood 1997: 10ff.

What happens in the music workshops?

What is learnt and what does this mean for the development of those involved?

These questions led to sub-questions addressing issues of what needs to be in place in terms of organisation, partnerships and shared understanding in order to gain quality in the project and also the question what needs to be taken into account when transferring the practice, e.g. to another country.

During a preparation phase preceding the in-depth research of one particular eight-week project, the practice of Music for Life was investigated, starting by researching existing material and holding interviews with founder Linda Rose and Padraic Garrett, staff development practitioner at Jewish Care; the observation of separate workshops and interviews with various musicians engaged in the project throughout the years.

In the autumn of 2010 a particular Music for Life project was researched, which took place in a brand new residential home in London, managed by Jewish Care, which we have called the Emanuel Zeffert House. Three musicians were part of it, they included Matthew, the workshopleader and oboist, and the supporting musicians Anneliese (harpist) and Fiona (cellist). Also the care staff development practitioner Brian was involved in the research. Field notes were made consisting of observations of each workshop; narrative interviews took place, consisting of thematic interviews with the three musicians as a group and expert interviews with the workshopleader and care staff development practitioner following each weekly session. In addition, throughout the project reflective journals were kept by the three musicians and the care staff development practitioner.

Informed consent[18] was sought from all participants involved, including the families of the residents with dementia who took part in the music workshops. In order to secure the privacy of the participants, their names are shaded in this book.[19]

The contents of this book

Chapter 2 comprises a conceptual framework which aims at providing important background information related to the researched practice. It consists of three parts that address the three areas of 'music and dementia', 'communication and participation', and 'learning and leadership'. Relevant information on dementia informs what needs to be known in order to connect responsibly to the context of engaging artistically with people with dementia and their carers in the institutional environment of a residential home. The person-centred approach underpinning this practice, together with key

---

[18] See also Garrett 2009.
[19] See Appendix IV for an overview of the protagonists.

learning processes and styles are described, as well as the role of (applied) musical improvisation as a tool for various forms of communication.

The third chapter focuses on the methodology of the research, describing 'grounded theory', in which the theory generated through coding of data and reflection can inform the development of practice. Grounded theory is explained both historically and as a method, and finally we address the way we worked in this particular study. The most substantial part of the study, chapter 4, consists of an analysis and 'thick' description of the data, which by means of the coding results in identifying the four main themes of Identity, Communication, Participation and Development. Conclusions and a discussion close the study.

The book contains five appendices, meant to support the reader in thinking about putting the project into practice. The first appendix deals with detailed information about the project Music for Life in the UK. In the second appendix project founder and developer Linda Rose gives a comprehensive overview of what is entailed in the project management of musicians engaging with people with dementia and their carers in residential homes. It includes a pragmatic and reflective framework for the management of the project, a wide-ranging analysis of the roles and responsibilities of a project manager, observations on monitoring and evaluation, and a description of three realistic scenarios illustrating what management might look like in practice. In the same appendix, reflections on project management are given by learning consultant Peter Renshaw, based on interviews with several practitioners involved with the Music for Life project.

The third appendix consists of a biography of Linda Rose and her work in the context of this study. The fourth appendix gives an overview of the protagonists and finally a list of instruments, constituting the fifth appendix, informs the reader about the musical instruments that are used in the practice.

2

…music, and only music, can do the calling

Conceptual Framework

Once one has seen such responses, one knows that there is still a self to be called upon, even if music, and only music, can do the calling.

Oliver Sacks[20]

2.1   Music and Dementia

Each Music for Life project is a unique reflection of the interactions and identities of a converging group of participants, situated in relation to the environmental and organisational culture in which the activity takes place. Each project is the sum of its characters, its context; projects may involve similar logistical and creative processes, but at heart, projects are about the people involved, their learning journey and the connections they make with each other through engagement in communication and participation. The project, as Jewish Care staff development practitioner Padraic Garrett describes in an interview, is "how you are with people, what you do for people, what you are with people (...) every Music for Life project is a project in itself, that's independent and is different."

The profile of staff and residents in participating care settings in London often reflects the broad cultural diversity of Greater London. Emanuel Zeffert House, the setting in London at which this research took place, reflected this diversity in its overall staff profile. In this Jewish Care managed setting, there was a large contingent from South East Asia, Eastern Europe and Africa, alongside staff from throughout Great Britain. Within this staff group, there was a mixture of educational backgrounds, socio-economic status and religious beliefs. This diversity was at counterpoint with residents at Emanuel Zeffert House – many of whom were generally of European origin, long-term residents within the UK, relatively affluent and with highly educated backgrounds, all united through their practice of Jewish faith. A commonality within the setting was gender, with a high proportion of both staff and residents being female.

In this particular project transition was a key motif. Emanuel Zeffert House had recently opened as a flagship care setting in the heart of the Jewish community. Most of the residents and staff were drawn from two homes which were closing for redevelopment; homes in which many had established long-term connections, relationships and associations. The relocation had been managed sensitively within Jewish Care, with an awareness of the impact of potential emotional issues that could be invoked by a very physical transition; including fracturing of relationships between

---

[20] Sacks 2008: 385.

staff and residents, insecurity or confusion due to lack of familiarity of environment.

Transition was also present as an issue in terms of the managerial context of the home. Some staff had left the organisation during the relocation, resulting in a situation where some staff members were relatively new, or still being recruited, with existing staff working hard to ensure that an excellent quality of care was still being delivered. The physical layout of the new home was very different than in the previous working environments, fracturing existing configurations of staff teams, alongside the personal and professional relationships that underpinned these teams.

At the time of this project, there was a sense that immediate impact of the relocation had been reduced, and a growing sense of security was developing for residents. However the project was seen as a real opportunity for further integration into the home and the development of meaningful relationships, looking towards enabling a sense of celebration within the home. Staff development practitioner Brian reflected on the unique opportunity for interaction and engagement that the starting Music for Life project could present, saying, *"My sense of the home at the moment is that it's pretty calm in terms of residents (...) I think they have that calm at this stage; considering what they went through, I think that's a really good thing (...) But maybe what there lacks at the moment, there needs to be a bit more stimulation (...) And I think we're doing that with Music for Life."*

It is important to also consider the impact of the research on the project. Participation in the research, prior to and during the project, was perceived as a positive opportunity by those involved; an opportunity to broaden the existing reflective practice of the delivery team (i.e. musicians, staff development practitioner and project manager) through participation in interviews and reflective journals.

The person-centred approach

Dementia, as an umbrella term, is used to describe progressive impairment of the brain structure and chemistry as a result of a range of specific diseases and conditions. Common expressions of dementia are difficulties in communication and language skills and in processing, interpreting and recalling information. These difficulties can manifest themselves in a variety of ways: engaging in and interpreting verbal language; verbal expression including words for objects, names; remembering and recalling recent events; taking in or focusing on new information; remembering and recognising people; experiencing a 'different reality' from others.

The experience of dementia is different for each person, related to the nature and progression of their neurological impairment, the state of their physical health, their life history, character and identity, and the attitudes and behaviour of others in their social context. Thus, dementia transgresses its status as a medical condition; it is a complex disability with tremendous scope to interact with and impact on the emotional and social fabric of a person's life.

In the past, traditional definitions of dementia centred on a medically oriented, pathological perspective of the condition, largely ignoring the social aspects and impact of the condition on the individual. A modern culture of ageism, enhanced by concepts of progression and a drive for productivity in all aspects of life, created an environment of stigmatisation and misunderstanding.

Even today, the picture painted of dementia is often one of ultimate suffering: where the person with dementia lacks the capacity for well-being and self-awareness, their identity and capacity for self-growth is stripped away; "a death that leaves the body behind".[21] The reality of dementia can potentially be difficult for others to cope with; for instance, the attempts to communicate with a person with dementia could be perceived as 'challenging behaviour', rather than an expression of that person's lived experience and an opportunity for others to understand the person with dementia's subjective reality and develop meaningful communication in a way that enhances their well-being. Individuals around the person with dementia may experience a variety of emotions and negative attitudes, which, if amplified in their relations with the person, can lead to the development of a *malignant social psychology*, a mode where the person with dementia is depersonalised, excluded and oppressed; their personhood undermined.[22]

A paradigm shift in the way dementia is perceived and how dementia care is approached was pioneered by Tom Kitwood in his seminal publication 'Dementia Reconsidered: The Person Comes First'.[23] Kitwood's perspectives transformed this bleak outlook into a more positive ethos in which the *personhood* of the person with dementia is at the forefront. Personhood recognises that the person with dementia transcends their condition; they are a *Person with dementia* rather than a *person with Dementia*, with needs just like any other person.[24] It embraces the uniqueness of all persons, highlighting that all persons are of value, that we all deserve recognition, respect and trust, and possess the need to feel loved. It acknowledges that the psychological needs of comfort, attachment, inclusion, occupation and identity are important aspects in the well-being of a person.[25] These tenets

[21] Kitwood 1997: 37.
[22] Ibid: 47.
[23] Kitwood 1997.
[24] Ibid: 7.
[25] Ibid: 81-83.

10

form the cornerstone of a person-centred care approach, in which emotional well-being is enhanced, and the unique personhood of a person with dementia acknowledged, valued and celebrated. Within the project Music for Life, the personhood of all participants – people living with dementia, care staff, musicians – is valued as a central tenet, creating the conditions for an egalitarian learning environment and equality in relationships.

In enhancing the personhood of a person with dementia, there are ways in which the carer and person with dementia can interact, *positive person work*, which centres on curating a socially and psychologically positive environment for emotional well-being. Kitwood outlines the importance of holding, validation and the recognition of the value of the person with dementia, which can act together to provide a sense of emotional security and belonging. He emphasises the need to create opportunities for fostering states of timalation[26], relaxation, and celebration to be experienced, thus enabling the person with dementia to engage meaningfully in activity through facilitation, negotiation and collaboration, alongside a space where the person with dementia can interact with others freely and on their own terms through the acts of creation and giving.[27] Brian highlights the importance of a sense of faith in this regard; in order for these positive interactions to occur, an attitude of belief in the potential of the person living with dementia must be present: "*Celebration is important. Music for Life is planting a seed of belief in our ability to celebrate and enjoy life with the residents at Emanuel Zeffert House.*"

In order to 'believe', to truly enact person-centred care and meaningfully connect with the person with dementia, the relationship between carer and the person with dementia needs to be authentic, and the carer must possess empathic qualities, strong motivation and a sense of curiosity and discovery.[28]

It is important for care staff to be able to become 'present' in their awareness of the reality of the person with dementia, evolving from a 'state of doing' to a 'state of being', which may mean letting go of their assumptions and anxieties, and valuing subconscious experiences and intuition. Brian reflects on the importance of his role as staff development practitioner in endorsing the importance of emotional reflection and enabling opportunities for this type of reflection to occur: "*For me the value lies more in being able to feel the project and the sessions and it is only in this way that we can allow it to do its work. When one experiences something powerfully, it leaves a deep and lasting impression. As the staff development worker on the project, I want to safeguard staff members' opportunities to allow the experience sink deeply within them. Words are often not the*

---

[26] Interaction where the prime modality is sensuous or sensual (Ibid: 90).
[27] Ibid: 90-92.
[28] Rogers 1961.

vehicle for this. Time to allow the feelings to integrate and motivate are of ultimate importance."

There are challenges in developing the conditions for person-centred care in care organisations at a macro, meso and micro level, and it is possible for the concept of person-centred care to become rhetoric. Social and political values, human and financial resources, the organisational culture, the complex, high-energy nature of the work, and the personal attributes, skills, experiences and intrinsic motivation of staff all have an impact on the ability of organisations and individuals to engage at a person-centred level.[29] Brian recognises these challenges as endemic issues faced by many care homes and care organisations within the UK, acknowledging the complex nature of care work and the great need for change of attitude at a societal level, stating, *"I sometimes reflect on the expectations put on care staff generally. We provide them with training and raise their awareness of working in person-centred ways. However, they invariably work in care home situations where they often feel under pressure to have time to do their work according to person-centred principles. The greatest tension is trying to work according to the pace of the person with dementia. This is very difficult in homes with a ratio of one staff member to four residents. Our society hasn't yet been prepared to value people with dementia as deserving a higher ratio of staff."*

Brian makes a clear call for the development of a different attitude and approach from society at large if care is to become truly person-centred. At the heart of the person-centred movement is a fundamental respect for personhood; if we value and believe in the ability of people living with dementia to develop and sustain meaningful, interconnected relationships with others, a sense of shared vision entailing respect, love, compassion and understanding must become vital and valued tenets for everyone involved.

From person-centred to biographical approach

The concept of personhood is, according to Kitwood, underpinned by three types of discourse: those of transcendence, considering life as 'sacred', those of ethics, considering that each individual has the right to be valued and those within social psychology. The latter addresses issues like self-esteem, the place of an individual within a social group, the performance of given roles and "integrity, continuity and the stability of the sense of self".[30] The definition of personhood derived from these discourses reads: "a standing or status that is bestowed upon one human being, by others, in the context of relationship and social being. It implies recognition, respect

---

[29] Kitwood 1997: 103 -116.
[30] Kitwood 1997: 8.

and trust. Both the according of personhood, and the failure to do so, have consequences that are empirically testable."[31]

Within the context of personhood Kitwood also addresses the recognition of the many ways in which biographical knowledge can be incorporated into care planning and practice: for example based on care staff consulting with family members on the life histories of people with dementia.[32] He furthermore states that "In dementia the sense of identity based on having a life story to tell may eventually fade (...) When it does, biographical knowledge about a person becomes essential if that identity is still to be held in place."[33] Kitwood suggests that it is essential to regard personhood in terms of relationships, if we are to understand dementia: "Even when cognitive impairment is very severe, an I-Thou form of meeting and relating is often possible."[34] Thus, even in this context the position of Giddens is relevant, who describes self-identity as the self as reflexively understood by the person in terms of her or his biography and where the capacity to use 'I' in shifting contexts, is the most elemental feature of reflexive conceptions of personhood.[35] Giddens argues that,

> The existential question of self-identity is bound up with the fragile nature of the biography which the individual 'supplies' about herself. A person's identity is not to be found in behaviour, nor - important though it is - in the reactions of others, but in the capacity to keep a particular narrative going.[36]

Projects like the current one under study are concerned with finding, or rather 're-finding' the person behind the dementia.[37] Musicians engaging with people living with dementia and their carers aim to facilitate this process through music. The practice of finding the person behind the dementia through music can be underpinned by the words of George Herbert Mead on identity, where he states that "Both aspects of the 'I' and 'me' are essential to the self in its full expression."[38]

For the musicians themselves biographical learning and knowledge is also at stake. Daniel, a Music for Life musician who was interviewed in the initial stage of the research, observes:

> Doing this work has been a way for me to connect my musicianship with a deepening sense of who I am in this world, brought about by extraordinary interactions with extraordinary people (...) This work continues to teach me who I am, and is a benchmark against which I judge everything else I do. It's

---

[31] Ibid.
[32] Ibid: 56.
[33] Ibid.
[34] Ibid: 12.
[35] Giddens 1991: 53.
[36] Giddens 1991: 54.
[37] Kitwood 1997: 10ff.
[38] Mead 1934: 199.

extraordinary how working with people whose version of reality is so vague can in fact be the ultimate reality check!

For everybody involved in the practice, musicians, residents and care staff alike, the concept of *empowerment* is vital. Empowerment refers to "an experience that changes an individual's understanding of him or herself and/or the world."[39] It strengthens the notion of 'agency'.[40] The core of empowerment can be found in a *participatory* approach, which includes two interconnected aspects: the transformation in the individual's self-definition and the transformation of the social environment through participation.[41] 'Disempowerment' within participation occurs often in this practice: residents can feel disempowered as a result of their advanced stage of dementia and care staff can feel disempowered because they do not feel knowledgeable enough about music which can lead to feelings of strong anxiety and vulnerability. We also see disempowerment amongst musicians, where low self-esteem is often connected to high perfectionism in musical performance.[42]

Music as a new way of communication

Music belongs to a spiritual sphere, it is a timeless art expressed in a meta-physical language. Words can only capture one dimension of its ephemeral and spiritually resonant nature; music can communicate where words fail, expressing gestures that may never fully be able to be conveyed in words. Author Marcel Cobussen proposes that,

> The world in which music exists is a spiritual world. Music is an art in time, flowing in a bodiless world. It surpasses the borders of the universe of bodies. We cannot grasp music in the same way we touch and feel matter in our world. Like air, music does not show itself... Not only do we need our ears to hear music, the musician needs his body as an instrument to awaken music. Ears, drumming hands, stamping feet, the bow that moves the strings of the cello: these are all part of a bodily world. Music is born in a space that connects a spiritual and an embodied word.[43]

Relating to spiritual realm.

Music is often perceived as a transcendental language which we can all tap into intuitively through listening and music making, acting as mediums through which music flows, and inducing spiritual, trancelike states at an individual level. In this trancelike state, achieved through musical communication, it is possible to feel deeply connected to the experiences and feelings of others at a spiritual level. Matthew describes how in improvisation a sense of collective consciousness and recognition of a shared human experience can be attained: *"I'm again thinking about*

---

[39] Antikainen et al. 1996: 91.
[40] Antikainen 1998: 228.
[41] Ibid.
[42] Smilde 2009a.
[43] Cobussen 2008: 45.

14

Rebecca and singing with Rebecca, I can't think of anything that I've ever done in my life that's anything like it. You know, of kind of losing myself so much in the essence of another person (...) it's a real connection with their spirit, I think."

Musical language is at its essence inclusive, a language we can all access and understand, a language beyond our material world. It makes no demands of a person, except to listen. Listening entails not just opening your ears in a very practical sense, but also abstracting meaning from the music, interpreting the purity of what the music is trying to communicate.

Music is truly a celebration of life at its essence, reflecting who we are exactly as we are, complete with all of our imperfections and vulnerabilities. Music not only allows us to express aspects of our deepest emotional and spiritual selves, it also illuminates our self, our 'I'; a pure, truthful self separate from our social self. Gary Peters proposes:

> Art does not express the self, it meaningfully configures it. Where autonomy aesthetics (popular amongst improvisors) has a tendency to *assume* the self that, within the aesthetic realm at least, is free to act, both the Hegelian and the Heideggerian models understand art as a situation, a predicament, a "clearing" within which the self approaches itself from out of the darkness of misrecognition into the "lighted space" of recognition.[44]

This is particularly relevant in Music for Life, where communal participation in the creation of music can illuminate the person behind the dementia in a beautiful, meaningful and connected way, as Fiona describes: *"I felt very moved while playing for [this resident], just very connected to her somehow and after the session I had a really special conversation with her (...) She kept saying 'I played, I played' so I finished the sentence with 'Beautifully' at which point she said 'Really' and 'Lovely' (...) She was away from her default counting and I saw a very gracious, affectionate lady (...) It was music that had formed a connection, and made way for a personal interaction."*

This relationship between being engaged in music and awareness of identity is explored in Oliver Sacks' study on music and the brain.[45] He speaks of improvement of cognitive functions, mood and behaviour in people living with dementia, which, after they have been activated by music, may last for hours or even days. Sacks observes that,

> The perception of music and the emotions it can stir is not solely dependent on memory, and music does not have to be familiar to exert its emotional power (...) I think that they can experience the entire range of feelings the rest of us can, and that dementia, at least at these times, is no bar to emotional depth. Once one has

---

[44] Peters 2009:14.
[45] Sacks 2008.

15

seen such responses, one knows that there is still a *self* to be called upon, even if music, and only music, can do the calling.[46]

Here Sacks refers to the potential of improvised music in reaching people living with dementia. Improvised music, "the art of thinking and performing music simultaneously"[47]; music created in 'real time' and literally "unforeseen"[48] until its emanation, forms the basis of musical communication within the Music for Life practice. As music is, at heart, a social language, the creative process in musical improvisation is social and interactional; it is the product of an active and experiential participatory communicative process. A musical creation therefore cannot be reduced to the inspiration of one person and develops its own identity, intrinsically linked to and separate from its creators, whilst still belonging to the community in a state of shared ownership.[49]

When using improvisation as a metaphor for meaningful social communication, it is crucial that each moment in improvisation is invested with freshness of response and a sense of openness to dialogue, to collaboration, and to honesty.[50] Like improvisation, the development of social relationships between people is also an interactive process; relationships take time to develop and grow in an organic, non-linear fashion, they require genuine, ever-changing dialogue and negotiation between individuals. Therefore authenticity and a sense of 'connection' in musical communication is an integral value within the practice, as described by Fiona: *"I know that I often want to play something that would be just right for the person I am playing it for and I always ask myself: 'How can I reflect who you are and how you are in the music I play for you? How can I play music that you can own? What is your sound?'"* Reflecting on the context, it can take great skill and courage on the part of the musician to find the 'right' type of music, particularly when working with vulnerable people with a fragile sense of self-identity, who may not be able to communicate explicitly what the 'right' type of music is for them.

Achieving authenticity in musical communication in this context, coupled with the inherently emergent and uncertain nature of improvisation, therefore involves a high level of risk-taking in communication and participation, a sense of "surrender" to whole-hearted creative 'play' in the moment.[51] In order to surrender, to create a genuine dialogue, trust is a key element: trusting yourself and trusting others can only happen in an environment where a sense of safety is felt at a fundamental level.

[46] Ibid: 385.
[47] Azarra 1999: 22.
[48] Benson 2003: 24.
[49] Sawyer 2000.
[50] Peters 2009: 17.
[51] Nachmanovitch 1990: 142.

Surrender in improvisation, at a collective community level, entails negotiation, listening and collaboration in communication. It requires the musicians to find each other as a team, as people, to find the 'right' type of musical communication. It requires a conscious effort from all participants to build an environment of trust, an exploratory 'play' space, safe from fear of judgement and preconceptions.[52] Surrender in improvisation, at an individual level, requires emotional strength – confidence and courage, and a movement towards collectivism at an individual level.[53] Musicians, as 'experts' in the area of musical improvisation, have a great responsibility to perform in their creative and musical leadership within this context. This can involve a high level of personal risk-taking, a leap of faith. Surrender can lead to a host of emotions; it can enact self-enlightenment, a sense of collectivism and creativity, but can also expose vulnerability, expectations, pre-conceptions and lead to self-censorship.[54] Matthew recognises the crucial importance of musical communication as a way of validating creative surrender: *"Having a great team who recognise what is happening, and are there with solid, affirming playing really makes this possible – almost as though they are the safety net, or the people 'watching your back'. They feel the moment, and aren't afraid of the intimacy. 'Yes', their playing says, 'go on, go on.'"*

2.2 Communication and Participation

Musicians, staff and residents

The musicians, staff and residents were all selected carefully in advance of the project. The three musicians involved, Matthew (workshopleader, oboist), Anneliese (harpist) and Fiona (cellist), were relatively experienced within the practice, with between five to fourteen years of experience, and regular inclusion in projects. A fourth musician, Harry (flautist), was involved for one session, midway through the project, due to the absence of Fiona. All musicians have very different musical backgrounds and experiences within their overall practice. They were selected for their complementary personalities, and taking into account instrumentation that would work well together in a chamber music context.

Matthew has been involved in the practice of Music for Life since 2002, initially as a supporting musician, but gradually he developed into the role of workshopleader. His practice centres on his work as a freelance creative music workshopleader for a variety of arts organisations in which he interacts with a diverse range of people, together with performing in chamber ensembles and contemporary bands, and his work in arts

[52] Ibid: 69.
[53] Ibid: 51, 142, 155.
[54] Nachmanovitch 1990: 23.

17

management at a music academy. He also volunteers, programming interactive music events for a community festival in London.

Anneliese is very experienced in the project, having been involved since 1997, through a training programme in collaboration with the now defunct chamber ensemble 'Sinfonia 21'. Originally from Austria, she relocated to the United Kingdom for music study. She is a professional harpist, performing as a freelancer mostly in opera orchestras, alongside instrumental teaching and her work in the project Music for Life, which forms the basis of her creative workshop experience. Anneliese's inclusion into the practice was a case of being in the right place at the right time: "*I just fell into it (...) I stuck with it, because there was something that I really, really got out of it that I didn't get anywhere else.*"

The third musician, Fiona, is engaged as a freelance cellist mostly in chamber ensembles, alongside instrumental teaching and her work in Music for Life, complemented by other work in arts and health contexts. She became involved in the project Music for Life through the Dementia Awareness training programme, in 2007. Fiona describes her driving motivation behind her practice stating, "*I think for me, since being really small I knew I loved music. I knew I wanted to do music, but I've always had this conflict of wanting to work with people and wanting to help people. I went to music school when I was twelve, and before I went I had this huge dilemma as to whether I could do music and still help people, or work with people (...) And through my time there I needed to find another outlet, because I knew I was a performer, I could feel that there was that. But there was just this other bit of me going, you know I believe in music, and I love performing, because I love when it touches someone, I love when you communicate something.*"

Lastly Harry, who replaced Fiona for one of the project sessions, is a professional flautist. Alongside Anneliese, he became involved in the project through the Sinfonia 21 training programme in 1997. Like Matthew, he also acts principally as a workshopleader within Music for Life, a role he has enacted since 2009. His performance work is mostly as a freelancer for chamber orchestras, musicals and contemporary dance, alongside instrumental teaching and his work in Music for Life.

Matthew, Anneliese and Fiona had all worked together on Music for Life projects before but not all on the same project simultaneously. Fiona reflects positively on the composition of the musician team, saying: "*I definitely felt a sense of support but also look forward to learning how to really support and work together better over time.*"

The team of musicians was supported by the work of the project manager Deborah, who engages in a variety of responsibilities, acting as the chief liaison, logistical manager, team mentor and debrief facilitator. Brian, staff development practitioner, facilitated reflection with staff in debriefs, complementing the work of Deborah, and also acted as a liaison within the home. Both undertook an observational role during the music making.

Four staff members and one volunteer from Emanuel Zeffert House participated consistently in the project. Diallo, in his job as care assistant, interacts directly on the 'frontline' with residents, through one-to-one social contact. This is sometimes of a very practical nature, for instance, socialising with residents at meal times, and of a more social nature at other times, alongside delivering personal care, such as assisting residents with getting dressed or having a bath. Anne, as a nurse, supports the work of care assistants, through providing nursing care for residents and acting as a team manager. In this role she is responsible for managing the activities of care assistants on her unit. The project also included representation from two senior managers; Helena, a new staff member with responsibility for developing and enacting staff development initiatives within the home, with an emphasis on an outcome of enhancing resident care, and Samantha, social care coordinator, responsible for developing, managing and delivering a range of social activities with and for residents, involving staff and volunteers. Both Helena and Samantha had been involved in Music for Life projects before at other Jewish Care settings, and Helena was a lead logistical contact during this project. In addition, although volunteers form a large part of Jewish Care's strategy for integration within the Jewish community, it was unusual practice to include a volunteer within the project. Rachel had been donating her time at other Jewish Care residential homes for a few years, and in her role as a volunteer, she would principally provide opportunities for social contact, either formally, such as helping out in the beauty salon, or informally, for instance, sitting and talking to residents in resident lounges.

All of the staff were well-educated; some, for instance Helena and Samantha, had been involved in dementia care for many years, in contrast to Diallo, who had only been involved in dementia care for a short period of time. In addition, there was peripheral involvement of the registered manager of the home, Carrie, who observed the first session, and was initially involved in setting up the project. Sessions were also observed by a senior figure within Jewish Care, demonstrating the reach and value of the project within other areas of the organisation.

Staff development practitioner Brian reflects on the value of inclusion in Music for Life projects for staff, regardless of their position within the home: *"I see that it is equally important for each of these people to be in the group. Regardless of the role somebody has in the home, really for me it's about that person getting to know themselves, and getting to know, I suppose, what they want to give and what they have to give. And I don't see that it's that much different whether you're the manager of the home or you're the person who's cleaning the bedrooms, really... For Helena it's a great chance for her as a new member of staff to get to know a small number of residents intimately and a small number of staff quite intimately. It's a great thing to happen for a social care coordinator like Samantha; in the whole role of exploring how to engage with people it's very important to have access to somebody creative. And for a new volunteer in the home, to be part of a team and help build that person's skills. Whereas the other two frontline staff and the musicians are probably more used to hearing and understanding the reasons why they might be involved, which is often about being able to engage with that tension between task and being with people. Is it about what you do, or who you are with people?"*

Ten residents, including two reserves, were recruited in advance of the project through a selection process that involved eight staff from the setting, five of whom were participating in the project, plus three additional care assistants, alongside Matthew, Deborah and Brian. This followed the usual project format for selecting residents, as described in more detail in Appendix I. Initially, twenty-three resident names had been identified in a long list of potential candidates, prepared by staff in advance of the selection process, a higher number than in other projects – indicating a strong desire and need for inclusion in activity for residents at Emanuel Zeffert House. The rationale for selecting residents focused on what specific impact the project could potentially have on their well-being, with the key question posed by Deborah, "what would this project give to that person that other activities can't?" as well as an opportunity to develop relationships and understand more about the resident. Residents were profiled against this rationale; staff at the meeting took an active role in making the case for particular individuals, sharing understanding of the impact and manifestation of their dementia on their social and emotional well-being and their state of physical health. The staff involved experienced difficulty choosing the final group of residents, with each candidate being ranked highly in terms of their need. A high proportion of females were identified initially, with the eventual group consisting solely of female residents, drawn from various different units. There were existing relationships between some of the residents and staff participating in the project, for instance Diallo and two of the residents, Abigail and Jessica.

Many of the residents identified and selected showed characteristics of advanced stages of dementia, with increasing frailty and dependency on others for most aspects of their personal care. They were all withdrawn in their own way, experiencing confusion and a sense of isolation as a result of their memory loss and difficulty in communication, with a need for stimulation and positive social contact. Two of the residents liked to walk about, often showing signs of anxiety. Fragility was also present in the physicality of the group, with six out of eight residents confined to wheelchairs and needing to be transferred to other chairs by staff, in some cases through using a hoisting machine. One resident, Hannah, was partially sighted, and most experienced a level of hearing loss. Some residents could often be quite sleepy, whilst others had a tendency to call out repeatedly or react aggressively. During the meeting, the concept of balance in the group dynamic was discussed, with Matthew stating that a group with "*extremes (...) can be tricky if there's not a spectrum; very different needs can pull the group in two directions.*" This balance was a major factor in the project, as Matthew reflected during the project, "*Although we are a group, and there is a sense of group, it is fragile; it comes and goes as the residents slip in and out of that awareness.*"

Widening professional and local perceptions

The special feature of this researched project, however, is the consensus that the music sessions were consciously observed from different professional angles. Participatory research does not look for any simple 'truth', but rather for research results that have been discovered communicatively. There is the experience of the musicians who realise with subtle musical sensitivity the interactive situation with the residents with dementia. There is the knowledge of the care staff who know the residents and their idiosyncrasies. There is the remarkable overview of staff development practitioner Brian whose institutional experience and worldly wisdom are indispensable. And finally there is the perspective of the researchers whose job is to link these different professional views and to widen the horizon of each approach. Cooperation and communication between the different ways of looking at and interpreting social situations – and this means learning collaboratively – constitutes the basis of our project.

2.3 Learning and Leadership

Learning in transition: biographical learning, transformative learning and situated learning

The sociologist and philosopher Zygmunt Bauman stresses that in no previous time has the necessity for making *choices* been so prominent, one reason being that people fear to be 'left behind' or excluded because of failing to commit to new demands.[55] This has major implications for education and learning, also in music. Learning, Bauman says, should indeed be lifelong, because lifelong learning equips us to make our choices, and it especially helps us "to salvage the conditions that make choice available and within our power".[56] Lifelong learning and its implications range from the *macro* level of society at large, to the *meso* level of the institution and learning environment, and the individual *micro* level, relating to the individuals in society.

---

[55] Bauman 2005.
[56] Ibid: 128.

The concept of learning clearly changes and within this shift we can see that biographical knowledge and learning play an important role. Biographical learning includes people's experience, knowledge and self-reflection, their learning about transitions and crises in their lives; in short everything people have learned throughout their lives and have absorbed into their biographies. From biographical learning a new understanding of people's learning processes can emerge, both in terms of emotion and cognition. We therefore speak not only of lifelong but also of *lifewide* learning, both horizontal throughout the lifespan as well as vertical.

Thus a new understanding of people's learning processes can emerge from biographical learning, in particular when it concerns *transitional knowledge*, where reflexive learning processes take place within the individual but also depend on others within a social context. A biographical approach to learning has the capacity to change both the individual and the context in which the learning takes place and can thus be seen in contrast to 'conventional' education. Through the biographical approach, learning processes can become "voyages of discovery" for learners and inform us about how we deal with transitions in life.[57]

Seen from this point of departure, we can say that of central concern for musicians engaging with new audiences, like for instance people living with dementia, are the *transformative processes* that the musicians go through, based on increased moments of insight through reflective practice. Transformative learning is based on gaining new understanding emerging from critical reflection on one's own assumptions and presuppositions[58], or as Kegan simply terms it: "knowing differently".[59] Jack Mezirow argues that transformative learning creates the foundation in insight and understanding essential for learning how to take effective social action.[60]

Catherine, a musician who has been doing work for Music for Life for years, and was interviewed in the initial stage of the research, says:

> I take what I've learnt and then I take it to the next context and then the cycle becomes bigger (...) Obviously I developed as a musician through this work: it made me who I am. I teach classroom music, lots of singing. I think the skills I've learnt within Music for Life have made me good at that too. Because you look for different things. You're looking for signals of engagement, personal engagement from a child; even in the context of a whole class you're trying to look for those small little signals which indicate that particular individual and what you might do for them. To encourage their involvement, to encourage their musical development, that might be not for right now, this minute, this task, but for their life. For endless development in the future.

---

[57] Alheit 1994: 293, see also Alheit 2009.
[58] Mezirow 1990.
[59] Kegan 2009: 45.
[60] Mezirow 2009: 96.

Transformative learning relates to the learning of an individual person, but what Catherine describes here goes beyond this as it also relates to changes in the longer term in a process between herself and her pupils through interaction and communication. Therefore we can consider it a transformative process in which the learning at stake can be termed *transitional*.

For musicians and care staff alike, 'learning in transition' underpins the practice. Transitional learning is linked to biography, because it shows people's awareness of structures that have underpinned their life course 'up till a moment' and their realisation of the possibilities of changing it. It is a process that changes both the learner and her environment. This may also apply to a person living with dementia. When a member of the care staff changes her relationship with a resident as a result of an interaction through music, she has learnt in transition.

In terms of the development of the musicians, we can argue that the learning of the people with dementia and the care staff needs to be mirrored in the competences required by the musicians in order to engage with their audiences in a meaningful way. The musicians must be able to reflect on their practice, on their roles, and be responsive to what they perceive. Critical reflection, as defined by Schön[61], is central to the way in which practitioners cope with different situations in practice, where they have to connect to the social or institutional context. According to Schön, critical reflection can give the practitioner the opportunity to make a new sense of situations.[62] Reflective inquiry is therefore of importance to the musicians. They have to be *reflective practitioners,* who have the ability to reflect 'on' their action as well as 'in' their action[63] (i.e. reflexivity), in the latter case drawing on *implicit* or *tacit knowledge.*[64] Schön gives the example of improvising jazz musicians, who reflect less in words than "through a *feel* for music."[65]

When the musicians reflect, their implicit knowledge gradually becomes explicit which can then lead to insight, the development of learning strategies and input for training. Only through an increasing awareness of emotional and implicit practice can the cognitive and explicit emerge. Thus the practice as researched relates both to *lifelong* learning and to *lifewide* learning. Because whoever is the learner, she always carries her biography with her.

Fiona's reflections after the project has finished mark the beginning of her transitional learning: *"I think we created a place of belonging that did enable*

[61] Schön 1983; 1987.
[62] Schön 1983: 63.
[63] Schön 1987.
[64] Polanyi 1966.
[65] Schön 1983: 56.

the residents to feel safe and I believe these moments of well-being have helped to create change, even for a few moments or perhaps long term. It has been tough and challenging and I have felt very affected by being part of the project and by spending time and connecting with the group. I also feel like I have been left with something unquantifiable in terms of a human/spiritual experience. I feel like it has left a mark in the tapestry of my life and I like to think whether it is 'remembered' or not by the residents that it has had a similar impact on them. I feel this at the end of every project and feel very rich from the experiences Music for Life allows me to experience."

The 'place of belonging' which Fiona refers to, relates to the concept of a 'community of practice', which is critical to learning as a social group process. Central to communities of practice as described by Etienne Wenger[66] is *situated learning*, taking learning as "an integral and inseparable aspect of social practice" as point of departure.[67] Wenger's study focuses on learning as social participation, where he distinguishes four interconnected components: *meaning* (which is learning as experience), *practice* (learning as doing), *community* (learning as belonging) and *identity* (learning as becoming). A community of practice integrates these components.

The concept of *legitimate peripheral participation* is pivotal within situated learning, where the learner learns through participation starting in a peripheral position, gradually reaching a more central position, and finally achieving full membership of the community. Lave and Wenger point out that this is not always the case: "(...) there may well be no such thing as an 'illegitimate peripheral participant'. The form that the legitimacy of participation takes is a defining characteristic of ways of belonging, and is therefore not only a crucial condition for learning, but a constitutive element of its content."[68] In addition, the authors argue that 'central participation' in a community of practice does not exist: "Peripherality suggests that there are multiple, varied, more- or less-engaged and -inclusive ways of being located in the fields of participation defined by a community (...) *Changing* locations and perspectives are part of actor's learning trajectories, developing identities and forms of membership."[69] Lave and Wenger therefore warn against the notion of linear development within a community of practice, where there is in principle no periphery. Peripherality is empowering; being in the periphery is disempowering.[70]

Wenger points out that learning transforms who we are and what we do and speaks in this context about a "transformative practice of a learning community" as one that offers an ideal context for developing new

---

[66] Wenger 1998.
[67] Lave and Wenger 1991: 31.
[68] Lave and Wenger 1991: 35.
[69] Ibid: 36.
[70] Ibid.

understandings.[71] "It is that learning – whatever form it takes – changes who we are by changing our ability to participate, to belong, to negotiate meaning. And this ability is configured socially with respect to practices, communities, and economies of meaning where it shapes our identities."[72]

The social perspective on learning is summarised by Wenger by the following principles: "learning is inherent in human nature; is first and foremost the ability to negotiate new meanings; creates emergent structures; is fundamentally experiential and fundamentally social; transforms our identities; constitutes trajectories of participation; means dealing with boundaries; is a matter of social energy and power; of engagement; of imagination; of alignment, and involves an interplay between the local and the global."[73] And above all: "Communities of practice are about content – about learning as a living experience of negotiated meaning – not about form."[74]

The creative music workshop and artistic leadership

The styles of learning described above play a role with regard to an important given required for today's musicians engaging with new audiences: that is the ability to respond artistically to changing societal contexts.

'Community musicians', as such musicians are sometimes termed, devise and lead creative music workshops in health care, social care, in schools, in prisons and the like. These creative workshops are *participatory*, underpinned by the notion that the improvisational nature of collaborative approaches in workshops can lead to people expressing themselves creatively, instilling a sense of shared ownership and responsibility both in the *process* and in the final *product* of the creative workshop.[75] Exchange of ideas and skills among the participants ('participatory learning') is an integral part of the process. As Gregory phrases it: "The principle is the notion that you are with a group of people, that you encourage them to come out with their own ideas (...) The key part is that together you develop something into something else."[76]

In order to function as a musician engaging with new audiences, like for instance people living with dementia and their carers, a musician needs to be able to exercise leadership. Leadership can have meaning at an individual level. Drawing on the work of Max Weber[77] we can say that

[71] Wenger 1998: 215.
[72] Ibid: 226.
[73] Ibid: 226-227.
[74] Ibid: 229.
[75] Gregory 2005.
[76] In Smilde 2009b: 279.
[77] Weber 1947.

leadership is dependent on having authority and the ability to exercise authority. Within musicianship we can speak of *shared authority* through collaborative artistic practice, which is underpinned by qualities like informed decision making (sometimes in an implicit way), adaptability, flexibility and committed values and attitudes.[78] The ability to lead by example and attitude, while developing and using transferable (life) skills and social skills is highly relevant when a musician wants to connect as an artist to different cultural contexts. This can be termed generic leadership. It requires a lot of reflective practice and the ability to act in the moment with an implicit reflective stance (in other words: to be reflexive).

Within the creative music workshop both artistic and generic leadership play a role. Artistic leadership skills include "having the skill and judgement to create and frame a project that will work, knowing how to enable the participants to hear, see, feel and understand the connections that are integral to the creative process."[79] Generic leadership skills include "creating an inspiring, enabling environment that encourages participants to build on their strengths and acquire the confidence and skills to explore new challenges and extend their musical skills."[80] It therefore involves a practical understanding of the relevance and impact of learning styles and learning environments, in which the concepts of 'space' and 'pace' play a key role. Attention to the overall pacing of activities and tasks and to curating and sustaining a creative 'space' – including the physical environment, is paramount. The combination of artistic and generic leadership is encountered in creative workshops or "laboratory environments in participatory arts"[81]:

> The key (...) is to lead by following and to follow by leading. Leadership is about listening and responding sensitively without negating one's own knowledge and expertise.[82]

The notion of the 'artistic laboratory' thus becomes clear. Within an artistic laboratory the workshopleader needs to switch between various roles, know how to 'read' a group, develop antennae for what is fit for purpose for a particular moment, realising participatory learning whilst facilitating the exchange of skills and ideas amongst the participants. In such artistic laboratories the boundaries between performing and composing disappear, and we can subsequently observe *shared leadership*, both in an artistic sense as well as in a social sense.[83]

---

[78] Smilde 2009a.
[79] Renshaw 2007: 33.
[80] Ibid: 34.
[81] Gregory 2005.
[82] Ibid: 293.
[83] Smilde 2009a.

Shared leadership within the context of musicians engaging with people with dementia requires more than reading a group and having a radar for what is appropriate for a particular moment. Daniel, the Music for Life musician quoted earlier on in this chapter, says:

> (…) it requires individual freedom, and not to be so fixed in what you're doing, but to be very flexible to go with somebody else's ideas. Because the balance is very fragile. And in the rehearsals and the preparation hour we always do some playing where we have to develop our sensitivity to each other and a sort of responsibility about where the music is going. It's very easy to just improvise freely, and just sort of let the music go wherever, but when you have a particular agenda, you have a person who is playing that music with a particular resident, you have to incorporate them into what you're doing. So you can't just think, 'o well, I feel like playing it like that'. Because then that's *your* thing, you know? So it's really floating, we float around each other in that way, and that is why the people we have in the project are really special.

Workshopleaders are responsible for taking the initial leadership. They can however take up their role in different ways, as Linda Rose points out in a preliminary interview: "Some workshopleaders are very upfront, others will make a decision that they want it to be very democratic and they will work out who is going to do what. But they hold responsibility for the team, and for the team development as well." Being a workshopleader in this particular dementia context is very different from other community settings, and needs a lot of generic skills, insight and experience; according to Linda:

> (…) if they hadn't worked with people with dementia they wouldn't understand the particular issues there are in working with that kind of group. In terms of use of language, in terms of the need for repetition, in a way that isn't patronising, the ways of addressing people, the attitudes of staff, the difficulties of bringing people even into the room, what to do if somebody is aggressive or upset, or is talking about something they can't relate to in the past. They say: 'oh, it's so nice to see my son again', when talking to a musician. And [the musicians] don't know how to handle that, 'what do I do?' I don't think you can bring somebody straight into that, it's too scary.

Applied musical improvisation

Improvisation, as a process, can be 'applied' within particular contexts. For instance, the particular context of Music for Life is in dementia care settings, through which musicians aim to use improvisation in a manner that not only communicates meaningfully with their 'audience', in this case, people with dementia and care staff, but also acts to engage them in the music-making process. Applied improvisation entails a variety of approaches that seek to 'tune in' to the group in order to create music that authentically reflects the group and its constituent members, with musicians drawing upon a body of shared repertoire – approaches, discourses, concepts – developed through a history of mutual engagement and negotiation within this shared enterprise.

Musician Catherine reflects in the interview in the initial stage of the research project on the importance of 'attention' within the creative process, asserting that the underlying focus of the improvisation is connecting to the present moment, stating,

> It is mostly intuitive. I don't really think we have any definite don'ts or definite do's (...) Sometimes it's possible for us, it's easy to drift off to our music making (...) and that can become something that is separated from its context. I suppose the only rule is to keep it really, firmly rooted in the present, in the absolutely present moment of those people.

In order to achieve communicative potential, or develop this state of 'attention', it is important for objectives in improvisation to be clear, although the realisation of them can be intuitive: "in planning we focus attention on the field we are about to enter, then release the plan and discover the reality of time's flow. Thus we tap into living synchronicity."[84] The beliefs, attitudes and ethos of the musicians, formed and influenced through prior learning, may affect the way that they may interpret another person's communication and participation. These frames of reference are present in both reflexive, tacit approaches as well as in critical reflection and explicit collaborative planning.

Music therapy or not?

Although there are a number of correlations with principles of music therapy from a musical viewpoint, it is important to note that the Music for Life practice is divergent from music therapy, where the intent is on achieving specific clinical, therapeutic outcomes through the application of therapy-based methodology. In music therapy, the music is a vehicle, secondary to the therapeutic interaction; clinical outcomes are the aim, and a trained therapist delivers and assesses the intervention, which is primarily focused on the people receiving therapy. The focus of the project Music for Life is more akin to a creative workshop approach, in terms of artistic and social ethos and outcomes.

In the practice of Music for Life, the music is the central point from which communication, participation and a sense of community all emanate, underpinned by learning through action and reflection. The improvised music is a creative, intuitive, spontaneous reflection of the personalities and character of the group, an artistic response. Professional musicians act as a creative resource in the sessions: artisans, skilled in engaging others in a shared participatory artistic experience with strong professional identities as performers, music facilitators and educators. These musicians have built up specialist knowledge in this context, alongside a diversity of musical background and skill sets, developed primarily through engagement in the Music for Life practice, in contrast to skills developed in therapy training.

[84] Nachmanovitch 1990: 21.

Importantly, the project creates community by celebrating a mutual sense of discovery and a sense of inclusion and belonging in a shared musical and social experience, of which the group has shared ownership. The practice aims to establish a non-hierarchical community of equals: where people living with dementia, care staff and musicians are all of equal status and importance. The practice also takes place within, and reaches out to, a wider community – recognising the importance of care staff as vital instigators in sustaining and developing the learning, relationships and engagement initiated through participation in the project.

Guiding principles within the practice

Although the identity and content of each improvisation is unique in character, there are some guiding principles often employed within the Music for Life practice, that give a sense of shape, form and coherence to improvisations. These principles have much in common with musical principles used in music therapy, although they have emerged through engagement in practice rather than being underpinned by a theoretical basis or formal training. They are conceptually approached and assessed in ways that differ from those in music therapy.

The musicians use *musical frameworks* within the sessions in order to invite and inspire communication and awareness of others at a group level, whilst simultaneously aspiring, at an individual level, towards an inclusive environment in which the pace of communication is personalised for each individual. A sense of musical structure can develop through developing musical frameworks; musical structures that entail a degree of flexibility in content and delivery, designed to stimulate further musical development and additions. Some frameworks may be loosely pre-developed frameworks, for instance, those that are developed in the planning and preparation phases of the project and are a consistent feature of each session, and those that evolve naturally and spontaneously as a result of interactions.

Within these frameworks the musicians use powerful processes for enabling musical dialogues include mirroring, imitation, turn-taking, matching, reflection or translation and a 'hammer' approach. These are all natural steps that fluidly interact as part of an evolving process, applied as a leadership response based on interpretation of the needs of individuals within the group and the group as a whole. Therefore, frame-working involves a high degree of responsiveness: the structural architecture of the frame occurs in real time in response to the evolving character of the musical elements and social scenario. These processes include creating a sense of invitation, leading to connection, conversation and ultimately, community.

Three particular pre-developed frameworks consistently serve as cornerstones within the researched Music for Life sessions: a 'framing piece' that both introduces and begins each session; a 'welcome song' in which all participants' names are sung, and an activity in which hand percussion instruments are introduced through passing them around the circle, from participant to participant. These frameworks all vary in terms of how structured they are, for instance the framing piece and welcome song, although very different in execution, consistently contain similar processes and involve *extemporisation*: improvising on familiar musical material, and/or evoking the unique identifiable characteristics of a style and genre.

This contrasts to the framework of introducing the instruments, which may begin in a similar fashion from week to week, but becomes fluidly responsive to the resultant exploratory actions of the group. This 'passing instruments activity' acts as a bridge into more fluid frameworks, inspired by the communication of participants. Throughout these frameworks, the responses of participants are interpreted and validated through a number of communicative techniques such as modelling, mirroring, imitation, matching and translation, all of which lead to musical communication and participation, and the production of emergent musical forms.

Repetition is often key in strengthening an evolving framework; for instance, within an improvisation, a simple motif – melodic, rhythmic or structural i.e. drone or phrase structure – may be repeated, varied and extended, with space for musical dialogue and development to occur. Repetition in musical language is a key asset in developing a slower musical pace, giving musicians the opportunity to interpret and relate to others. Repetition is also present in the verbal and non-verbal communication in this context. Often in verbal language, instructions are framed, re-framed and modelled, using a variety of body language, including gestures, to reinforce the verbal communication. For instance when musicians introduce an instrument, they will often contextualise what the instrument is, stating its name, some ways it can be played, as well as showing and playing it clearly.

A type of *scaffolding* occurs within activities, in which prior elements are repeated, but then gradually extended through adding another simple developmental step each time the activity is repeated.

In addition to this, *modelling* is an important process in enabling the musical and social communication and participation of staff and residents in Music for Life sessions. Non-verbal gestures, often reinforced through repeated, simple verbal instructions form the basis of this technique. Modelling occurs at a multi-sensory level, combining visual, aural and tactile elements, and thus appeals to kinesthetic, visual and aural learning styles. It often precedes a musical interaction, for instance, introducing a hand percussion instrument or baton, directing or instructing a particular musician to play. It occurs both explicitly and implicitly when instruments are initially chosen or passed around. Frequently, musicians and staff will verbally introduce the instrument and then give a suggestion for how it may be played, followed by modelling this action physically. This becomes implicit modelling during framework activities such as passing instruments around the circle; as the activity repeats, it begins to set up expectations of future actions. The previous modelling begins to become more internalised, leading to more exploratory experimentation with the instruments, and the emergence and development of a wider musical language.

Musical textures are often homophonic, for example, the combination of a melody and accompaniment, or involve an interaction of a few simple melodic and rhythmic ideas. Silence has a strong impact within improvisations, and can serve as a frame before and after improvisations, a space for recognition of achievement and engagement. Closely related to silence are the concepts of *pace* and *space*. Project founder Linda Rose reflects on the learning of musicians, early in the history of the practice:

> It was very challenging for the musicians. One of the things they needed to understand was the pace at which they needed to work, which was much, much slower (...) Also it was very important to make sure musical textures weren't cluttered when three or more musicians were playing. People could focus maybe on one or two musicians playing. Musicians had to be careful about dynamics, be aware, because maybe people's hearing might be impaired. They had to understand the kind of space you could use, be aware of how near you could go to a person without worrying them, use a lot of eye contact.

Several techniques seek to connect with participants, in this case, participants living with dementia, as well as care staff, through close observation of their body language and assessing how it relates to their musical contributions. For instance, *mirroring* may be used as a technique – simultaneously copying the musical motifs of the participant as well as mirroring their body language, as a way of meeting that person at an empathic level.[85] A similar technique to mirroring is *imitation* – where the musician subsequently repeats an exact copy of the participant's contributions.[86] Matthew describes why he might incorporate mirroring in a session: *"Mirroring is if, well particularly if somebody is doing something that is different; you know, showing a different side of themselves, then yes, mirroring is a great thing to do. A great way of reinforcing what they're doing."*

Closely related to mirroring and imitating is the concept of *matching* – creating congruous music that may not exactly mirror or imitate the participant's musical contribution technically, but acts to enhance it through a match of style and quality. *Reflecting* is also an important component of applied improvisation, whereby the musician reads the participant's mood, focusing on creating music congruent to that mood or underlying communication, even if it contradicts other aspects of that person's communication.[87] Further to this, two other concepts discussed by the

[85] Wigram 2004: 82.
[86] Ibid: 83.
[87] Ibid: 90.

musicians include 'translation' and the 'hammer'. *Translation* involves validating the communication of an individual, including their musical communication, but transitioning over time to another type of musical communication in order to enable a different type of communication to occur. The *hammer* takes translation one step further; it involves a more immediate 'breaking' of the prevailing communicative atmosphere in order to create a different sense of overall energy and group dynamics.

Improvisation within a Music for Life session may involve transitioning through a series of frameworks, for instance, moving from a *turn-taking dialogue* where there is a sense of a question and answer dialogue, to a *free-floating dialogue* where simultaneous overlapping musical conversations occur.[88] Within these evolving frameworks, these processes of mirroring, imitating, matching and reflecting are all fluid in the way they interact together, sometimes occurring simultaneously.

Additionally, music can act in a *holding* capacity; as Fiona refers to it, as an 'anchor', essentially giving a sense of form and shape to participant contributions and experiences, through grounding the music via rhythm (i.e. pulse or rhythmic sequence) and/or the establishment of a tonal bass and harmonies.[89] Fiona reflects on this process, and how it can sometimes be difficult for a musician, perhaps experiencing a different sense of pace and form to the participants, to deliver: *"The welcome song also was repeated many times, so many that I wondered if we were doing it too many times. It felt very laborious, which in retrospect seemed to reflect the energy of the group. However I actually think this was so important in anchoring the group. They needed the repetition to enable them to understand the process and it really helped to establish a sense of group."*

These types of musical interactions all take place within the Music for Life practice but more or less in an intuitive, responsive and fluid, organic way, with an emphasis on drawing out musical communication and participation. Inclusion of the participant(s) at the centre of the improvisation, and engagement in a musical experience through communication and participation are the motivating forces behind these approaches, rather than a clinical outcome as in music therapy.

Reflexivity and responsiveness, guided by intuition and experience, are hallmarks of the musician-approach in improvisation within this practice. The medium of improvisation, coupled with its application within the context demands instant decision-making and a decisive attitude. Coherence of form and decision-making is only revealed upon retrospective reflection.

---

[88] Wigram 2004.
[89] Ibid: 97.

3

first-hand observations

Grounded Theory - Methodology

... one thing more is needful: first-hand observations.

Robert Ezra Park[90]

3.1   Introduction

When addressing the methodological approach which we preferred in our analysis, it is useful – as with a lot of important insights in this book – to tell a little story. To put it more accurately: it is not about a simple 'method', but rather a new *research style*, formulated by Anselm Strauss, one of its inventors. Both he and his co-author Barney Glaser have at their time called it (empirically) *grounded theory*, and they wanted to mark a new and innovative start in social science research.

When the two presented the concept in 1967 for the first time in their book 'The Discovery of Grounded Theory', they had quite polemical interests. Glaser and Strauss planned to challenge the ruling sociological research of the post-war period in the US with an alternative research model. The mainstream research was based on a precarious division of labour of so-called 'grand theories' on the one hand (the most influential has probably been the system-functionalism of Talcott Parsons)[91], and 'hard' quantitative social research on the other. Empirical research completed primarily henchmen services, 'proletarian work' so to speak, for the producers of grand theories who behaved like 'theoretical capitalists', as Glaser and Strauss ironically formulated. The result was very disillusioning. The grand theories went further and further away from social reality. But also the empirical research lost contact with everyday life, because it usually proved hypotheses which were derived deductively from the grand theories, examining artificially isolated variables that had nothing to do with real processes.

It seemed forgotten what one of the leading figures of the Chicago School of Sociology, Robert Ezra Park, had written in the 'register' of American sociology in the 1920s:

> (...) one thing more is needful: first-hand observations. Go and sit in the lounges of the luxury hotels and on the doorsteps of the flophouses; sit on the Gold Coast settees and on the slum shake-downs; sit in Orchestra Halls and in the Star and Garter Burlesk. In short, gentlemen, get the seat of your pants dirty in *real* research.[92]

[90] Cit. in Burgess 1982: 6.
[91] See Parsons 1951.
[92] Cit. In Burgess 1982: 6.

This tradition, which benefited from the work of the important American pragmatists – from the grand philosopher and educationalist John Dewey (1896, 1917, 1938), from George Herbert Mead's social psychology (1934) which is still current, also from the innovative ideas of the logician Charles Sanders Peirce ([1903] 1991) – was the basis of Strauss' and Glaser's thinking. They were just not interested in testing well-known hypotheses, which they considered unfit to reconstruct and understand social change. Rather, they wanted to 'generate' new theoretical knowledge. And such knowledge they discovered through intensive analysis of empirical reality. Thus the vital relationship between theory and empiricism was at the core of their considerations.

That is why Glaser and Strauss were not just interested in theory 'as such', but in its importance for practice. Their findings should be key concepts for professional work – especially in the field of medicine and care, but also in education or politics. Therefore their research was always very practical: for example the interaction with dying people, the scope of action for professionals in a hospital under the conditions of modern medical equipment or the strategies of action in high-risk pregnancies.

Despite this openness and curiosity of the setting, the grounded theory approach is not an optional procedure. It can be understood as a theoretically legitimated 'advancement' that reflects and controls its own learning process. The actual procedure itself has changed over the course of its practice[93], particularly with respect to its objects of research. However the basic innovative impact still persisted. First, nevertheless, we want to describe the theoretical background of this respective 'research style' (Strauss) in more detail.

3.2   The pragmatist background of grounded theory

Glaser and Strauss developed an idea of the research process, in which the amount of new knowledge is not coming directly from one conventional stage to another – hypothesis generation, method testing, data collection, data analysis, verification or falsification of the hypotheses – but it also takes place *during* the research process. It can be considered a continuous dialogue between theoretical assumptions and the data obtained, as it were "a spiralled reciprocation between theoretically based ideas and empirically based facts."[94]

This willful back and forth that might be misinterpreted as indecisiveness or randomness has a philosophically and methodologically interesting background in the action concept of American pragmatism. Already at the beginning of the 20th century, Dewey and Mead had severe debates with the

---

[93] See Kelle 1994.
[94] Dausien 1996: 93; translation by the authors.

then emerging behaviourist psychology about their rather simple model of behaviour.

In an epoch-making article about the so-called 'reflex arc model' of 1896 it was John Dewey who plausibly showed that human activity does not function in the simple way as shown in the following scheme:

Fig. 1: The 'reflex arc'

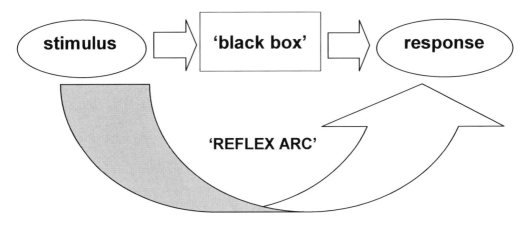

Instead, he made it clear that action must be taken as 'a *holistic* process' in which certain 'stimuli' as such are principally perceived. This led to the idea that usually not a *stimulus* determines an action, but – conversely – the running process selects the relevant stimuli, as has also been described by George Herbert Mead in 1903 in a little-known essay about the *Definition of the Psychical.*

We can illustrate the plausibility of this astonishing notion with a relatively simple everyday life experience. If we are involved in a particular affair, as to try to convince our little daughter why it makes sense to tidy up her nursery, then her defiant foot-stamping or her objection that the father himself does not keep good order at his own desk, are quite relevant stimuli for the next action. The noise of a police car on the road, a just discovered grease spot on the wall or the music from the radio in the kitchen are irrelevant stimuli and do not play any role for the progress of the plot. This means that the action itself, as a 'holistic', continuous process selects the stimuli that are relevant for the progress of action. Only when a 'stimulus' calls the entire context with which we are currently engaged into question, for example, if an earthquake causes our house to cave in, we are forced to make drastic changes of our action plans. Once this is done, we again perceive only those stimuli that are relevant for the actions at issue.

The pragmatists, however, go a step further. Even the idea that action is usually purposeful, intentional action, they perceive as problematic. The idea that a particular aim of action has been set by the consciousness 'as such', is not compatible with empirical procedures. "Naturally, action is only diffusely teleological"[95]: that means, normally we act with a certain basic intention; the concrete purposes of the action however usually appear during the process itself and may cause even the revision of the original intention. Let us take again our example of the educational situation: certainly, it was the intention of the father to stop his daughter's disorder, but the educational communication shows that there are good reasons to change his mind. This can be seen for example when the child convincingly demonstrates that she seeks her bathing suit in vain after reluctantly having tidied her room, whilst she usually finds things in her creative mess. The educational experiment has taken the sequence of action in a whole new direction. Ideal-typical purposive action is not usually the case, and especially in educational situations, not really eligible. The pragmatist plan of action differs significantly from the behaviourist one:

Fig. 2: The pragmatist alternative

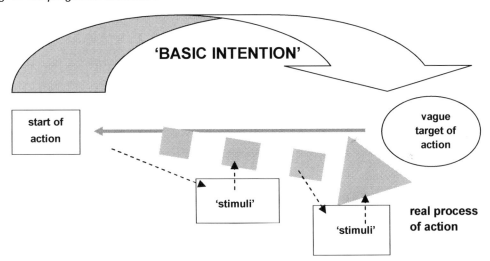

A very similar plot idea enhances Glaser and Strauss' strategies concerning the research process. When we enter a new field of research that is still relatively unknown, or if we want to look at seemingly familiar research landscapes with totally 'new eyes' because we do not trust any longer the well-known results, our action process reacts in a very similar way, "diffusely teleological" as in unforeseen everyday situations. We have a tentative idea

---

[95] Joas 1988: 423; translation by the authors.

of what we could expect, but we want to make discoveries and therefore have to be open for everything that could happen to us.

However, we are researchers. Our particular way of doing things differs from usual everyday behaviour, as we have to account for our line of action. Our research, no matter how it may differ from conventional design, should be 'reliable'. Therefore the 'openness' with which we meet the new field has a methodological limit. If we would enter the field totally unprejudiced, we would face two serious problems:

a. We could easily overlook that our alleged 'openness' is in fact not enforceable. At least our everyday experiences cannot be turned off in new situations. Their intuitive knowledge structures are prepared to compare each new situation with already known ones. They are based on a 'typification' of the social world that is accessible for us.[96] This process is not a conscious one. It takes place as it were *a tergo,* which means 'in the back' of someone. Whether we like it or not, we always have 'pre-judgments' about new 'worlds' that we come across.

b. The complex new constellation usually does not present itself in ways we can immediately perceive. From the data we collect in the ideal case 'without reservation'; new theories do not 'jump up' automatically. Certainly, the 'alien' also has its rules and orders. But how should we perceive them if they are totally unfamiliar to us? That means, we have no chance to handle it if we refuse to compare. We can understand the 'strangeness' only if we relate it to the known field. Any empirical research, any form of generating theory needs the *comparison.*

After all we touch here on an almost philosophical basic problem of empirical research: if important new conclusions about social reality – logically and practically – cannot be gained by uninfluenced observation (the logical conclusion preferring this way is usually called *induction*), if it is likewise problematic – as we have learned through the mainstream criticism of Glaser and Strauss – to gain empirical judgments about expected social reality through testing hypotheses derived from known theories (the logical conclusion of this process uses to be called *deduction*). What alternative then is left over?

Let us remember once more the idea of the pragmatists: Social action is usually, as we have seen, *'diffusely teleological'* (Joas). That is, it does have a vague idea of what is to come out of the action. However, the everyday experience shows that the action process itself can change its original intention, perhaps even revise it entirely. Action, we could say, has a 'target-oriented openness', a 'directed flexibility'.

[96] See Schütz and Luckmann 1979.

Exactly this quality is what grounded theory is aiming at in research: a 'planned flexibility'. 'Planned' in so far as certain hypothetical assumptions are necessary and useful, also about a new research field; 'flexible' and 'open' because these presumptions can change during the research process. From the first contact with the field, the hypotheses are enriched and extended with new information, and in the end, if anything, they may postulate the opposite of what they had originally believed in. The logician of the pragmatists, Charles Sanders Peirce, who had already developed this idea in the beginning of the 20th century, describes it as the astonishing accomplishment to put something in relation to what "we never have dreamed about before"[97] and he calls this process of a logical conclusion 'abduction'.[98]

The appealing idea that research could systematically be related to creativity, however, must now be somewhat limited. Every artist knows that creativity is based on the utmost discipline. Only when the tools of the sculptor or the piano virtuoso, the composer and the poet are developed and deployed by really intense experience, then a new aesthetic quality can be found. Very similar tools offer the grounded theory process a method to facilitate that abductive 'discovery' of theories. This approach is not a rigorous procedure and has developed variations during the application and refinement. We will describe below our own approach a little more concretely. It is our object of research – 'music and dementia' – which had a special effect on our proceeding.

3.3 Our own methodological approach

As we saw, the discovery of a new field of research and the development of a theory about this field is a complicated process that never runs in a linear way, but mostly in 'knowledge-spirals', in the continuous confrontation of theoretical assumptions with the data obtained. Some of the assumptions or open hypotheses – grounded theory calls it the *sensitizing concepts* – we have already mentioned: for example that music is a very special form of communication which reaches people with dementia perhaps more easily than verbal communication, or that there is something called the 'person behind the dementia' which could be discovered through music. Just to find this out, of course, we had to generate data that could give us clues whether our hypotheses were plausible or whether entirely different results appeared much more convincing.

We have therefore made two preliminary decisions which fit to the tradition of grounded theory:

---

[97] Peirce [1903] 1991: 404.
[98] See Kelle 1994: 143ff.

a. We have chosen a *qualitative* approach. Qualitative methods are in contrast to quantitative methods not based on numerical accuracy. It is not about an 'objectivity' which is backed up by measurable distribution of distinguishing marks.[99] Rather, it is about *subjective* perceptions of social situations that interest us[100]: for example, the attention of the musicians who work with people with dementia, the valuation of care staff who have observed the interactions between musicians and people with dementia, but also the expressions of the residents themselves who act out their feelings.

b. We have deliberately worked with various methodological approaches, for example with field notes, with focused interviews, with reflective journals (of the musicians and staff development practitioner) and with group discussions.[101] The interviews were *narrative*, set up as a biographical interview, meaning that we aimed for the interviewees to tell their stories, holding back ourselves, giving them the possibility to reflect, not feeling led into certain directions.[102] The resulting qualitative data has been *'triangulated'*, as method experts use to say,[103] that is, we have systematically documented the material and created a dialogue between the different data just to find patterns which are able to make the complex situation graspable.

We have decided on a practical approach that is described in the tradition of grounded theory as *coding*.[104] Strauss and Corbin suggest a triple step of 'open coding', 'axial coding' and 'selective coding'. Strictly speaking, however, it is neither about procedures clearly distinguishable from each other nor temporally distinct phases of coding. Rather, there are various ways of dealing with the data material which researchers use and vary, go back and forth if necessary, and look for relationships between the coding procedures.

During *open coding*, the first step, it is important to 'break off' the data, to find key words (concepts) and identify first 'codes' or 'categories'. Strauss and Corbin write:

> Broadly speaking, during open coding, data are broken down into discrete parts, closely examined, and compared for similarities and differences. Events, happenings, objects, and actions/interactions that are found to be conceptually

---

[99] See Flick 2009: 383ff.
[100] See Alheit 2010.
[101] See Flick 2009: 333ff.
[102] Alheit 1993.
[103] Ibid: 443ff.
[104] See Strauss 1987; Strauss and Corbin 1990.

similar in nature or related in meaning are grouped under more abstract concepts termed 'categories'.[105]

Axial coding as a next stage is a more systematic form of coding. Here subcategories are identified, associated with higher-order categories, using a 'coding paradigm model' (see below). The model is relatively simple but generalisable: not just phenomena are compared and separated systematically, also the reasons that have led to the particular phenomena, the contextual conditions and the consequences which derive from the phenomena are taken into consideration in the analysis.

Fig. 3: The paradigm model (taken from Flick, 2009, p. 311)

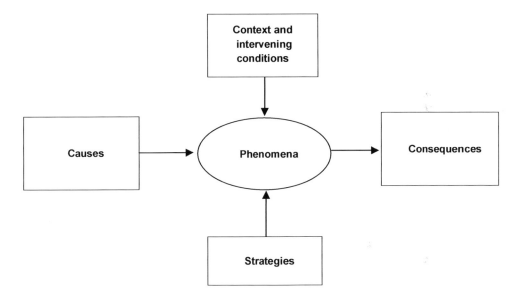

Strauss and Corbin write:

> Axial coding is the process of relating subcategories to a category. It is a complex process of inductive and deductive thinking involving several steps. These are accomplished, as with open coding, by making comparisons and asking questions. However, in axial coding the use of these procedures is more focused, and geared toward discovering and relating categories in terms of the paradigm model.[106]

Selective coding as the third step continues the axial coding on a higher level of abstraction. It depends on identifying so-called 'core categories' and on telling the *story of the case*, so to speak. The result is a theoretical idea about what 'is the case' (in the field). In our analysis, four core categories very soon moved into the centre of the research, in which the importance of

---

[105] Strauss and Corbin 1990a: 102.
[106] Strauss and Corbin 1990: 114.

the interaction between musicians and people with dementia became immediately clear: *'identity', 'communication', 'participation'* and *'development'* (see the following chapter). The relationship between these four key variables displays a (learning) process which makes the events in the investigated field highly interesting: for musicians, for caregivers, but also for the way society deals with people living with dementia.

4

What does the song hope for?

Analysis

What does the song hope for? And the moved hands
A little way from the birds, the sky, the delightful?
> *To be bewildered and happy,*
> *Or most of all the knowledge of life?*

W. H. Auden[107]

4.1   Identity

"'Dad, do you know who I am anyway?' The question made him shy, he turned to Katharina and said jokingly with a gesture of his hand in my direction: 'as if that were so interesting'." [108]

Identity is a critical issue for everybody involved in this practice, musicians, care staff and staff development practitioner, but also for the residents. Many of the stories can be summarised as relating to, sometimes unstable, identity: issues of anxiety, self-esteem, integrity, vulnerability, personhood, responsibility, recognition and acknowledgement play a role. A good feel of the 'identity struggle' of the three very different musicians can perhaps be obtained by how they speak amongst themselves in the group interviews that were held.

Matthew, the music workshopleader, struggles with his leadership and one of his big challenges throughout the project is to gain confidence and give space to other people involved. His quiet colleague Anneliese is focused on collaboration and shared leadership with Matthew and Fiona. Fiona is a sensitive musician who has a wonderfully intuitive way of connecting with residents and through that with herself. Finally there is Brian, the staff development practitioner who brings 'head and heart' together. He gently confronts the musicians with the reality of what it means to live with dementia.

Threatened identity

There is a lot going on amongst the musicians which we can interpret as components of a sometimes 'threatened' identity. The learning process of the musicians during the project is starting in an uncertain and unconfident way. Throughout the project there is often a feeling of disconnection and anxiety, especially just before the weekly workshops. It appears that the preparation hour preceding each session is crucial for the musicians to gain confidence and a sense of control. They cannot have anybody present at

---

[107] 'Orpheus', from *Another Time* (1940).
[108] From Arno Geiger (2011): *Der alte König in seinem Exil*. München: Hanser Verlag. Original text: "'Papa, weisst du überhaupt, wer ich bin?' Die Frage machte ihn verlegen, er wandte sich zu Katharina und sagte scherzend mit einer Handbewegung in meine Richtung: 'Als ob das so interessant wäre'." (p. 74, translation by the authors).

this time as they need this hour to get rid of their feelings of being rushed, and instead obtain a sense of space and peace and quiet. It is very valuable for the musicians at that moment to make music 'without an agenda' and connect, just before they start the session. Setting up chairs together, trying out instruments for the residents, practising together, 'getting sorted', feeling ready and confident is important, and sometimes it seems nearly magical in order to create a feeling of being potentially successful. Bringing in the residents early, when the preparation is still taking place, can therefore be experienced as a disruption.

This particular project was challenging, due to the fact that the home is brand new and the residents sometimes still felt unsettled, but also perhaps due to the fact that this project was being researched. Fiona was one of the first to notice a sense of unsettledness. We will first introduce Fiona in a bit more detail. In her reflections Fiona often connects the work in this practice with her own personal growth and development: "*you're constantly challenged and you connect with the people you're working with, and you also connect with more of yourself, I think. Because you're constantly looking at yourself as a musician and as a person. So it's a very rich kind of place of work, I think.*" Fiona shows bravery in addressing her feelings of responsibility and vulnerability. She is highly sensitive, and often writes about 'picking up' a feeling or atmosphere. She reflects on the feeling of anxiety preceding and during the first session: "*I think there was a general sense of anxiety that everyone wanted it to go well and perhaps this was tangible, even to the residents as well as the staff and us as a musical team.*" She comments on the atmosphere in the home as being 'unsettled and unsure', saying: "*not sure how much of that I was picking up on that too.*" Fiona points out that the work the musicians do can reflect broader emotional issues of residents and staff.

Clearly the musicians had to get to know the residents. Gabriella was one of the first they noticed from the beginning. Gabriella is every inch a lady, sometimes utterly lucid, at other times totally locked into her dementia. She is heard repeatedly, and almost without pause, counting 'nineteen, twenty, nineteen, twenty'. When a member of care staff addresses her, she looks into their face, and smiles momentarily before she lapses back into folding the tissue on her lap. Gabriella is quite disturbed and restless during the first session, and at some point this leads to annoyance. This brings Matthew out of balance, and makes him very critical about the musicians' achievements: "*The session lacked a sense of having clear, defined pieces, with good beginnings and endings. Maybe this contributes to a sense of unease within the residents, a lack of 'satisfaction' – Gabriella's frustration, 'Go on, go on, stand up and sing'.*" Matthew feels that "*it can potentially create a feeling of anxiety for the residents as well, if there's no resolution ever (…) I thought, yeah, we're not playing. We're filling in the background and nothing is happening.*"

This interpretation seems to mirror Matthew's lack of confidence as the music workshopleader of this project. He recognises the fact that he tends to want to be very much in control and he can even bring this back to biographical experiences, where he always needed to be the one in control of his rebelling younger brother. Matthew's big challenge throughout the project is to let go of this sense of control, to give space to other people involved and trust them to do things in their own way. He is very aware that a lot of this happens tacitly, through implicit knowledge.

Bringing this awareness into practice however, is not easy. Gabriella is not the only resident who makes Matthew feel unconfident and uneasy. Fear for people uttering their dementia in various and sometimes unexpected ways plays a role for him. Matthew is aware of his uneasiness with another resident, Rebecca, who right from the start of the project began seeking a lot of attention. Rebecca is, apart from Esther, who will be introduced later on, the only one of the participating residents who is able to walk. She paces the corridors of the home with a sense of urgency, back and forth, searching endlessly, an unarticulated desire compelling her. When she encounters others, she stares wordlessly at the faces of those around her, taking a long time to read their expressions. Sometimes she takes an outstretched hand and shakes it vigorously and rapidly. Other times she shows delight through close eye contact, knocking her forehead gently against that of care staff. Often she appears isolated, and susceptible to any small changes in her physical environment, unable to relax, living in a different rhythm to those around her. Matthew feels very uncomfortable with Rebecca: *"I feel her frustration and anger at being 'locked in' by her dementia. I find it very upsetting, and I am actually afraid of her – that she might 'freak out', strike me or someone else, grab my oboe."*

Clearly the residents are very different, the situation is new and uncertain; in addition a lot of expectations can exist preceding a project and this can be stressful. However, miracles cannot be expected, and it is important to strive for realistic expectations of care staff. Managing these expectations can make Matthew feel insecure. At some point he feels criticised by Helena, a new staff member at the home, responsible for enhancing the care quality of residents. Helena is new to the setting, very experienced in dementia care and works alongside staff and residents. Her remark that Rebecca is not being paid enough attention makes Matthew feel judged and he takes it badly.

This is where the importance of the work of the staff development practitioner comes in, where staff development practitioner Brian plays a pivotal role during the project. Brian aims to serve as a catalyst between musicians, residents, care staff and, more at a distance, the management of the home. He is very knowledgeable about all sorts of dementia. Brian describes himself as "*somebody who quietly goes around just to check to see what is happening and what isn't happening.*" He confronts the musicians more than once with the reality of what it means to live with dementia and through this brings about a learning process in the musicians.

Brian often stresses the big importance of critical reflection for care staff who work with people with dementia; they need to be allowed time and space to do that. He emphasises what people living with dementia can bring to others through mutual engagement: *"My sense is for people with dementia, that the people who are working with them don't get enough opportunities to reflect on how the work is impacting on themselves and their own growth. They don't get enough chance to understand what people with dementia are giving back to them in their lives. And on a day to day basis just to think and to be in their work, I don't think they have enough facilitation. So I try to do something, that's what I want to bring in (...) I try to be the voice that says that's so important. Because if you have a happy, fulfilled worker you have a good chance that the residents will also be happy and fulfilled. And I think that's where Music for Life comes in (...) Staff have an opportunity to observe and see and be with people and to experience people and to rejoice alongside people and to reflect on that."* Brian tends to take a key role in managing the logistical aspects of the project, *"I try and act as a liaison. I suppose I always have a certain amount of anxiety that different aspects of it are not going to happen."*

We find such a heightened sense of anxiety preceding the second session, where it feels like the musicians more or less clash during the preparation hour with Deborah, the highly experienced and long-term Music for Life project manager. Together with Brian, Deborah is the integer spider in the web of the project. She is knowledgeable about music and dementia, as well as care contexts, and also serves as a mentor for the musicians. At this particular moment the musicians and Deborah clearly have a different set of priorities. Deborah encourages the musicians to start playing, whereas the musicians feel they should take time to have a good discussion about the seating in the circle.

The second session was demanding anyway; more or less hijacked by Sarah, a resident who keeps calling out loudly for her mother. Sarah is a petite lady, who often sits with her head in her hands. Her hands will quiver as she places them in her lap and looks around the room, then raises one shaking hand to her head, her body slumping into the chair, crying emphatically 'Mummy! Mum'! Other residents around her often appear startled by her cry.

Such behaviour of residents inevitably leads to unpredictability which can cause a lot of anxiety amongst the musicians. At some point during the same session Rebecca slapped Fiona's hand very hard. Fiona afterwards shared her anxiety in the debrief, showing that she clearly let the residents' distress in. Later on Fiona reflects: *"I really felt in my gut a sense of desperation that I believe I was picking up from the residents. I don't think I have seen it or felt it in such a tangible way before, so this was quite challenging but also terribly sad. I think as a team we dealt with it very well and the music that we provided walked a very narrow line between reflecting this desperation and taking the group to a more hopeful place."* Matthew admired her, saying after the session: *"there's courage, there's real courage in facing things like that and to keep playing. And that's the extraordinary thing, Fiona just kept playing. How on earth do you do that? You know, when you're in real pain yourself and you keep playing for the good of this group of people it's extraordinary. It's a really courageous thing to do."*

Despite the feeling of desperation related to the calling out of Sarah which Fiona writes about, Matthew feels that he has been successful with Sarah, because he felt he connected with her. Matthew relates his own difficulty of asking for mental support if he needs it, like for instance after this particular session. He can only accept such support if someone offers it him on his or her own initiative. Matthew continuously struggles with his lack of confidence, and with issues of power and leadership. He clashes again with Deborah at the beginning of the third session, where they clearly have separate agendas and priorities. He writes: *"I was very aware of Deborah's anxiety today about the set up of the room etc., and this did impact on how I was feeling during our preparation hour, that I was struggling to retain leadership, and not transmit that anxiety. There was a clash of agendas – mine being to connect with the musician team, and Deborah's being to get the practical stuff done."* It continues as Matthew feels that he and the other musicians are not granted the time and space to prepare. He feels distracted and stops playing. When Deborah tells him that this is the best they can do, Matthew does not really believe it, sensing that the musicians' need for privacy during the preparation hour is not really acknowledged: *"my suspicion is just that, 'oh, it's just okay if I just slip in and get this, oh and they've got these screens up so they can't see us walking through'. There's just, it feels, I know Deborah has said this is the best they can do and I don't believe it, I suppose is the bottom-line. But if that's where we're at, then fine. It still niggles away at me a little bit, I suppose. That kind of space doesn't feel secure and safe for us in that first hour, really. And I think that affects the playing."*

Anxiety is not only an issue for the musicians, it also exists within the care staff. An example is the incident that takes place between Matthew and Rachel. Rachel is a volunteer with a Jewish background. Her role as a volunteer differs from that of the other staff employed in the home, with a primary social focus on spending one-to-one quality time with residents. She is very well spoken and highly articulate, assertive and clearly full of life, curiosity and has a strong interest in, and love for classical music. During the passing of instruments in the welcome song of a session, Rachel spontaneously starts handing out instruments, but she is told by Matthew not to do that. Rachel reports during the debrief that she felt very embarrassed by this. Matthew shows surprise during the interview after the session:

"I was just so struck (...) everybody is so vulnerable, the staff, the musicians as well as the residents. You know, somebody as confident and willing and intelligent as Rachel, it felt like she just wanted to curl up and die about it. Somebody even like her is so personally affected by that." In his reflective journal Matthew writes: *"I do really want to let the music 'take off' at some point soon. I think this will be the next stage on bringing the group together, move us all onto the next stage, particularly the staff, who are held back by their anxieties about 'doing the right thing'. This was voiced by Rachel, who was upset that I asked her not to hand out instruments. I thought I had done this so gently, I thought I said 'Maybe not just now' – I thought I had been so careful, but she still took it so badly, and it has completely knocked her confidence."*

In one of the group interviews the musicians come back to the incident with Rachel. Matthew says: *"And I said really quietly to her, 'maybe not just now'. And she was devastated by it, came back in the feedback afterwards. 'Oh god, I'm not going to, I'm gonna wait to do what I'm told from now on, I'm just gonna wait.' And I was like, nooo! And I thought, this is somebody really confident, with high self-esteem..."* Apparently Matthew takes Rachel's high self-esteem for granted, but of course that may not be realistic.

Anxiety throughout the sessions can lead to many feelings of vulnerability. During the fourth session Matthew reflects on an interaction between Fiona's one-time replacement, flautist Harry, and resident Abigail. Abigail is often sleepy, drifting through periods of dozing and periods where she seems very alert, suddenly animated and energetic. She is friendly, polite and down to earth with others. At times, she seems to have a strong sense of self-awareness, but at other times appears very confused, and puzzled or distressed by the behaviour of others around her, withdrawing from contact with others. Harry interacts with her.

From the field notes:

Matthew has been playing the soprano chime bar[109] near Abigail. Anneliese sometimes echoes him and it is a lively motif. He then sings "Abigail" and asks Abigail if she would like to play them: "can you try playing these, can you have a go with these?" Matthew asks her to pass the hand chime[110] to Helena. Abigail begins to play, a bit slower than the piece before, but Anneliese quickly locks into her pulse. However, it continues to slow down as she explores the chimes – Anneliese stops playing. Matthew then asks Abigail with which musician she would like to make a piece. "Abigail, would you like to make a piece, either with Anneliese...

---

[109] A tuned metal bar mounted onto a wooden resonator box. The sound is produced by striking the metal part of the chime bar with a beater, most often a beater with a soft rubber head, or a wooden head. The set used in this project incorporated a chromatic pitch range between the notes g' to g'''. Soprano chime bars are generally in the range c'' to a''', and alto chime bars in the range of c' to a'. See also Appendix V, 'List of musical instruments'.

[110] Tuned square tubes with an external clapper system, rung by hand, and similar to handbells. The hand chimes used in this project were pitched at c', e' and g'. See also Appendix V, 'List of musical instruments'.

Harry... or it could be with me?" She "hmms" yes after each name and it's not clear whether she understands. "Do you want to choose one of us...Anneliese or Harry?" She heartily agrees by saying "Harry" and looks at him. Harry asks whether he can come and sit in front of Abigail and asks "Okay, do you want to start?" She starts playing repeating notes. Harry sits on the floor in front of her and starts to improvise on it very gently. He almost immediately joins in with her. It is a lively piece in D major, a duo between Harry and Abigail, which Anneliese slowly begins to underpin, ever so softly adding some harmonics to it. The improvisation begins to peter out, so Harry and Anneliese stop playing. Harry asks Abigail if she would like to try another note, pointing out that by that she can make lots of different sounds. "Abigail, can you try one of the other notes, how about that one... you've got lots and lots of different sounds... Yes, that's great." Abigail picks this up and as of that moment produces different notes. He lets her explore for a bit, then joins in again, improvising over it. Harry continues, Anneliese knocks the harp softly. The piece moves through a variety of tonal centres – G major, E minor, D major. The piece then becomes less harmonically stable and the duo seems like musically impenetrable until Harry plays a lively figure in the higher register, with which Anneliese is able to join in with a repetitive accompaniment figure in D Major. As Harry starts to energise the rhythm, Anneliese's involvement becomes stronger. Hannah immediately responds by engaging more strongly as well. At the end Harry says "Thank you Abigail, that was lovely" and Matthew echoes "well played". Harry remarks: "there was a lot of energy in that piece" (laughter). Matthew says "Yeah, there was - you gave him a work out" to which Abigail responds "Yes". Matthew: "you made him work for it." Harry agrees: "I played a lot of notes there" and Abigail replies "good!" There is laughter between her, Helena and the musicians. Harry says "Can I have a rest now" and Abigail says "sure". Matthew asks if he can takes the chime bars off her lap "not so comfortable is it?"

Harry tries to encourage Abigail, inviting her to use another note, giving her the time to explore, before he joins in with an improvisation. He has a good sense of the slow pace that is required for Abigail, and at the same time approaches this as an artist. This helps to develop a musical piece which moves through different tonal centres. Abigail's piece is an example of an episode that unfolds with a clear beginning and end. There are two moments of disengagement which are dealt with by the musicians, verbally, by exploring, and also by strong physical and mental support of Harry: he sits on the floor just in front of her so that an intimate atmosphere is created which leads to Abigail's confidence.

Matthew feels the vulnerability that can be at stake in such interactions and puts himself in Harry's place, observing: *"So when you're really out there, like Harry making a piece with Abigail today, you don't know what's going to happen. Anything might happen. She might react amazingly and play a fantastic duet with him, she might hit him with the beater. It's entirely possible. She might be very upset. And he's got nothing, no music to hide behind. He's just there with his flute."* Harry is just there with his flute; the resident is not the only one who can be vulnerable and feel exposed, as Matthew continues to reflect: *"I suppose there's a kind of heightening of your awareness of the person you're working with. You're making them and yourself more vulnerable, I suppose. Hopefully you're gonna make a strong connection with someone that's going to be seen by everybody else. Everybody's going to watch this. And so it's very exposing to do that. To go kneel in front of someone, get very close to somebody and make a piece with them or play for them. Yeah, it's very exposing."*

Anneliese senses this. She feels *that "Harry's piece with Abigail felt quite strange. Was she just locked into playing or did she respond to his music? She surprised us all with this gesture of 'we did it' at the end. We all laughed."* Harry is an outstanding musician and very experienced in the practice of Music for Life, where he is one of the long-term music workshopleaders. He is confident, cheerful and humorous, creating an atmosphere of lightness around him.

Despite appearing calm and quiet, Anneliese can also feel very unconfident. She is a real collaborator and longing for a shared leadership with Matthew and Fiona. In her reflective journals she shows her anxiety by describing clashes related to this between Matthew and herself. For Anneliese, safety and risk-taking amongst the musicians are big issues, as it shows more than once, like for instance in the following discussion amongst the musicians:

Anneliese: *"(...) you have to be able to function as a group and I think that feeling of safety is just paramount, isn't it? Because you're not going to take risks, because this work is full of risks, musically and in every other sense, and if you don't have that nice, you know, padding around you, then I would never have returned to do this work again."*

Matthew: *"No. It's potentially far too..."*

Fiona: *"Yeah, costly."*

This is a key statement for a good working community of practice, where safety is a social fact and not an individual feeling. It requires the whole group. 'Costly' is used by Fiona as a word which can be recognised as possibly underpinning its impact if the safety is not provided.

Notwithstanding the fact that improvising is the core skill connected to this practice, it can nevertheless create a deep uncertainty. Improvisation is deeply related to individual and group identity. It is always an open process, and can contain a feeling of much risk for the musicians involved. There is in this sense a high amount of uncertainty and self criticism from the side of Anneliese when she says: *"I find that the striving to say something meaningful musically, I find that hard. And we found again and again that when we say something with our music, then things fall into place. Quite often we have been able to save situations with music. It always comes back to the music again. The other things have to be there too, we have to have lots of skills, but if the music is – if you look at it from the other side – is sort of superficial, sometimes we can amble along, and we sort of don't quite know where we're going, I certainly don't, and then very often the focus isn't there, there isn't any direction, yeah, I find the two of them go so together and I personally find the musical side hard. Yes, that's my challenge, actually."* At some point Anneliese even addresses strongly the relationship between improvisation and identity, arguing that, "*if the music doesn't work, then as a person you're also not going to function in the same way in this group.*"

An important learning point for the musicians in order to release their anxiety is not to take things too personally. Often musicians tend to connect perceived failure in performance to low self-esteem.[111] Matthew, Anneliese and Fiona are no exception, as we can hear in the following discussion:

Matthew*: "(…) And so we identify ourselves with our playing."*

Anneliese: *"I played well, I feel good."*

Matthew: *"I played well, I am a good musician, I am a good person."*

Fiona: *"I'm ok."*

Matthew: *"I'm ok."*

Fiona: *"I play badly, I'm a disaster."*

Matthew: *"Yeah, with our identity, is so."*

Fiona: *"It's all tied up, isn't it?"*

Matthew: *"And we judge people and people judge us on that. Like, he's a rubbish player, he doesn't play in tune, dadada, and that really lowers your status as a human being."*

The musicians tend to experience a similar feeling as soon as they sense their connection with a resident has failed. High expectations therefore need to be managed and be realistic; a resident can walk away due to dementia, and that has nothing to do with the quality of the musicians' performance.

Fiona raises the question of the relationship between the sense of failure in performance and low self-esteem in her reflective journal when she comments that a Music for Life session reveals how you are feeling yourself. She experienced having a hard time when some instruments were rejected by residents, even during the very first session. She says: "*I was just aware of how unsure one can feel about what one is offering and aware of how to deal and handle this well. How personal this can feel!*" The latter phrase is telling. This is not just a job. Fiona clearly experiences it as a personal failure if residents refuse an instrument, whereas this might require 'detachment' from her side, realising that a person's response may well be the result of the dementia itself. This is what makes the work of the staff development practitioner so important.

---

[111] See also Chapter 2.

Another example of fear of failure is the moment when Fiona accidentally 'reads' Matthew differently: at some point in a workshop she has the feeling that the tune of the framing piece has started, indicating closure of the session, and she continues to work it out, but Matthew stops her. It is similar to Matthew stopping Rachel handing out instruments discussed earlier on. Different interpretations of this 'misreading' incident are given: Fiona herself thinks this miscommunication is related to the fact that she felt uncomfortable throughout this session and this has to do, she feels, with the session reflecting the 'larger issues' in the home. Fiona's high sensitivity picks up on the feelings of unsettledness in the home. Anneliese however, shows annoyance with the way Matthew handled this and connects it to a lack of leadership. She writes in her reflective journal: "*Reflecting back on the situation I am wondering about the old question of leadership again. We have failed time and time again to make these sessions work in a 'democratic' manner. In this particular situation I wonder if Matthew would have been more open and receptive to other ideas and clues if he, as the leader, did not have so much else to consider? Fiona was left feeling she had made a mistake (...).*" Anneliese feels that Matthew's style of leadership should change into a more shared form of leadership. She implies that this incident was damaging for Fiona's self-esteem.

Matthew feels he knows very well how things are related; he reflects in the interview after the session that for the musicians the definition of 'success' in the context of this project is, that "*a resident takes an instrument, a piece is made and musicians feel they have done a good job. And so the desire for [the residents] to play an instrument can be very much tied up with our own feelings of success or not.*"

In a comparable way musicians find it hard to cope with resident Esther. Esther is a very active and statuesque lady, and appears to be quite vibrant, energetic and social. She talks a lot and engages in a very free and excitable way with staff and visitors. She often speaks of going to visit and caring for her mum, needing to do this and that, and seems fixated on tasks, jobs and actions, appearing to live in a remembered past. Relationships with other residents are fractious; with some there is even an element of intimidation, verbally and physically, though usually short-lived. Together with Rebecca, she is the only one of the eight residents who can walk. Esther is also very musical. Esther's continuous walking out of most of the session is interpreted by Matthew as there 'being no progress'. Thus there is clearly a feeling of personal failure when a resident walks out! Matthew realises however at some point that a lot is connected to feelings of self-esteem and self image.

Brian also reflects on the musicians' tendency to take things personally. He realises that criticism coming from the care staff about what happened and what did not happen in the session can contribute to this. However he also feels that the musicians might be a bit too sensitive to that. He reflects:

"I think people's relationships with one another are quite sensitive within the group, I think it's quite an exposed sort of place for everybody, musicians, staff and residents. I think people can feel quite exposed, or feel very sensitive to how other people react to them." Brian can play a strong role in helping the musicians coping with this; however there are also moments where he feels that he fails or where he feels 'the system' fails.

The sixth session was experienced by the musicians as a breakthrough, where a real connection was made between Rebecca and Matthew. This was very empowering for Matthew.

From the field notes:

Rebecca is very still (...) During the welcome song Matthew sings to Rebecca first and smiles after her name, waiting for her response and acknowledgement (...) she focuses on him intently, and after a few seconds beams a smile to him. She appears engaged throughout the piece. Matthew plays the metallophone bass bar[112] at the end of the welcome song and then asks Rebecca "would you like to...?" He looks to Rebecca and indicates for her to play it. She does – hitting it very rapidly. He waits and indicates for her to do it – when she doesn't, he says "can we hear this sound again Rebecca?" she again plays rapidly – this time a little longer than before. Matthew copies the intensity of this immediately in singing, and Fiona echoes his interpretation with a short cadenza. Rebecca then hits the bass bar once, all the time she is very focused on Matthew and her body arches towards him. Matthew sings very strongly – it's very bold, dramatic and fiery. It could almost be described as 'toreador' like at this point, and finds a harmonic centre of D minor. He waits again – she doesn't play, so he continues singing a little whilst keeping very strong unwavering eye contact. Matthew's singing is underpinned sensitively by a drone from Fiona, and occasional interjections from Anneliese on the harp. His singing softens a little, it's a very dark tonal quality, almost cantor-like in execution at times. He holds the bass bar for Rebecca and adjusts it where necessary to enable her to hit it strongly. She keeps her eyes on him except for when she looks down at the bass bar to play. The music becomes very gestural – phrases full of breath and space, waiting for an answer. Fiona continues with a drone and Anneliese plays very crunchy chords with sixths. Occasionally Rebecca plays the bass bar – always very strongly and just the one strike. Near the end she plays some quick notes and Matthew immediately imitates it in his singing. The piece has a Jewish atmosphere. There is a coda where Fiona and Anneliese play vibrantly. When it ends Matthew waits at least fifteen seconds before saying "thank you Rebecca... thank you for playing... really lovely piece. I love your strong playing, very powerful. You inspired us to make some really important music." Rebecca shakes Matthew's hand and smiles broadly. The others in the group are drawn into this piece.

---

[112] Bass chime bar, metallophone, or bass bar: A chime bar metallophone is a tuned metal bar mounted onto a wooden resonator box, in the pitch range of G to a. The sound is produced by striking the metal part of the chime bar with a mallet or beater, most often soft mallets with a wool-wrapped head or hard rubber. An alternative version of the bass chime bar metallophone is the bass chime bar xylophone, where a tuned wooden bar is affixed to a wooden resonator box. See also Appendix V, 'List of musical instruments'.

Rebecca's Piece (session 6)

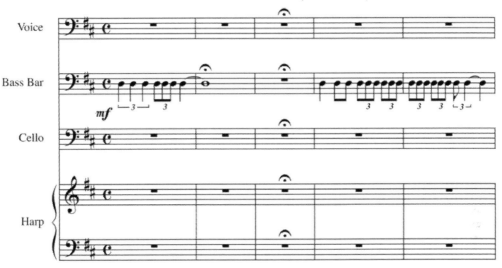

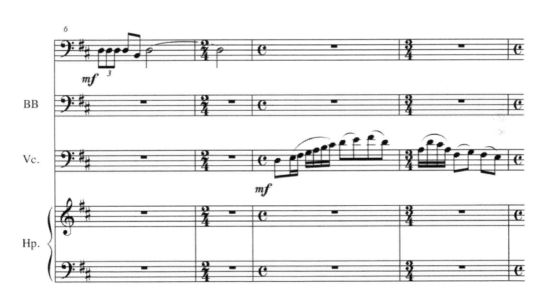

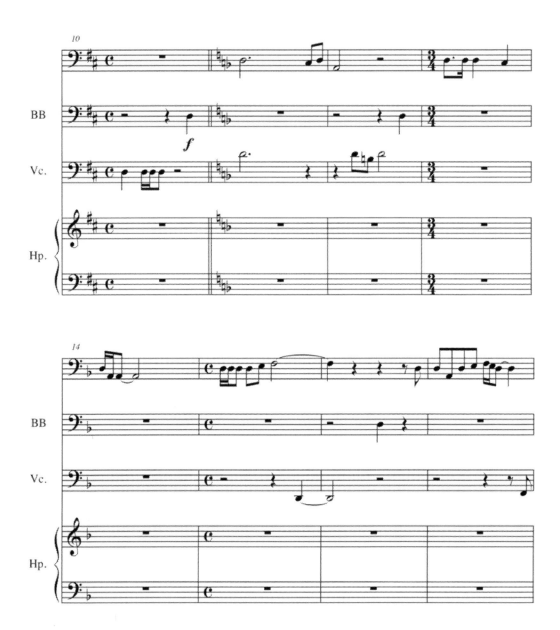

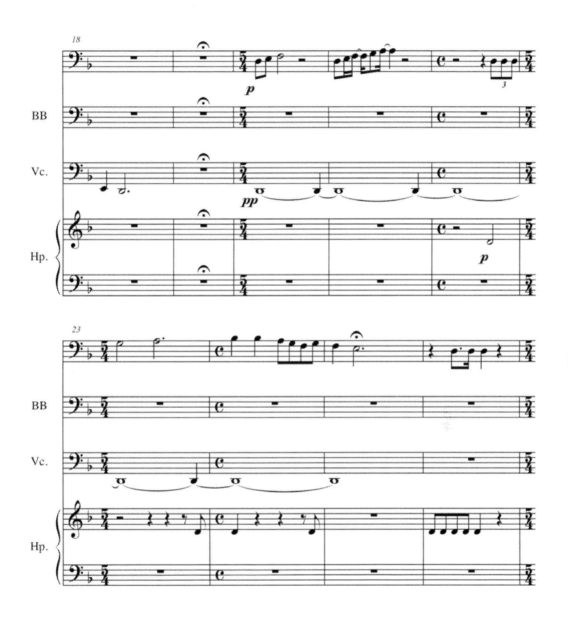

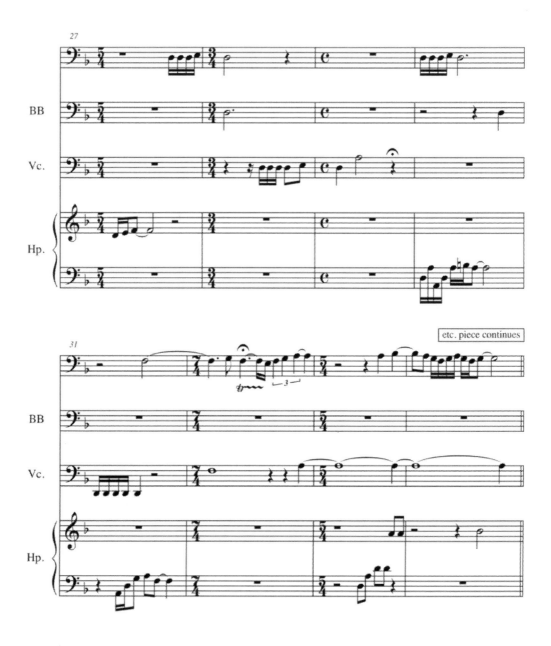

Matthew comments on his inner voice, which he calls 'the Snark', that keeps whispering to him, lowering his confidence and self-esteem and which he tries to silence: *"The Snark went into overdrive, 'you aren't a singer! It's an easy trick to sing Jewish sounding music for Jewish old ladies – you aren't even Jewish yourself, you have no right!' But as the responses came from Rebecca, and I focused more and more on my singing, trying to make it as beautiful as I could, the Snark got quieter and quieter, silenced eventually."*

The piece that evolved in dialogue with Rebecca is described by Matthew as a 'ceremony', in which *"Rebecca would ring the bell and then the music would happen again until it died down and it was back to her and she would ring the bell again and initiate the next wave. And it felt very, very serious. And that was what was in her face as well."* A turning point was the moment where Rebecca stopped playing aggressively and turned to the ceremony-like approach initiating each musical phrase. Matthew gives a brilliant insight into the reflexive practices that are key to this practice when he says: *"When that piece started I had no idea that it was gonna go the way it did. It was a very unthought-of thing, to sing to Rebecca wasn't what I'd imagined. The absolute reaction in the moment about, I suppose really tuning in with a resident, almost split-second actually, a very unplanned piece. Just seizing that moment. I think that was a real moment of reflecting, actually, in which you just reflect back exactly what you see. And I suppose you just have to trust your instinct on that one and think, this is what I'm seeing and this is what I think you want. And just going for it."*

Feelings of vulnerability were not only raised by the Snark; they also showed after the session during the debrief, when Anneliese burst into tears after Matthew praised her for her playing. Matthew's recognition of Anneliese's musicianship was highly connected to the experience he had just had through connecting with Rebecca, which was partly made possible by Anneliese's support. His reflection that musicians are all caught up in their own private thoughts and words, wondering 'what the other thinks of you' and 'whether the music is any good' is well-known amongst musicians. Realistic self-esteem however also exists amongst the musicians in a group interview where Matthew considers that having more courage and taking more risks may have to do with growing older, having a different perspective on things and being a bit more experienced.

For the care staff there are obviously comparable issues at stake. An important observation is made by Brian about the relationship between the learning of the staff and self-esteem: *"I think it reaffirms what I believe myself, that people are motivated by their connections with other people. Staff get motivated by the achievement of the residents that they're with. I think staff have great abilities to actually feel on the level of the person and to actually share the person's emotions. And I think they have a great sense of shared identity. And a sense that the residents' accomplishments are like their accomplishments. More than anything else it confirms my belief that staff really want the best and will give the best they can."*

Clearly, the feeling of 'threatened identity' can be healed. However, this appears not to be a learning achievement of the individual, but rather a communicative procedure that includes all participants involved.

Recognition

'Recognition' is a major part of social identity and it is an important concept in this practice in different senses. Recognition is related to empowerment, for all learners involved. Residents are recognised in their music and they are in particular acknowledged very consciously when they are thanked for their piece.

The most clearly directed recognition happens during every session in the 'welcome song', a song in which the workshopleader goes around the circle, singing every individual name of the person in the circle and continuing to do so until the participants feel recognised and acknowledged. This is visibly a very powerful tool; it makes people often lucid, aware and happy. Brian points out that it leads to a sense of equality and respect. Below follows a description of the welcome song from the fourth session.

From the field notes:

Matthew uses a c hand chime. The song starts with Harry, whom Matthew has just introduced. Matthew sings: "good morning Harry" and Harry sings: "good morning everyone. Thank you for having me here." Names are sung twice around the circle with short cadenzas after each name. Matthew then makes groups of three individuals, then calls names across the circle, then finally ends by singing "good morning everyone." The song is very vibrant in parts. There is a slight sense of urgency when Harry's djembe[113] comes in and the tempo picks up, however, people are responsive when their names are sung just the once and when Matthew cross-picks people they are quite awake. Abigail appears very engaged throughout the name song. Her replies are very happy and responsive, and the musicians immediately embellish beautifully. At the beginning of the song she joins in singing, and this continues fairly regularly throughout the piece. After her name is sung for the first time Abigail says "Good morning." Matthew responds by saying "Lovely to see you" and Abigail replies "to you, all of you."

After Helena's name Abigail says "Good morning everybody." When Harry begins to play the drum later in the piece, she nods her head in time to the pulse. She appears to enjoy it when Matthew recognises her at the end of the song – motioning towards her with a strong physical gesture "good morning, good morning!" Gabriella seems to be asleep but Matthew wakes her up (and Harry on the flute). Gabriella

---

[113] Also known as djembé, jembe, jenbe, djimbe, jimbe, or dyinbe. Originating from West Africa, the djembe is a goblet drum with a skin head, often made of hardwood and untreated goat hide. The skin head is attached to the drum with rope, and the drum is 'rope-tuned' through a weaving process. A variety of sounds can be produced using hand strokes, a rich bass tone through striking the centre of the drum, and drier tones near the rim. In the project, a large, soft wool-headed mallet was used to produce a sound. See also Appendix V, 'List of musical instruments'.

appears happy. She mouths the song when her name is being sung and says "thank you" at the end and laughs as Matthew says "you're very welcome." Matthew and Rachel stroke her arms. Gabriella then sings along in full voice to Matthew's name and her face is alive, with a large smile. She smiles regularly and looks around the circle, and sometimes even laughs. She sings along in a very engaged way "good morning all" whilst Rachel strokes her arm. Sarah seems to be in a generally good state of well-being. She listens quietly. Samantha, next to her, looks shy when it is her turn. Sarah sings "Morning" during Abigail's name and then Rachel's name. Helena waves to Sarah across the circle when Sarah's name is sung. Later, when her name is sung again, she smiles. Anneliese is actively beaming a smile to Sarah, and this echoes the music at that moment, which is very vibrant. Jessica has her eyes closed during the name song, but she mouths along and sometimes sings very softly. Harry brings Rosamund's attention to Rachel's name as Rachel's name is being sung, by gesturing towards Rachel. The high pitch of the flute, during Sarah's name, appears to affect her. She twitches and moves slightly forward as if getting ready to get up. She responds to Harry's "Good morning" but appears to be a little ill at ease. The first time round, Hannah starts to sing her own name, in the right key and with the right melody. The musicians gift her with a big improvisation. Later, Hannah doesn't appear to register when her name is being sung and the musicians give an extra moment of space and hello at the end of her name for her to respond – she doesn't. Rebecca stares at Harry when her name is being sung. She notices but remains distanced. Soon after, when Matthew's name is being sung, she taps Helena's hand very hard, then gets up immediately and leaves with resolve.

Welcome Song (session 4)

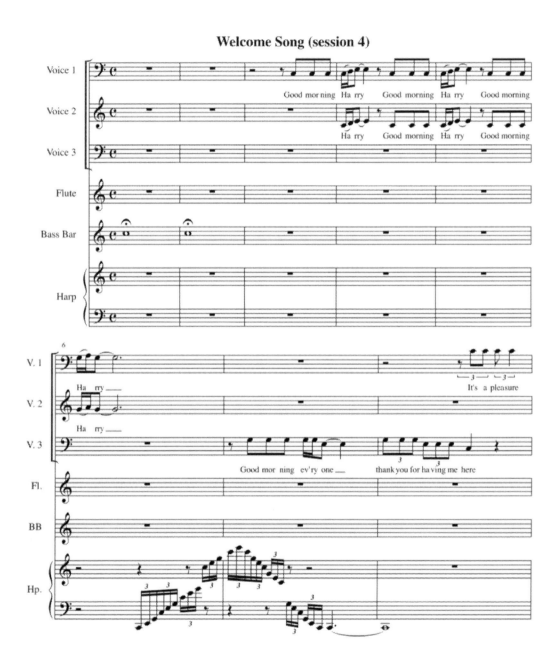

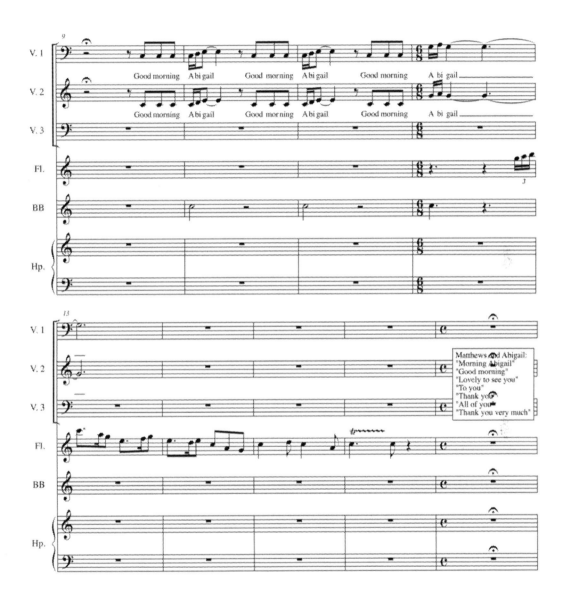

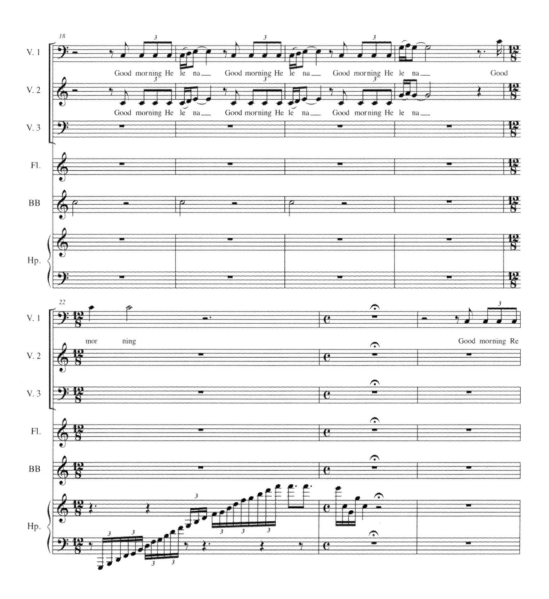

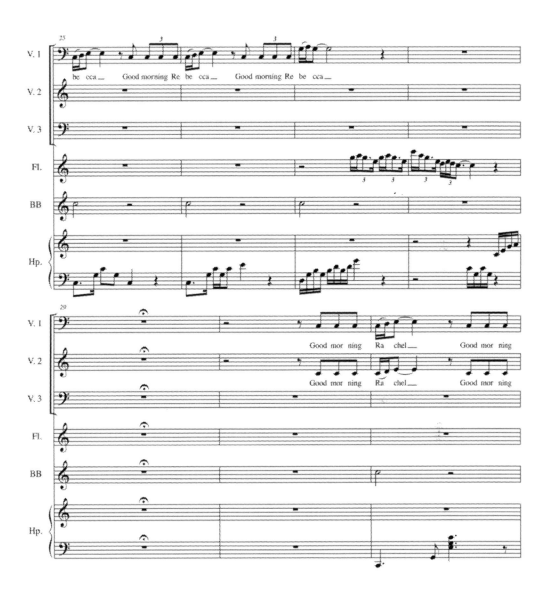

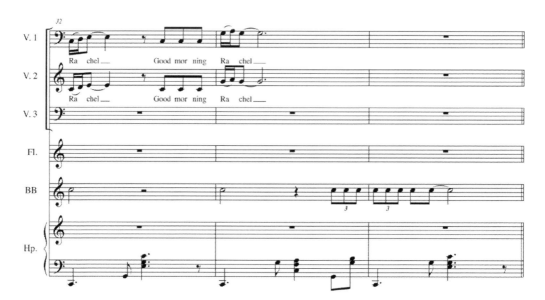

In the description of the welcome song we met Samantha, Social Care Coordinator within the home. Samantha is well spoken, professional and polite, and appears to be very thoughtful and sensitive, she is also a bit shy. Quietly, modestly and diligently she delivers her work.

There is recognition of the needs of residents and endorsement of where they are 'in the moment'. If a resident chooses to leave, this needs to be recognised as participation is free. It is sometimes a tough process for the musicians to accept when a resident chooses to leave, as is often the case with Esther and also with Rebecca. Acceptance and recognition are also sometimes needed in the circle, e.g. when a resident does not want to pass an instrument. Fiona reflects on 'choice', which is to her mind one of the few things that can be offered to residents in this context. She says: "*Choice is a huge part of this work and I was really reminded of how each person has autonomy. The residents are in so many ways powerless at this stage of life, particularly in a residential home. They are without many choices and that is something we can offer. Although we can encourage someone to take part, knowing what the benefits are, it is always crucial to remember that ultimately we are there to empower and support the residents, whatever that looks like.*" When Esther leaves during the session, some of these feelings of Fiona are endorsed by Brian who reflects that Esther left "*with a definite sense of being in control and a sense of adult responsibility with important things to do.*"

The musicians and staff development practitioner spend a lot of time immersing themselves into the different approaches that may work in order to recognise each individual involved. Brian acknowledges the personhood of residents by looking at the perspective of each individual person. He reflects for instance about Hannah, who is one of the residents who has not yet been introduced, although we have already briefly met her. Hannah loves making music, and is mostly very actively engaged. Despite being partially sighted and hard of hearing, Hannah appears to be relaxed in her environment, is well spoken and able to assert herself around others. These strengths mask a level of confusion; outwardly Hannah appears able to comprehend others and her environment, though occasionally this mask slips and the reality of Hannah's experience of dementia and a sense of confusion is exposed. When Brian reflects about Hannah's role, he says: "*I think Hannah held that place in the group today as the affirming, calm appreciative person. I think it comes from a very true place within herself. I think that it is an affirming group for her. But I also think it is her giving, giving out. I strongly believe that people do take roles and that's the role that she took today.*" This is a typical comment for Brian, where he puts himself in the place of the person with dementia and 'speaks for them'. He empowers the person in that way, by making sure that personhood is recognised.

The musicians often report in their reflections on 'the person behind the dementia'[114], when for example Anneliese reflects at some point on resident Jessica. Jessica is quiet and very softly spoken, and appears very frail, often drifting in and out of sleep. She appears comforted by her relationships with others, though appears distant and withdrawn for long periods. She clearly enjoys the sessions. After Jessica had engaged very actively in a piece of music and even told the musicians that the music was about 'a forest', Anneliese felt that : "*we got to see the real, dignified Jessica who is still residing in there.*"

It can be very confronting for the musicians to recognise a resident's pain, like for instance Sarah's crying out for her mummy. Fiona reports about the distress and how the music tried to reflect this desperation, and at the same time taking the group to a more "*hopeful place*". Fiona also acknowledges what support she needs in order to deal with this. It reflects her biographical learning when she says: "*After the session I realised that it had reminded me of a close family member who had a severe breakdown several years ago. At this time she regressed to a child-like person that was very difficult to see. Somehow Sarah's crying out had reminded me of this. I was very grateful for the support of the team and Deborah's offer to chat things through if needed. In this case I didn't feel the need, however I wanted to mention it as I do feel that in this work, the support network that you have is*

---

[114] Kitwood 1997.

67

so vitally important. It is very human work - you bring not only your musicianship but your humanity to this work, and there can be very real emotional issues that you come into contact with in the residents, and in your own life. In order to do this work well, good support and the ability to share this is so important."

Sarah's distress and the possible release of it is recognised through music in the second session.

From the field notes:

Matthew pauses for a moment before heading directly for Sarah. He touches her upper arms and comforts her, saying her name – "mummy" becomes tinged with sadness and slightly lower in pitch. Matthew asks Sarah "Can I play a piece of music for you?" to which she replies immediately "yeah, but it's not easy." There is a pause before Matthew asks "Can we try?", – immediately – "Yes". Matthew: "Will you help me?" He looks for the baton on the table and asks for the musicians' help in finding it – they instantly spring to the front of their chairs. Matthew: "will you help me Sarah?" as he passes it to her. She begins to look downwards and then holds her head in her hands. She lets go of her head and Matthew attempts to recapture eye contact with her by kneeling closer to the ground – she re-engages with him. At the end of the piece Matthew says "thank you so much... wonderful... wonderful, thank you..." and Sarah has a smile on her face. Matthew: "Thank you for making that piece of music with me...Thanks also to Fiona who was playing with you" – he gestures to Fiona who says "really lovely" and smiles at Sarah – and then over to Anneliese "and Anneliese." Matthew stays with Sarah for a few moments more, and there is a long silence afterwards.

Matthew asking for Sarah's help is parallel to the way he is 'helping' Sarah: this feels a significant episode in finding the person behind the dementia at a deep level. The musicians appear to recognise the importance of this in their speed of response. They discuss Matthew mirroring Sarah's body language, which then led to her sitting upright in the end.

It is interesting to observe how Matthew looks back on this episode with Sarah: "*I demonstrated to her that she is there and she matters and that her presence is important.*" Matthew clearly needs recognition himself: he comments that he wants the staff to see these big moments and that he needs them to feel good. He adds that he needs to make sure to make a balance between knowing what the residents want, and pushing and challenging them.

Brian reflects back on the episode with Sarah in a different way: *"So that was a very human two-way relationship that happened, and perhaps that's, that was a very important thing that it was two-way. That she was given the affirmation that she had given and contributed. There's a danger I think, that perhaps she may feel like she's always receiving rather than giving back. So I thought it was a very adult encounter. Sarah, it affirmed her as an adult. The complexity of that, that you have the child calling for mummy and this adult of eighty, ninety-something years of age, and I thought that was handled really well in the group."* Here Brian speaks again 'on behalf of the resident.' The key reflection on recognition in this particular episode comes from Fiona: *"Sarah was very distressed throughout the session. She was constantly calling out 'Mummy' throughout. The only time that she stopped was when Matthew offered her the baton and she created a very moving piece. Her words after were 'It's very difficult'. I felt the music provided an outlet, and broke the cycle of her calling out. I felt her words showed that we had engaged with the real Sarah, not the little lady who called out Mummy, but an articulate lady who was expressing how frightened and painful her existence is – 'It's very difficult.'"*

Fiona also relates about the recognition of Esther, with whom she had a connection on a deeper level at the beginning of the session; Esther left soon after that. She feels she really connected with Esther, not just by engaging in quick and busy rhythmic gestures, but in slower, focused and more open gestures. Fiona says: *"I really felt for these few moments that she slowed down, and I was able to see and sense the softer side of her. More than that it was just a lovely moment of connection."* 'Slowing down' is at the core here, and also the recognition of the fact that it is up to Esther to leave the circle. Brian acknowledges the legitimate character of a role in the periphery, when he reflects that to his idea Esther really felt welcome, but left out of choice and with dignity, without any feeling of having done something wrong. Thus the agency of individuals is highly valued. If someone wants to leave, the choice is up to her. The only thing of importance is that someone should leave still feeling wanted. Fiona describes it likewise, when she comments on Esther's premature leaving, saying that *"It would be wonderful if she felt able to stay longer next week, but equally I felt she had a few moments of well-being and was able to exercise her choice to leave."*

A wonderful example of engagement and recognition takes place between Gabriella and Harry. They make a cheerful piece of music together and Gabriella becomes very lucid. This lucidity shows through how she engages musically, how she makes contact and it continues throughout the discussion after the piece has finished, where she shows a very humourous side of herself. Gabriella and Harry improvise on texts: 'That sounds good, sounds really good'. In the following part of this chapter, on Communication, a musical transcription of the interaction can be found.

From the field notes:

At the end Harry says: "Gabriella...that sounded really good." They laugh. Matthew says "Gabriella, how was the music?" and she makes a joke "it sounds really good." Matthew: "Would you like to hear some music on the harp at all?" Gabriella agrees. Anneliese starts the closing theme. Matthew says "we're kinda actually almost out of time" to which Gabriella says "no...!" and Matthew replies "Afraid so." Gabriella makes another joke "that is not so good!" They laugh.

Many interesting things happen here: initially Gabriella starts counting when she is asked to play, but soon leaves it and becomes very lucid once she is engaged in the music. The dementia and the 'real' Gabriella both show up and in the end Gabriella's personhood is on the foreground. She not only picks up rhythmically, related to musical language – 'that sounds good, sounds really good' – but also in terms of communication and verbal language.

Some residents are really difficult to read. An example is Rosamund, briefly mentioned in the field notes of the welcome song. The musicians often wonder who she is and how she can be reached. Rosamund interacts little with other residents, preferring to speak only to visitors and staff, often appearing distrustful and disdaining towards other residents. Often her piercing eyes will scan the room, contradicting a mostly impassive expression on her face. Sometimes she finds the nature of objects confusing and appears to have difficulty talking fluently. During visits from her children, Rosamund appears to come alive with joy, perhaps resonating with her earlier life as a homemaker, in which she enjoyed solitary activities, such as reading and playing the piano. Matthew feels challenged because Rosamund will sometimes not take part in the process of passing instruments, however one can also wonder if Rosamund does not understand and may feel embarrassed about that.

Rosamund is thus often an enigma for the musicians and they try hard to understand her better. The musicians need to recognise that her dementia clearly exists and this happens in a struggling way. Fiona relates about a conversation she had with Rosamund where Rosamund disclosed that she felt she is living amongst 'old fossils': "*It was at this point that I felt the sense of connection and trust that we had built had helped her to feel that we were equals. It was a real insight into how she felt in the home, and a very typical problem of people being frightened of the dementia, old age and illness that they see around them. I think our task is to try and integrate Rosamund as much as possible through the music. I felt we really turned a corner with her this week, especially as she commented to Anneliese about the 'beautiful music and the wonderful singing'.*" Matthew reflects insightful on Fiona's disclosure saying: "*Somebody who's feeling that she's having to accept I have the same disease as these people. Yep. That's hard, that's hard.*" Then followed by: "*But it sort of gives very clearly a way forward that it's not the music that she's resistant to, that there's other things that are stopping her.*"

Matthew summarises in an excellent way the recognition of the group in all aspects, partly in the interview and partly in his reflective journal: "*There was a sense of well-being within the group, and I have been thinking about where this comes from, and how 'symbiotic' it is:*

Residents can be helped to feel it when the music is 'right', when it touches something within them, when they participate (however that might look – making choices, listening, responding, leading (...).

Staff feel it when they 'know what to do', when they act reflexively, when they feel connected to the musicians, when they make music that is theirs.

Musicians feel it when they make strong playing connections together, when they see responses from the residents and staff.

None of these happen without the other things – it is a three-way cycle that happens simultaneously. It is about being in relationship. And so a kind of virtuous circle is created, that is about each person being in relationship successfully with the rest of the group and finding their relationship with the group and with each other. And with their own sense of themselves as well. The session being an opportunity for that to be expressed for them musically. And also for them to be able to express themselves in a way that they care for each other within the group, is an expression of oneself as well, you know, to show you care for somebody else. And it was all of these things being able to come into play. It kind of builds really, and generates what is seen as a successful session, I think."

Integrity

It goes without saying that integrity is a core value in this practice. During the group interview preceding the project the three musicians spoke about it a lot. Matthew shared a story on that occasion, equally powerful with dignity, integrity and personhood at the core: *"I'll always remember, I was making a piece with a lady who had a woodblock and made loud noises on this woodblock constantly. And I was making this piece with her. I'd come up close to her, was kneeling in front of her and was totally sort of locked in this thing. And she was locked in with me and we couldn't stop you know, because she kept driving me, I kept responding to her. She was stuck either, because of the dementia, she was stuck in a pattern, or she was keeping it going for me because I was playing, so she had to keep playing and we were totally stuck. And I tried to stop the piece several times and it didn't stop, she kept going and the way out of that was a musical solution in the end in that one of the other musicians joined the piece and then began to change the piece from inside. And that was what unlocked the thing, and I was able to step back. The woman stopped her repetitive playing and it all just shifted. And kind of everyone's dignity was preserved. Do you know what I mean? There wasn't this kind of... cause when somebody's stuck in a pattern like that, the anxiety is, how do we get out of this, without stopping her physically or it becoming embarrassing. You know the rest of the group are aware that she's not playing appropriately, you know, the dementia is being highlighted."*

Integrity is interwoven with recognition, responsibility, dignity and personhood. Musical integrity is an important given as we can see through Matthew's example. Musicians are very conscious about concepts as mirroring and translating, imitating and the like. Important is that the music needs to reflect on the resident's self, but *not* reflect back the resident's dementia. An example is Rebecca, who can be quite aggressive, slapping other people, and likewise slapping instruments. Matthew comments on this: "*there's almost a cruelty in reflecting back to her this kind of movement which would be ridiculing her. You know, you don't want to mirror back somebody's dementia at them, do you know what I mean?*"

The overall attitude of the musicians is one of high integrity and a very conscious awareness of do's and don'ts when making music with people with dementia. The musicians take responsibility to make everybody involved to feel welcome and recognised, even in small detail, like making a compliment on how someone looks, or asking if a person would like to be addressed by her first name or surname. The musicians make a real effort to try and find out more about a particular resident, in order to find ways to reach her musically and give her a sense of belonging. Hannah for example is often taken into consideration; the musicians sometimes wonder if she really has dementia, however Brian confirms this. The musicians ask themselves how they can 'stretch' Hannah, how to bring her into contact with her creative self and what instrument and what music fit her. The musicians likewise try to find out about Rosamund, what is behind her reluctance to participate? Why does she seem so isolated: is she bored or is she just not feeling safe? In short there is a lot of integrity and effort going into recognition and personhood.

An important incident with Rosamund occurs in the sixth session and is a big learning moment for the musicians. Rosamund is brought in and she is not able to get from the wheel chair into the arm chair. In the end she needs to be hoisted. This feels as a very 'exposed' thing; musicians feel embarrassed by the openness of this activity. Fiona and Anneliese try to distract the observers by playing. How the musicians react is very significant. Fiona accounts: "*At the beginning of the session Rosamund was unable to get out of her wheelchair into her arm chair and so the staff had to wheel a 'hoist' into the centre of the circle and very publicly use it to transfer her into her arm chair. Rosamund was actually fine throughout this process and seemed very calm. Anneliese and myself played gently in the background just to try and create a calm atmosphere and also to take the focus off of her. However, in the debrief there was a general feeling that this had been distressing to see and seemed a very public and maybe de-humanising thing to have happened to Rosamund before the session. During this part of the conversation I was really struck by Brian's insightful comment. He simply said; 'I hear what you're saying but I think it's important to remember that this is a very real part of every day for the residents. We often have to use*

the hoist and many other similar procedures that are difficult to see and experience for the residents. But this is the reality... This is their reality.'
I was really struck by what he said and realised how important it is that a Music For Life session operates out of this sense of reality. We are wanting to help people to feel as comfortable as possible, to be as real as possible – to express how they are in the moment and also we need to be able to find a way to incorporate this practical reality into the session, and as a musical team be as comfortable as possible with some of the harsh realities of the resident's life. This can be really difficult but is as important in the practical layout and set up of the sessions (...). " Fiona then continues with a key observation about the practice: *"I think the amazing thing about music is that you can be 'held' in the moment, or taken to a new place. You can provide a safe place in music that accepts each person as they are in that moment, or you can help to transfer them out of their current emotional /mental state to a different place, even for a moment. I was really pleased that Anneliese and I had played during this procedure; I think the music helped to 'hold' this difficult moment and also made the incident simply a part of the session as a whole."*

Matthew reflects in a similar manner, saying: *"To us it appeared humiliating, frightening, intrusive. Brian pointed out that this is part of who she is now, and she brings that to the group. All of the feelings and thoughts I had about witnessing it are mine to own. As Brian said, there is a deeper dignity, which comes from seeing beyond my own feelings and upset, and which remains connected with the person, honouring them whatever their situation or difficulty."* This is a very significant observation, key to the values of this practice, showing a lot of insight and also showing an interesting profile of the staff development practitioner, who is not only a dementia facilitator for the care staff, but in this way for the musicians as well. Brian shows that dignity is based in reality. Through that he actually establishes the dignity for people. This is the reason that Brian also points out that he finds it important that musicians build up a sensitivity to what a care environment is and that this environment is challenging.

In a group conversation the musicians come back to the hoisting incident with Rosamund; a dialogue between Matthew and Fiona comes down to Matthew's summary of what he learnt from Brian, confirmed by Fiona: *"And Brian was pointing that out really, and was saying, this is who she is, that's what she brings to the circle. He was talking about dignity and just about how dignity is almost something which is given to people, rather than people having to maintain it themselves. Because they're in circumstances where that isn't possible. You know, what we imagine as being dignity is just not possible. And so therefore, it's given to them. And by us witnessing that, seeing Rosamund being mechanically hoisted, we maintained her dignity. That is an incredible learning process."*

The musicians reflect on the necessity of being authentic and to be really who you are. This entails risk taking and the decision to be brave. Fiona points out that a big responsibility for the musician is to 'be real' as a person, to be grounded and open. She is convinced that residents will pick up if you are not. She says: "*There has to be a real honesty from within yourself, if you're expecting the people you're working with to feel safe to express musically or in however way they are. And they will pick up if you're not being authentic, I think, this is maybe the right word. So your music has to be authentic and somehow I think we're all a bit human, and a bit broken and not able to do this all the time. But to kind of find that authenticity within yourself and to be brave enough to be who you are... And I think Deborah really instills that as a value, has really instilled that as a value of the project, so it's very person-centred, and then the music comes from that. And as the music is an expression of who you are it also has to have the integrity.*"

Fiona also points out that you always have to realise that you are in another person's space: "*I kind of feel like I'm over there, I'm in the other person's space. It's like you almost have to rely on what you've established in the first hour. Because your awareness can't be between the three of us, your awareness is suddenly on the other person.*"

Like Matthew earlier on, Fiona gives a wonderful example of musical integrity in the form of a story from another project she was involved in. She relates: "*And I had one moment, on the last project I was with we had an older man, quite, I think he was in his eighties, he'd been in the army, very rhythmic, very military (...) and all of this. And Harry was the group leader and [this man] asked him to create a romantic piece and he asked me to play for him. And suddenly his gesture changed. It had been very up and down with the baton, and suddenly he kind of did this, very soft movement. And I started to play the emotion he was giving and he keeps stopping me, o wow, there you go, that was very nice. There you go, you've heard it now. And we kept carrying on, because it was almost like he was wanting to say something else. There was more than this military (...), there was this other part of him. So eventually I think it took three attempts of him. He kept kind of joking about how he didn't want to stop, and then suddenly just he went for these huge, huge motions with the baton. I found it a really intense moment, actually, because I felt he was really giving of himself. And I don't really remember what I played, but I just remember so being with him and wanting to follow, not just the motion, but the conviction and feeling of what he was, it was quite an intense moment. But I wasn't physically going, oh, I'm gonna go high now or I'm gonna try this, or, you kind of go with this moment. I think that's why the sessions are so exhausting, because you're using every, it's like your antennae are all over your body because you're picking up on senses and then you're playing. And then there's your own spiritual and emotional reaction to what's going on. It's a really unusual process. For me it's a little bit like how I feel in chamber music. When you're really engaged with people, and you're playing off what someone else is playing to you, but it's kind of intensified even more, because you're trying to be someone else's music for them."*

Responsibility

Feeling responsible and being responsible are two different things and the musicians sometimes struggle with this. This shows in their learning process where they slowly find out where they can make a difference, and where they have to let go, taking their own boundaries into account. Dementia cannot be changed, but music can serve as a strong tool to create a better environment for people living with dementia.

There is a lot to learn from Brian in this respect. Brian feels very responsible, in many aspects. His role is that of a connector, for instance within logistic issues, seeing to it that everything is in place, but he has also the role of creating awareness: "*I try to help the team to understand the many challenges the home is facing on a day to day basis, and many of them being of an unplanned nature.*" Brian often shows an enormous sense of responsibility for making the connection between music and the care situation. He says: "*I sometimes feel that the culture of the creative arts world and that of care are very different. This can create a tension, but in my view, it is a helpful tension that can be enriching for life in the home. I hope it can also bring about growth for the team of musicians. Perhaps it is because the creative arts world has a different culture that it can be of benefit and enriching to the care world. Maybe this is at the heart of the project.*"

There is a delicate balance between wanting to reach people with dementia and to let go and accept when a resident does not want contact. This has to be respected and understood. Fiona describes the eye contact which she tried to establish with Rosamund in the first session, where she came too close and Rosamund moved away: "*I was just reminded of the need to have a highly attuned awareness of people's need for space in this work.*" Brian endorses these processes by stressing that trying to give too much support can actually lead to disempowerment. He points out the important condition that a critical aspect of the practice is "*slowing down, letting things go at the pace of the person with dementia.*" 'Time', 'space' and 'pace' are key words in this practice, and responsibility and integrity are therefore highly interwoven. Brian is sensitive to residents, tries even in detail, to 'crawl under their skin'; he realises for instance that it is hard for the residents to have to leave their normal breakfast area when it is used for setting up the session on the Monday morning. He feels it impacts on the residents.

There is also a balance for the musicians between respecting the reluctance of a resident to participate and trying to engage with this resident, however always preventing a sense of 'exposure'. It is important to create a feeling of trust and an atmosphere of safety for participation. Matthew learns about himself in this sense, where he realises that Rosamund's reluctance to participate in the sessions may have much more to do with her own anxiety than with his performance.

Brian argues that when you do not know how to respond you cannot support a person living with dementia. It is a sense of puzzlement which everyone can have throughout the project. On the other hand however, musicians can have a hard time finding the balance between feeling responsible and drawing the line for self protection. Matthew frames this by saying in his reflective journal: "*We fear going to that place where we are made to look hard at things. By keeping things moving, we can avoid the feelings of discomfort that might arise, or of looking too closely into the reality of the people with dementia.*"

Brian reflects retrospectively on realism which is required within his personal sense of responsibility and wanting to be in control. He realises that he needs to balance the control on the one hand and the moments where he has to hold back and just support the staff on the other hand. He says "*...we all have our observations and you probably feel it more than anyone this time. And it is important to be aware that there are times to hold back, definitively. It's ongoing development.*"

However for Brian it is unimaginable to hold back by leaving behind his sense of responsibility and not be part of the debrief as is suggested at some point by Matthew. Brian responds to this by taking up his role as staff development practitioner. When he reflects back on a newly tried out set up of the debrief, where Matthew acts as chair and he and Deborah take the backseat, Brian observes a genuine effort of the musicians and staff to understand the residents. Nevertheless he remarks: "*I also feel that there was an interpretation of residents' actions and behaviours that did not accept the reality of dementia in their lives. I wonder if this will change over the coming weeks or if it is too painful to enter into this harsh reality. A lack of understanding can lead to the projection of our own feelings and realities on to people with dementia.*" He continues to say: "*I feel that we are beginning to reach the point where we can meet people as they really are and accept dementia as part of their lives. Perhaps we are coming to a point where we can meet each other with our differences including dementia and this meeting can be on more equal ground.*" That is a very crucial observation, relating to personhood and equality, identifying a critical element of the role of the staff development practitioner and giving the evidence why his presence is required in the debrief.

Matthew considers the balance between creating music that reflects how the residents are feeling and on the other hand that as a musician you can feel 'trapped' in reflecting the low energy that can exist. Hence it is important to sometimes break this atmosphere through music. Matthew also becomes aware that he needs to keep a realistic lead over his own thoughts related to how residents might consider him. He is actually afraid of Rebecca and Rosamund; of Rebecca in terms of what she might physically do to him unexpectedly, and afraid of Rosamund in terms of what she might think of him. However this is of course not very realistic. Matthew writes the script for Rosamund, thinking that this work is far 'below her', but he also slowly begins to realise that perhaps Rosamund is afraid that her dementia will show, and that is something very different. He says: "*I'm less afraid of her judgement now. Often she will express that, oh, it was all rubbish, all of this kind of stuff. But actually maybe, what's at the root of it is her fear of making a mistake. Which is much more in keeping with the sense of dementia, you know, with her dementia maybe and her covering up her confusion. It's much more of a depth of understanding her.*" This is a reflection which helps him not to feel responsible for the whole process and outcomes, which would obviously be impossible.

During the final session Hannah is invited by the musicians to play the harp. Initially she seems to enjoy it and then all of a sudden it stops. Of course this does not mean that the musicians have failed in their responsibility, it just shows the signs of dementia, where someone can suddenly 'tumble back'. After the last session the musicians have reached a shared feeling of where responsibility begins and ends: in the group interview they discuss that it is not about 'ticking boxes' nor about input and output, but more about being able to respond as an artist in the moment. That is a very crucial observation.

Brian reflects on the feelings of responsibility of staff members: "*I think it's always a matter of choice. It's about, do I choose to grow or not? And do I choose to remain in this kind of work or not? And if I want to choose, I mean, I want to say to staff in training sessions: make a choice to work in dementia care (...) it's too, I mean, if I'm just there doing a job, it's not enough. I have to make a choice and there's no point in complaining about, it's like this or it's like that. It's an elective choice, there are other jobs to do. And if you're choosing to work in dementia care one of the aspects is that you need to be able to love. You need to be able to relate to people.*" Indeed, within the social space of working with people with dementia, within responsibility, 'choice' is the hidden challenge.

Learning benefits

As we have seen, awareness of dementia and what it involves creates important areas of learning for the musicians, not in the least related to their own perceptions, their self-confidence, and their hidden wish for development in terms of 'progress'. The learning that takes place is different for every individual involved, but still it can be development or, as Brian calls it, 'growth'.

The musicians need to make their choices from an awareness and understanding of dementia. What instruments will they for example choose for the residents, how far can they push a resident that refuses to pass an instrument? Residents may not understand, feel disempowered and exposed and also motor issues may play a role. Nor should it be overlooked that care staff may feel vulnerable and insecure. They may not be knowledgeable about music, or feel shy or unconfident to participate. Musicians need to be sensitive to this and the role of the staff development practitioner is, once again, key in this respect.

Another part of dementia awareness is that the musicians need to learn to cope with the unpredictability of how things will develop. After the first session Matthew is very aware of his irritation with Esther's behaviour, and at the same time he feels compassion, realising that she cannot help it. He understands that he is frustrated with the situation, not the person, and that it is up to him to learn to cope with this, because nothing else can be changed. Also Fiona points out how dementia awareness needs to grow again during each project, she realises that initially she always experiences the situation as sad, whereas after a few weeks she is more able to see the person behind the dementia.

Matthew goes through an important learning process and he reflects a lot on his leadership. However his thoughts and ideas are not always put into practice during the eight weeks. Matthew is aware that he wants to be in control, and although he wants musicians to co-lead, he knows that he often does not allow them the space for that. He recognises that this position can be 'to drive everything'.

Matthew also learns about what he calls the 'balancing act' between cognitive and emotional learning. During the interview after the second session, where Sarah constantly called out for her mother, he explains that actually rationality and instinct go together, however in an informed way: "*I suppose I'm kind of struck by the balancing act of being rational and being instinctive within the session today. This was a session really based on gut reaction (…) And how much can be like that because there has been so much thinking and planning and talking. And things, you know, in the prep-session for years there's been, it's been digested and internalised which means the gut reaction works. And whether, without that, if you came and you just reacted on instinct constantly, I think it would be chaotic, I really do. I can think of sessions where I've worked with musicians where people said, 'I just felt this had to happen.' It isn't effective actually, because everyone's pulling in different directions (…) you know, it's within a context and an understanding. Within a knowledge, a framework, a very strong framework of knowledge.*" Matthew feels that through training you really need to gain knowledge, which you then internalise and re-use through a reflexive 'gut reaction'. In the end the experience leads to a gut reaction from the heart.

Not surprisingly Brian is very adamant on the emotional learning. He feels that being too analytical or intellectual about issues involved can distract from the chance to *feel* it. He says: "*So for me it's less in the head and more in the gut. I believe that's quite important. I often have a little bit of frustration that people go from the heart to the head too quickly in Music for Life. So I often feel the debriefs intellectualise what is happening and what has happened in the session without having the chance to feel it. I think sometimes that can be a defense mechanism as well where we protect ourselves from some of the depth of emotion that might be stirring inside of us. So we maybe escape to analysing.*" Brian senses that it is very important that this 'feeling' as an attitude is spread further into the residential home.

In some of the reflective sessions with the staff Brian tries an approach in which he wants to give this 'gut feeling' a place. He does this by means of making music together, like drumming or having staff choose words from cards and make associations: "*And people spoke about conscious connections, connections associated with their work, connections associated with their faith, their religion. And it led us into wider discussions as well of the music that the musicians made and what that stirs. So the point I wanted to make with the staff is that Music for Life is also for them. And that it is also a growth process for them. And yes, they are here to support residents and in some ways to support the musicians. I then asked them if they could each think of one resident that touched them, if there's something that they felt they wanted to communicate to the other staff team, to the rest of the staff teams. And I gave them that task in a way, that whoever that resident was, they would go back to that unit, where the resident lives and ask and speak and have discussions about what happened and why it happened. How it struck them and so on.*" This whole approach stems basically from the urge to create a real sense of belonging.

Nevertheless the learning processes of staff members can be tough, as not being knowledgeable about music can lead to a lack of confidence and disempowerment. This is very important to keep in mind. Care staff are used to a clear role and they know the job they have to do. As soon as they come into a Music for Life session they do not have a particular role, they are there as themselves and they are often not in their comfort zone. They have never expressed the issues that are encountered, nor responded to them and that is a huge experience. Brian feels it is very important to bear in mind that the journey for the staff is big, as it is for the residents. In his approaches, like drumming, or using little cards with words, he appeals to these processes.

This sense of lack of confidence amongst care staff brings us back to the incident with Rachel, described earlier on. Through this incident Matthew became more aware of the preconceptions, actions and reactions of care staff. He says: "*I have to remember that Rachel's reaction does actually signify 'progress' – it is the 'Music for Life Feeling', of not knowing what the best thing to do is. For me, it is from this point of 'not knowing' that brings me into the present, and into deeper relationship with the residents. But I only know this because it has happened so many times.*" Experience is key to understanding and interpreting the experience, and to understanding care staff reactions. It could be easy for the musicians, especially when they are very experienced, to feel removed from or forget the depth of this feeling of 'not knowing' of the care staff, even if they do recognise it as part of the process.

The musicians continuously learn about how to engage with residents in terms of reflecting back their identities through music. Fiona for instance ponders on reflecting back the gestures of Rebecca: "*Her intense gestures are more about her focus on you as a person/musician than actual musical shapes, so we are trying to find music that connects to 'her' rather than 'her gestures'.*" The focus is thus on personhood through music.

Regarding the learning processes required by the musicians, Brian strongly makes the case for the musicians to be aware of what dementia really means. People need to be met as they really are and dementia needs to be accepted as being part of their lives. Understanding about personhood must be deep: "*All we know is that in our day-to-day lives every day we're trying to, you know, it's about living our lives, surviving and facing up to challenges. That's what our brain does, our brain interprets our information and we're driven to move forward and understand what's going on around us and make our contributions. And the person with dementia is no different. But they are missing quite a lot of the connections we have. And so they're trying to make sense of that. But I think the person's sense of wanting to do and to be and to succeed are all there. All those feelings are still there. What I think I'm feeling is that drive, the drive to live is there. And so I think, how do we meet that person? And I think in day-to-day situations we do. I think staff are doing a fantastic job, and I think there are lots of human contacts all the time. It's about celebrating that and that's what Music for Life does.*" It is interesting to compare this with Matthew's struggle, when Matthew is actually pleading for letting go of a level of 'thinking', as it can be 'inhibiting'. However we can wonder in how far this plea is underpinned by his own lack of confidence, as he says: "*people are terrified of doing it wrong and we need to let it be a bit messier.*"

Despite his modesty and making sure that he remains on the background, there was a clash between Brian and Helena about their roles during the third session. Brian found out that Helena had put everything into place and Helena made clear to him that she wanted to be and to remain in charge of that. Brian had mixed feelings about it; initially he said in the interview that this is perfect and will give him less anxiety, also realising that she takes up her role on things where he always used to fill in the gaps. However in his reflective journal later on Brian admits that he has to let go and that this is not easy. He talks about this as 'the theme of ownership' that needs to be addressed.

The same contradictions can be found with Matthew in his relationship with Helena, when Helena told him that the musicians might not be aware of the needs of a particular resident. When addressing the topic in the interview, Matthew is rational and reasonable. In his reflective journal however he is angry with her, which comes down to a deep sense of insecurity: "*I think I would have been left with the feeling that she is unhappy with the project, and thinks we aren't doing a good job.*"

Matthew and Brian both work on their leadership, though from different angles. When, as mentioned earlier, after the third session Matthew wants to try out a new set up of the debrief session, preferably without the presence of Deborah and Brian, Brian reflects, like Matthew, on his wish to be in control, referring to the incident with Helena: "*I took it for my own growth and learning. There has been a certain sense of my own needing to make things okay. And needing to be in control and letting go of that. So last week it was with Helena, Helena told me to let go, this week Matthew told me to let go, so it felt a bit like, 'oh?' A bit like that. Nevertheless I feel quite strongly I have a role, and if I wasn't party to the debrief I would feel it very hard for me to continue next week and supporting the staff.*

In terms of learning benefits, the piece made with Rebecca in the sixth session stands out, at least for Matthew and also for Brian. As Rebecca apparently after this session started talking again, Brian feels that perhaps a bit of regeneration has taken place, which can happen in dementia.[115] He also connects it to an increasing sense of belonging in the home, which might lead to a feeling of more security for her. Brian makes a strong statement about what happened to Rebecca: ..."*What she was saying, meaning what she was expressing in her music making. The fact that she was in control, included other people and felt empowered is a big moment. It is beneficial for residents when musicians learn to be in the moment and adapt to the sense of pace that is required.*"

When at the end of the project the musicians reflect as a group about the landmarks of the past eight weeks, Rebecca also comes up. What happened with Rebecca gave them an awareness of their own roles, their learning process and their identity as a group. It is wonderfully phrased in the following conversation:

Matthew: "*Rebecca. For me definitively Rebecca. She's been my big moment, definitively. Just making that connection with her, such a breakthrough. For her and I think, no, not just a breakthrough for her, but a breakthrough for me as well. And I think we also spoke about this in the beginning of the project, being nervous of her actually. She seemed impossible, to read her, what she was feeling, what she thought. And she could hit you, you know?*"

---

[115] See also Sacks 2008.

Anneliese: *"A bit scary."*

Fiona: *"She's been so different. Actually I, and maybe this is really subjective, but I feel she's been different since that moment almost. Since that piece."*

Matthew: *"I think so. And maybe that's to do with how we feel."*

Fiona: *"Towards her maybe."*

Matthew: *"Whether it's changed how we feel towards her and then her response back to that, it's totally…"*

Fiona: *"Cyclical."*

Another interesting development is that the musicians increasingly start to realise that *they* learn themselves instead of observing 'a development'. In a debrief the following happens:

> From the field notes:
>
> Deborah also asks: "how have the changes in the residents affected us in any way?" Matthew answers that he was "struck today by the way Rebecca was, that grip of hers felt so different today." Initially he had found the grip "frightening" but "today it was a wonderful thing." He stops to find a word and Helena interjects "affirming" to which he agrees: "absolutely." Matthew questions whether there has been a change in her or if there has been "a change in the way I'm perceiving her… I interpret [the gripping and slapping] differently now."

It is important that Matthew wonders whether he has seen a change or whether actually *he* has changed. Also Fiona considers the change in Rebecca, which she seems to have perceived, writing: *"I simply asked her if she had enjoyed the session and she replied, 'We enjoyed it.' I do not think this was an accident. I felt that her use of 'we' clearly showed her awareness of the group that she was part of. This is just so great to see. I think that she is generally more settled in the home but that also the Music for Life project has come at a key time for her and has helped to integrate her into the community. This week, she was no longer an isolated figure wandering alone but part of the circle. I feel that her piece last week was a key moment in her feeling acknowledged and empowered and that her behaviour this week was quite possibly built upon this breakthrough, although that is of course, very subjective!"*

As we saw earlier, Rosamund is another resident who has been difficult to grasp, although Fiona definitely started to connect more and more with her throughout the sessions. Gradually we see a growing awareness amongst the musicians that they have to let go of the intention of involving everyone in the same way as they would like it to happen, or as they think is expected of them, and take things just as they are. Brian has an important insight on this when he says: *"And I think people's wish to have Rosamund participate in a different way was expressed by Rachel in the debrief. It was interesting that she hadn't been there for the past two weeks, and I think we've journeyed that journey in the past couple of weeks to come to an understanding about who Rosamund is. And what she wants to do and what she can do. And to live with her and to accept that. And maybe the acceptance of who she is and what she can do is more important than expectations of a different kind of participation. So it is more about presence than what somebody does, for me.*" Acceptance is, in short, a key word in this practice.

Anneliese and Fiona work with Rosamund especially during the last session. Rosamund does not want to be involved in the music making, but she consents to the idea of someone making music for her.

From the field notes:

Anneliese looks at Rebecca and says "Rebecca" three times – each time Rosamund responds as if it is her name. Anneliese asks Rebecca if she would like to play, but there is no response. Matthew says "Rebecca and Rosamund" as he looks across at Rosamund. "...Make some music," Anneliese says. Matthew says to Rebecca: "Anneliese could play the harp for you, how would that be? We could get her to play the harp for you... or for Rosamund?" He looks at Rosamund: "Could Anneliese play the harp for you?" Fiona helps by saying to Rosamund, "Would you like that? Would you like to hear that? It's really beautiful." Rosamund comments, "I'd like to hear it, not to play it." She chuckles. Fiona agrees, and Anneliese starts a very open motif in Eb major. Hannah has shaken her caxixi[116] and Gabriella looks as if she is about to shake her maracas[117], so Matthew goes over, and quietly and sensitively asks if they would mind if he could take their instruments as a piece is being made for Rosamund that he'd like them to listen to: "can I just take it for now, so we can listen to the harp?" Fiona starts to sing to Rosamund. It is beautiful and gentle singing, wordless; a counter-melody to Anneliese's playing. She uses her whole body in gestures and has a questioning and radiant face as she sings to Rosamund. They hold eye contact with each other at times. Fiona gently strokes Rosamund's hand as she sings. Fiona asks at a point "sing with me?" She continues to sing wordlessly, and then sings once "Rosamund, it's for you". Rosamund immediately responds saying, "it's for you" to which Fiona responds: "No, it's for you!" and laughs, saying "it's for both of us maybe." The piece finishes at this interaction. Rosamund quietly says, "That's lovely", and Fiona responds with "thank you". Fiona then says a little louder, "thank you for letting me share it with you" and Rosamund responds, "you're very welcome". Rosamund adds: "it makes me want to cry" and Fiona responds: "I know, it does make you want to cry, doesn't it?" Matthew affirms to Rosamund: "thank you" and then "thanks Fiona and Anneliese" nodding at them. It's a quiet end to a very gentle interaction.

---

[116] A woven basket shaker, with a flat bottom usually made from cocoa shell, and filled with seeds or other particles. It is associated with West African and Brazilian music. See also Appendix V, 'List of musical instruments'.
[117] The maraca (also chikita or egg shaker) is a native instrument of South America, traditionally made of gourd or coconut shells, but also commercially out of wood, plastic and leather, occasionally clay; the shell is usually attached to a handle for ease of playing. The sound is produced when beads or small particles inside the maraca hit the inside of the shell. Chikitas are small plastic versions of the maraca. Egg shakers work on the same acoustic principles as the maraca, are handle-less, and have the same size and shape as a chicken egg. See also Appendix V, 'List of musical instruments'.

Fiona reflects back in her journal: *"My time with Rosamund in the final session was so special and a real landmark in her journey. The session started with her blowing me a kiss as she was wheeled in and throughout the session she was very responsive to Diallo and myself. At one point Hannah and Diallo had played the harp and Matthew suggested, when Rosamund reacted to Rebecca's name (thinking someone was calling her own name), whether she might like to hear the harp at which point she said 'I'd like to hear it but not play it'. This was the first time she had ever accepted an offer of music and the first time she had made a clear choice. As Anneliese played to her, I was holding her hand and suddenly felt that I needed to sing to her over the harp's accompaniment to help her really know that the music was 'for her'. I'm really not very confident at singing, and was very nervous but somehow in those situations you just do whatever is necessary to connect! There was such a sense of intimacy in singing to her and I felt very close to her. I knew that on other sessions she had very occasionally sung herself so it just felt right. I was amazed as she really seemed to 'receive' the music for the first time in eight weeks. At one point I was singing a tune with the words 'la, di, daa..' or words to that effect at which point she looked at me and said 'la di daaa back to you'. There was a real sense of sharing in the music with her and I felt that we had broken through her isolation for the first time in the group context. This was really validated by the conversation that we had directly after the music. I said to her, still holding her hand, 'It's for you' at which point she said to me 'It's for you' and so I really wanted to validate this sense of shared experience and so simply said 'It's for both of us – thank you for letting me share it with you', to which she replied, 'That's alright'. I then asked her if she enjoyed the music and she replied with a real clarity that I hadn't seen during the eight weeks, 'I loved it, it makes me want to cry' at which point I think I did!! I was so moved by this experience. Just sensing the sense of connection that I had with her, and her openness to the group. In this moment she had chosen to receive the music and be open to both me, and the group as a whole; to see how the music had broken into her isolation was just so moving."*

In Fiona's reflective journal we meet Diallo, a member of the care staff, for the first time. His role within the home is as a care assistant, where he fulfills a number of duties directly with and for residents, including personal care. Diallo conveys a sense of relaxedness and warmth, as he cares sensitively for those around him, taking time to consult with residents, reassuring them gently in times of distress.

Also Fiona goes through an important learning process during this project, where at the end of the day she reflects: *"I was really struck by how in this work you just have to accept every moment for what it is then. There were no neat endings. The project seemed to reflect clearly what life in the home is like day-to-day, and perhaps life with dementia in general. There were good moments, moments of clarity and lucidity when the residents seemed to be able to show and communicate who they really were and really be part of the group. Then there were distressing moments when residents seemed to regress, when they seemed lost and isolated."*

Strong transitional learning can be seen in Matthew's final reflection which encompasses a huge learning process: *"During this project I think I have learned even more deeply the importance of allowing space for each person, and of valuing each person in the group; and that group consists of the musicians, the staff, the residents, the managers. Then beyond those people who have direct contact are the receptionists, staff who bring the residents to the group and transfer them from wheelchair to arm chair, relatives, cleaners... and so the list continues. And then, once the session is over and I have left the care home, something of that awareness seems to remain as I get on the tube and share that time with other strangers, as I go into a busy department store, and gradually I have to let it slip away, and adjust to being in the 'normal' world again, with its sharp edges, deadlines, and exacting demands for perfection. But I can carry what I have experienced with me, and try to remember to connect with it when I can, to value this life I have for what it is."*

Professional identity

Brian gives a very illuminating insight into what the project does with the professional identity of the care staff involved. They know who they are and what they are supposed to do; their professional identity is even mirrored by their uniforms. But then a project like Music for Life comes by, connected to an unknown world, it can lead to a 'threatened' professional identity: *"(...) they have a title and they have a job that they do. And they know at certain times of the day they have certain jobs that they're doing. And they know that the main job they're doing is being there and being responsive to residents at all times. And they feel they know how to do that by and large and they have control over the choices they make, to respond to somebody and to do something and to go with somebody sometimes. But then they come into the Music for Life session and they're not, first of all they are themselves, not their role. They're themselves as individuals, they do have a role to support the residents, but not in the same way. And they don't have the knowledge of where it's going and they're trying to discover what Music for Life is about in the first few sessions and they're not sure. And they have expressed this theme in previous sessions (...) they don't know how they're supposed to respond and it feels very strongly that there is a leader and a couple of other people who will lead along with the other musicians. And intuitively they know that's part of their role, to follow that person's direction like they do at work. But it's not worked out in the same way as the workplace, where you're asked: can you do this, can you do that?"* Brian realises that this gives a clear indication of the role of the staff development practitioner, especially in the debrief. Brian's role is to give structure to this and also to make sure that people can have a chance to say what they want to say.

Professional identity is a complex concept, especially regarding the musicians. In their pathways personal and professional development are closely interwoven. Professional identity relates to using your music, and hence your identity, in a professional way to reach the other. To Fiona there are two essential elements involved: to be meaningful, and secondly, to be meaningful through the music. She points out that you connect both with the people you work with and with yourself. This makes it rich. On the other hand, taking responsibility of your own boundaries is key. Fiona says: "*I just think that the work that we do can be at quite a depth. So you're dealing with the emotions and the complexities of the people's illnesses that you're working with, and a lot of the life issues around that. Which are quite big, heavy issues, I think. And people are in very difficult situations. And I think if that is not managed well, if the structure wasn't in place, you could compromise your own emotional health. And, yeah, I think it can be costly to you as a person. Just because you're dealing with very complex situations and then you're with people at a very intimate level, so there need to be good boundaries and there needs to be a good structure.*"

This is a key statement about identity and the vulnerability of the musicians. Fiona comments on "*the amazing privilege that it is to be able to communicate with people without words. And to find a sort of soul to soul connection that I think can happen, not all the time.*" This comment highlights Fiona's intrinsic motivation and the balance between her sense of artistic drive and responsibility. Music is her outlet, so she wants to use it to communicate with other people. She is looking for new ways to give shape to her love for connecting with other people. Doing this without words leads to 'soul connection'. It is not only about seeing someone else empowered, but also feeling that you have brought your two issues together: musical performance and helping other people. This relates strongly to Fiona's biography as a discussion between the three musicians shows:

Fiona: "*I was caught between this like really elite world and wanting music to be of a really high standard, I think that's it, and yet really wanting to work with people. But sometimes working with people and the music wasn't there and it was a compromise of your artistry, which sounds a bit, I don't mean that in a proud way, I just mean, you want to bring your best. And have musical integrity, I think, in what you're doing.*"

Anneliese: "*But we found again and again that without this musical integrity, you don't get that, you don't get the same depth and connection. I think there really is, there's a real truth there. If, you can't just go and play something to them, it doesn't work. It doesn't work in the same way, you don't go as deep.*"

Matthew: *"You don't go as deep. I think it's really interesting, I was just thinking about it now we're talking about it. And we always said it's about the quality of the music that makes the difference. And I wonder whether it's the quality that we bring to it, that ensures the quality in the music. Do you know what I mean? It's the commitment to it. It's what actually, it's the thing that makes the difference. And as a result the music is of a higher quality. That it's the kind of commitment that it takes to focus on the music. It's the thing, maybe."*

Fiona describes the two worlds she is in as a musician as a battle between the 'really elite world and wanting music to be of a high standard' and 'helping people'. She feels she is still in the midst of it. This is key to the debate on quality within community arts in general: it is important to consider broad qualities, including artistic qualities, whilst not 'compromising your artistry'. Musical integrity is the key word for both artistic quality and the quality within communication. Matthew adds the word 'commitment' to this: so all in all we can say that for the musicians high quality is achieved in a very holistic way.

The musicians often reflect on their artistic learning, which is deepened by the awareness to respond in the moment, in a non-verbal way. Fiona points out her motivation which combines the artistic and social side of the practice: *"I think for me it keeps me sane in the music profession to do this work because it reminds me of why I love music myself. It reminds me of the power of music, that it's a bigger thing than just, it's not just entertainment, it's a bigger thing that we have. And I think there can be a lot of cynicism in the musicians' world, sometimes in the professional world, and I feel really lucky to have these experiences sometimes. I just don't view it as my next pay check, it's something I can believe in and love. And so I suppose it fuels my love of music and my love of working with people and my belief in the chamber music aspect of it, the playing together, feeding off other musicians and the creativity of that. And I just love telling people about it. I was just on tour and telling people about it and they're so amazed at the thought of doing that with your instrument, other colleagues, and I feel really lucky. But it does kind of keep me sane because otherwise I wouldn't be able to do music if I didn't have the outlet to come and do this sort of thing."*

Throughout the sessions Matthew tends to nurture the hypothesis that the musicians need to get rid of their anxiety and insecurity by the 'evidence' that residents make progress. He thrives on the success with Rebecca in the sixth session. However his anxiety remains, and for him the beginning of every session is daunting: *"the moment the session is about to start you think, 'Oh can I do it?'"* Critical comments feel as *"a blow to the heart"* (...) *"I think as musicians we all felt vulnerable."* It is interesting to see how for Matthew on the one hand 'professionalism' does not help provide a sense of empowerment. This is because 'identity' is so vulnerable in this practice: any criticism can be seen as criticism of yourself as a musician and hence as a person.

The musicians find the question about how the work in the Music for Life practice feeds into their other professional activities difficult. Fiona and Anneliese struggle with addressing it. Matthew mentions some concrete outcomes, which are: respect, everybody's potential to be creative, or educational work being coloured by it. But also he feels that he learns to let go of having everything planned, that unpredictability need not necessarily be negative and 'slowing down' can lead to new developments.

Brian finally gives a strong statement: *"I think first and foremost it's always about residents and about giving residents the best, the best possible we can give. And sometimes that's hard on us. Sometimes we have to go out of our normal routines. And sometimes we're asked to give that extra bit to ensure that we can offer something special. And this is something special. And so for me it's about through the process of Music for Life that people will see that individuals, individual residents have had something special. And when people say they've had something special and they can rejoice in that, then it makes sense. And I think that's the level it works at. And my experience of staff is that no matter how overworked somebody is, or sometimes burdened with work, that when they see somebody that they're working for in the home, a resident, having a smile on their face or achieving something they haven't achieved before, that their sense of enjoyment and rejoicing just makes their job worthwhile. My belief is that the project makes it worthwhile and people see that."*

Conceptual summary

Identity is constructed in the practices of social communities, where, as Etienne Wenger argues, the participation not only shapes what we do, but also who we are and how we interpret it.[118] His identification of identity as "a way of talking about how learning changes who we are and creates personal histories of becoming in the context of our communities"[119] can seamlessly be applied to what we encounter in the practice of the musicians and staff development practitioner, residents and care staff.

Identity exists on a personal level as well as on a group level. The musicians' learning process and in the end their development towards 'acceptance' lead to an identity that is a constructed version of 'becoming' through learning, or to put it in simple words: we can observe how they are coping.

[118] Wenger 2009: 211.
[119] Ibid.

Identity as belonging and becoming

Matthew reflects during the course of the project: *"We've always assumed that it's the playing together what brings us together (...) I think that sharing in doing all of the things (...) is all part of the sharing of the responsibility and the planning and all of that. And when you play, you're starting playing from that point (...) Joint decision-making is important, negotiated with respect for each other and awareness of each other (...) The idea even goes beyond the musician team, it goes for the care staff as well."* This mirrors the image of a community of practice, where meaning is negotiated within the process of human engagement.[120] At the end of the project Matthew reflects that, *"I want us to feel connected at the deepest level (...) with each person accepted just as they are, recognised and honoured, fully dignified. The only way I can think of to even come close to achieving this is to try to be it myself. To still all the voices in my head, all the judgments, all the criticisms of others, of myself, and accept."* This is where Matthew reaches the stage which echoes Giddens' observation about identity, *"the capacity to keep a particular narrative going."* [121]

It is an important learning process for the musicians to realise that at one moment a resident can be a conductor, the next moment she can tumble back into the darkness of her mind. Lifelong learning is clearly *not* always about improving and developing, and the residents are lifelong learners as well. In this sense there is no development although there is learning: people living with dementia can realise their personhood and identity in the moment through artistic practice.

Fiona also reflects on the different forms of 'becoming' when she says: *"I've been thinking a lot about how music can be inclusive without people having to actively participate. Music can simply go to people, without people having to come to it. It is a wonderful thing about music, and as a performer you can even play for someone in particular without it being known or acknowledged and yet, something of that intention can be felt by the listener."* Periphery thus can be a new core, it is therefore that Lave and Wenger actually speak about legitimate peripheral participation.[122]

Identity and shared leadership

Matthew is moved by his colleagues, seeing how they use their musicianship in this practice and the trust it requires: *"It's moving to see people that you know and love playing anyway."* He realises that in a project like this it does not work to want to be in control of everything *"because the musicians feel thwarted by it, there is not an honesty in the relationship with them."*

[120] Wenger 1998: 53.
[121] Giddens 1991: 54; see also Chapter 2.1, under 'From person-centred to participatory approach.'
[122] Lave and Wenger 1991.

Matthew worked hard during the project on shifting this leadership into *shared* leadership. Stepping aside, he discovered that both Anneliese and Fiona can be leaders as long as they have the space to try things out and feel confident. He experiences the opportunity to let go as "*like being able to breathe.*"

The musicians need to work on their low self-esteem. Low self-esteem can even lead to notions amongst musicians that one has to give a brilliant musical performance in order to be a 'worthwhile' person.[123] They need to be prepared to be out of their comfort zone whilst at the same time inspiring confidence in the group.

Identity and sound: the artistic process

The person-centred musical improvisation in this practice consists of tuning in with a resident *and* oneself and can therefore be considered a musical metaphor for identity and connection, for I and Thou, as Fiona says "*you're trying to be someone else's music for them.*" Fiona asks herself the question what *sound* can reflect who the residents are at a particular moment: "*What sound can I try now to help either reflect who they are at this moment or what sound is going to connect? It's all about your observations about that person, rather than about what you're creating.*"

Reflection-in-action and sound are fundamental concepts in any creative music workshop in a community context. Sean Gregory observes:

> Things need to be said through music, through *sound* in the first instance (…) Saying things through music can contribute to how people interact, to how people feel about themselves, view themselves as individuals, and how they interact in groups. That is achieved through the fundamental organizational means of sound, like rhythm, harmony, textures, whatever. They are steered, created and manipulated even in response to what is needed at that moment.[124]

It is of critical importance to connect; the word 'connection' is used a lot in relation to identity. Sensitivity is therefore also a much used word amongst the musicians. As people with dementia are sensitive, Fiona observes: "*There has to be a real honesty from within yourself. Residents will pick up if you're not being authentic.*" Sensitivity amongst the musicians, 'feel' or 'knowing that the other knows'[125] is therefore key. Trust and extensive personal contact are conditional for the transfer of tacit knowledge and understanding.

Connecting through sound already happens in the improvised framing piece which emerges at the beginning and the end of each workshop.[126]

---

[123] Steptoe 1989; Brodsky 1995.
[124] In Smilde 2009a: 279.
[125] Smilde 2009a: 145.
[126] See also Chapter 1.

Identity and uncompromised quality

We heard Fiona describing the two worlds between which she felt she had to choose: that is the artistic 'elitist' world and that of 'helping people'. Actually there is no dichonomy, as long as 'quality' is seen as a collection of qualities, amongst which artistic quality is of central importance. Linda Rose writes about musicians engaged in this practice:

> At all times the quality of their music-making is paramount. For their music to communicate they need to be at the height of their musical skill. Their playing must matter and mean every bit as much as any public performance on the concert platform.[127]

It is important to consider this practice as a collection of interconnected qualities. Peter Renshaw phrases it as follows:

> In recent years many commentators have observed how the arts are seen to matter more and more in our present turbulent world. It therefore behoves all people working in the arts to ensure that their engagement resonates with the diversity of needs found in the many different arenas in which they work (...) engagement must always have integrity and quality at its heart. A commitment to people and to art goes hand in hand.[128]

Understanding the place of this practice as leading to 'belonging' can diminish debates on artistic practices as either 'elitist' or as 'social work'. When a musician engages with a social context she will never compromise her artistry in the work she delivers, together with others.

4.2 Communication

Communication is an interactional process of interpretation and action, expressed through language. When we communicate, we observe the communicative action of another and attempt to relate to it through interpreting and assigning meaning to our observation. Often, the meaning we assign stems from attitudes, assumptions, values and beliefs we have learnt through our biographical experiences, which also in turn influences what we wish to communicate, and the language we use in responding to another's communication. As we communicate, we learn; and through seeking to understand the perceptions of another person we find an opportunity to perceive our own experiences differently.

Language, as a system, has evolved over time to enable us to understand other's communication, and to be understood. Language may take multiple forms; within verbal language there are infinite numbers of ways of expressing oneself, all of which can be enhanced, reinforced or negated through interaction with our body language. Within any language, verbal or

[127] Linda Rose in Renshaw 2010: 223.
[128] Renshaw 2010: 118-119.

otherwise, there are a variety of dialects; we speak multiple dialects simultaneously in life, all of which we may interpret differently but in which we seek to find a shared understanding. Through this shared understanding we can begin to form relationships with each other, and in relation to each other. Over time, we learn and experience conventions in communication, for instance, taking turns in conversation, which may involve accepting, rejecting or embellishing someone's statements, asserting a new line of conversation and leaving space for another to respond. We also learn to interpret the meaning behind languages, especially through reading the body language of others, and the way by which they communicate verbally to us, for instance, vocal tone and pitch.

Musical communication uses a different set of languages to other forms of communication, however it takes place in a social context. Music is always produced and received in relation to an 'other', even in the most intimate settings, therefore it can be viewed a strong metaphor for social communication. Within the context of this researched Music for Life project, social and musical communication cannot be divorced; musical communication is both affected and inspired by social interactions and connections, and in turn, these social interactions, connections and relationships are sustained by, and through, musical communication.

Within this context, it is important to understand what the reality of communication for a person living with dementia is. It is still possible for a person with dementia to understand and respond to conventions underlying language, and to develop meaningful social relationships. However, interpretation and action within communication becomes more difficult, as a grasp on language and its application begins to erode. Similarly, understanding of another's use of language becomes affected. With language stripped away, the 'emotional landscape' becomes particularly relevant within a dementia context, with a greater tendency for a person with dementia to sense other people's emotions through their body language.

For a person with dementia, interpretation can become increasingly difficult, as they try to make sense of the world around them, and their relationships with others in the present. This confusion can manifest in the communication of a person with dementia, sometimes in quite extreme ways; for instance, verbally in the agitation and calling out of Sarah, as she cries "mummy" repeatedly, "mummy, where are you?" This communication challenges others in turn, who must not only accept it openly, but also try to understand what feelings and factors may be driving this type of communication, and what they can do in their own communication to address and alleviate this distress, as Matthew explains: *"You open yourself up a lot sometimes in these sessions and you make yourself very, very vulnerable, and you engage with the fact that somebody's really desperate and really in despair (...) She was really in pain there. And because of the session there isn't a way of looking away from it and you see it full on. It's a real harsh reality and that can be very upsetting."*

Brian reflects further, questioning how Sarah's communication may also impact on the well-being of others within the home: *"I suppose for me it's the reality of that, what it's like to listen to that for other residents who are actually sitting beside her. And I wonder where they think they are, how confusing it must be to hear somebody calling 'mummy, mom' all the time in quite a sharp pitch. I wonder what kind of places it brings them to? Do some people think that their children are calling out to them? Or do they feel like calling out for their own mom? Or do they just feel, well I can't stand this any longer. It doesn't feel like a peaceful place."*

For others living with dementia, a sense of confusion can appear in their communicative actions, for instance, Rebecca. Brian surmises that this is an expression of an underlying problem in interpreting the social and physical environment surrounding her: *"There's an urgency about things (...) I just think that the reality is that she moves very quickly from one way of feeling to another (...) My sense of Rebecca feels very lost, and that's what she's expressing all the time. And that's her challenge really, how we can help her not feel so lost. I mean, the loss obviously comes from her dementia, things she can't remember, situations she can't make head or tail of."*

Sustaining communication with someone living with dementia can be difficult as they can 'slip' in and out of awareness. Matthew details the amount of focused effort he was making in order to engage with Gabriella, and how the engagement was directly related to this effort: *"I was having to work very, very hard with Gabriella (...) I was really trying to connect her to the group through holding her hand and taking her along with me. And that felt great, because I could really see that the effort I was making was really making a difference with her, and that she was coming with me and that she was coming into the group, and she was singing with me, she was singing people's names, she was looking around the circle. It was hard work and the minute I stopped doing it, she went back into her counting pattern. The second I took my attention away from her, she slipped back (...) She slipped back straight away, as soon as I let go of her."*

For the musicians working in this context, the combination of these different styles of communicative action can create a challenge when trying to create a coherent sense of group, as the musicians discuss in the final group interview:

Matthew: *"Why did it feel so draining and such hard work? Was it to do with the residents and with the mix of residents? They were all quite isolated."*

Anneliese: *"I think it's definitively got to do with it."*

Matthew: *"I think we spent a lot of energy just sort of holding that group and that's just by willpower, isn't it? You can talk about, you know, the music has to be like this, dadada, but you just kind of have to ugh! You just have to be there and hold that group and that takes a lot of effort. The group doesn't hold itself. And I was very aware, so many times, just when you think, 'yes, yes, we've got there, we've got them in the group and you look around and you take your eye off the'…"*

Fiona: *"…Just for a minute."*

Matthew: *"Yes. And it starts to slip back. People slip back into themselves and the connections are gone and you have to work again to bring it all back again. It's hard work."*

Anneliese: *"You know, having two people out of six or seven or eight, who wander as a matter of fact, quite regularly just wander, that is already quite a high, tall order. When you've got somebody who will always repeatedly say the same word, supposedly automatically, we're not so sure about that, but the list goes on. It's really, I think the combination was really…"*

Fiona: *"…Challenging?"*

Anneliese: *" … Quite a tall order, actually. I really think so."*

As the musicians discuss, the energy involved in 'holding' the group, in maintaining connection through communication can feel draining and 'challenging'. This energy or 'willpower' is driven by a core set of values that enable the musicians to transcend the challenges inherent in this particular communicative context. It could be argued that these values are essential to building any sense of community, and paramount in building positive social relationships: values of unconditional love and acceptance, respect and trust, a genuine interest and faith in the unique personhood and capabilities of all people beyond disabilities. When these values are balanced with validation, empathy, invitation and authenticity in communication, a sense of community and communion can begin to emerge.

Interpretation and interaction

In understanding how dementia can uniquely affect the communication of a person, an act of interpretation must occur. Interpretation in a communication context is the act of assigning meaning to language, it involves observation of the communicative language and actions of another, perceiving the intention underlying it and making meaning of the situation. After interpretation comes action and interaction, ascribing meaning to, and acting in response to another's communication, resulting in the creation of a social dialogue. The way we interpret and respond to a situation is a product of our prior learning experiences. As mentioned in the previous part on 'Identity', the learning experiences of participants are holistic, experiences in which the rational 'head' and the intuitive, emotive 'heart' interact. In addition, some of these experiences may only have been processed at a tacit or subconscious level. Within the context of this project, observation of the communication of others is an important way of assessing levels of engagement in communicative processes, and in developing ways of communicating meaningfully with each other.

Key indicators of engagement may involve an individual making and receiving sustained eye contact, active participation in social and musical interactions, and a greater sense of alertness and concentration, appearing awake and aware. In Matthew's description of Jessica in session two, it is: *"Just to sense where somebody is and whether they're ready, as Jessica was today, absolutely ready. Last week I would never have worked with her as we did today. But she was really ready today. If she just woke up just really differently, I don't know what it was."* This understanding or sense of Jessica being 'ready' – demonstrated throughout the session through her sustained alertness, consistent active participation, and creation of a focused piece initiated by her, is also partially based upon a tacit understanding of what it means to be 'ready' to communicate and participate. This very sensual way of understanding the dynamics of the group is also relevant in Matthew's reflection on session one, where he comments on the importance of reading, responding to and curating the overall group dynamic in his role as leader: *"I think you have a feeling of balance. It's about trying to achieve equilibrium and an equality, to try and bring up the energy of some people and calm others, and then likewise with the musicians; to feel that they are connected and plugged in as well. I guess you constantly have that feeling of just, you know, the aim is that we function as a group. And so with that kind of overriding aim you can feel where the energy needs to be addressed at different times. And that way you do have a sense of everybody, I think."*

In order to sense the group dynamics, it is also about understanding that there are different types of valid participation within the session, and that sleeping for example can be interpreted in divergent ways: as a sign of disconnection as well as connection. As Brian observes, *"I think there may be a sense that people aren't really connected when they're sleeping or that there are different qualities of sleep, rest and participation."* In a group interview Harry reflects further on the ability to interpret the same signs differently: *"So often if a staff member is sitting next to somebody and they don't see them actively participating by playing a piece, they don't necessarily view the tapping on the chair or the foot going as a valid bit of participation. Whereas we do tend to think, well, that's okay, she's engaged."*

In addition to having a sensual understanding of when someone may be ready to communicate and participate, communication and leadership in this context also require an understanding of the potential steps involved in supporting someone to take the risk in communicating and participating. In the following reflection of Brian, support or enablement for an individual, in this case, Rebecca, is attained through an exploratory, emergent approach to interpretation throughout the duration of the project: *"Support is getting a greater sense of who the person is and then being able to understand what they're telling you and respond in the right way. I think it's about discovering: what does that person want? And I think we all have a sense of puzzlement, all of us, I think everyone has a sense of puzzlement, like what does Rebecca want from us, how do we respond? I don't think we know how to respond, therefore we don't know how to support. And I think if Music for Life can help us just to understand maybe a little bit more. I think it's a mystery, really, I think a lot of it remains a mystery to us. But I think sometimes we can stumble along some answers. I kind of feel that we will over the next six weeks get some answers, when we're through."*

There are always questions, and never answers; developing a spirit of exploration is key to the practice, as Matthew and Fiona surmise:

Fiona: *"You feel really unsure (…) cause there's always a risk even in a supportive role, there's very few times when you get: I really know what I need to do now, this is what I need to do. It's almost like, well, I need to do something, I'm not sure I'm gonna try this. And you're never sure."*

Matthew: *"I'll try this, yeah. Nearly always."*

Fiona: *"Always. I'm never sure. I never know. Never."*

Matthew: *"Yeah, you don't have a certainty."*

Fiona: *"No. And even afterwards, you kind of go, was that the right thing to do? It's always questions, always."*

Reflexivity and a sense of ongoing exploration in an interpretative approach enable the musicians to enact leadership choices in the spur of the moment. This is particularly effective when some windows of opportunity to interact with individuals, such as Rosamund, may pass very quickly, or when it becomes clear that an individual within the group needs more focused attention, such as Sarah.

Matthew details, in session six, his thought processes behind his decision to initiate a piece with Rebecca, as previously detailed in the analysis on Identity, 'seizing the moment' in a way that was initially surprising to him: *"When that piece started I had no idea that it was gonna go the way it did. It was a very unthought-of thing, to sing to Rebecca wasn't what I'd imagined. The absolute reaction in the moment about, I suppose really tuning in with a resident, almost split-second actually, a very unplanned piece. Just seizing that moment. I think that was a real moment of reflecting, actually, in which you just reflect back exactly what you see. And I suppose you just have to trust your instinct on that one and think, this is what I'm seeing and this is what I think you want, and just going for it. There was just one facial expression the whole time, which was this kind of very serious looking face. So her lips were tensed and pulled together, a very strong, very direct gaze into my eyes. And that was what I was interpreting, just this kind of seriousness. And then in terms of how the phrases went and when it came to end a phrase, that was I suppose my instinct, to bring a phrase to an end and invite her and start the next one off. So I don't think I was getting that from her. That was to do with when I was feeling it was time to bring a phrase to an end and then let her start the next one off, if she wanted to. No change of expression, just this fixed really serious expression all the time. The only time she looked away was to look at the chime bar to then hit it."* Here, Matthew details the whole process of interpreting and reinterpreting Rebecca's communication and participation in the moment. As Matthew asserts, the approach within sessions is *"just not being attached, I think, to what you think should happen and able to see the possibility of straight away in the next moment."*

Spontaneity in approach is fundamental for the musicians in relation to their artistic identity – too much thinking or pre-planning can be stressful, and can create an environment where they feel inhibited as artists. In a creative workshop situation, creative freedom and spontaneity are of central importance, though, as Fiona observes in session five, this is sometimes difficult to enact due to the requirements of the communication context: *"As musicians it is great to have the freedom and confidence at times just to go for it! Often in these sessions one can feel very unsure and as if one is treading on eggshells but to have moments of musical freedom, and clarity as a team really gives you time to regroup and connect."*

Anneliese confirms this perspective, reflecting after session eight that executing a pre-agreed plan can sometimes sidestep spontaneity in interactions and musical communication: *"When you plan things in advance it does not work so well because it did not evolve naturally out of the moment as a response to what was happening..."* However, a plan can help to create an opportunity for individuals to communicate and participate. Often plans may be developed by the musicians during both the debrief and preparation hours surrounding the workshop, developing a set of 'play rules', both focused and general, that guide interactions within the session. However, it relies on the musicians to interpret the right moment at which to enact the plan, and to interpret exactly how the plan relates to the current communication situation, as the musicians discuss post-project:

Matthew: *"And so, just to have that [sixth] session where, we talked, we had kind of planned that [Rebecca] was gonna have her moment in that session, hadn't we? And we'd begun to talk about how we'd seen, you know, to take her seriously, like, 'I can acknowledge this power'."*

Anneliese: *"I think that's what we talked about. If she has some bad feelings or aggression or whatever, lets..."*

Fiona: *"Reflect it back..."*

Matthew: *"...Let it out."*

Anneliese: *"Yes, find a way that she can play something where she can show that."*

Fiona: *"Brian was very strong on that. He's like, what would happen. I think in the previous week or two weeks before one of the debriefs I think he'd said, what's so wrong about reflecting that back to, you know, doing something that really goes with that and see where that takes you. And I think you just took that moment."*

Matthew: *"Well we did. I think as a team we just kind of all felt it, 'this is the moment'."*

Fiona: *"I think it was like, 'lets jump off the cliff'."*

Matthew: *"Yeah, it really did feel like that."*

Fiona: *"It really did."*

Matthew: *"We all sort of looked at each other like, now is the moment."*

Anneliese: *"But you know, if you think about really planning something, it was a very open agenda. It wasn't like we said, oh –"*

Matthew: *" – We're going to make a piece like this –"*

Anneliese: *"– Or, try that instrument with her... and you just felt in that moment, 'let me try her with this chime bell' and it was just brilliant."*

Without sharing observations and perceptions of Rebecca's communication and participation, the musicians may not have collectively arrived at a new, shared perspective on how they might communicate with Rebecca in a generic and artistic sense. Through reflexive and reflective engagement in the project, the interpretative perspectives of each person begin to shift, as each individual learns more about each other's communication and relationships begin to build. For instance, understanding a person's communication may require some background knowledge of that person – which takes place primarily through reflective processes, including project debriefs; however this reflective approach is always married with an intuitive understanding within sessions, a reflexive interpretation and response in relation to another's potential current experience. Within the above dialogue we can see how, when shared, different perspectives of an individual begin to deepen, and influence practice within the music sessions.

In building learning around an individual's communication and participation, the reflection of others are important if one is to be able to develop, deepen or change their own understanding of individuals. For example, throughout the project, both musicians and staff seek to understand Rosamund's communication and participation style. This reflection enables them to develop a new perspective on Rosamund as a person; for instance, in session three, understanding her isolation as non-acceptance of dementia and rejection of her peers, 'old fossils', as detailed in the analysis on

Identity. This understanding is an important stage in guiding both future interpretations of Rosamund's communication and participation, and the ways in which musicians and staff choose to communicate and interact with Rosamund. For Matthew, validations of his own prior reflection in this instance *"gives very clearly a way forward: that it's not the music that she's resistant to, that there's other things that are stopping her."* However, this is not a fixed view, and we can see a shift in the way he interprets the subtleties of Rosamund's communication and participation choices, due to the perspective of Diallo in session five: *"You know, my thoughts about Rosamund were that she felt it was beneath her, this kind of work, making music in this way. But actually that's quite a different perspective that [Diallo] is observing, that she's afraid of making a mistake. And that can have a real influence on the way we work with her for the remainder of the project, actually. You know, I'm less afraid of her judgement now. Often she will express that, 'oh, it was all rubbish', all of this kind of stuff. But actually maybe, what's at the root of it is her fear of making a mistake, which is much more in keeping with the sense of dementia, you know, with her dementia maybe and her covering up her confusion. It's much more of a depth of understanding her."*

Here the reinterpretation Matthew attributes to Diallo is crucial, as it enables Matthew to develop new ways of understanding Rosamund, and approaching communication with her. This shared leadership in interpretation is also present in another interaction between Matthew and Diallo, in session three, when Diallo is able to share his experience of 'reading' Gabriella in order to enable Matthew to enact a leadership decision. Matthew details this interaction: *"I can't remember the exact sequence of events, but near the beginning, we were making a piece for Gabriella, I think she was conducting. And she kept saying she felt sick. 'I feel sick, I feel sick'. And I checked out with Diallo across the circle, 'is she really?' 'No, she's fine'. So, obviously it's great to have that reassurance from him. If she really felt sick, we needed to get her out of there, you know? One, it would be really distressing for her to actually be sick in front of everybody and also for the rest of the group it's really unpleasant. So that was interesting; to kind of keep her piece going for her whilst also wondering if she's actually going to be sick. Again, the input of the staff is vital, and their knowledge of the residents."*

For everyone involved, the process of interpreting another person's communication and participation, understanding what it means, and enacting a sensitive response, without the 'fear of making a mistake', can involve embracing a potentially risky approach, as Fiona phrases it, *"jumping off the cliff"*. For Matthew, it's about *"stepping into the unknown. It's when you're stepping into something and you don't know how it's going to play out, and you're doing things which you haven't planned to do."* It challenges everyone involved in the interaction to move beyond their comfort barriers.

Interpretation may seem a risky venture due to a number of factors. The nature of dementia means that validation and interpretation by staff and musicians may involve some guesswork, particularly if the communicative actions of the person with dementia are fragmented or incoherent, or seem out of context. There is risk taking in the processes of matching, translation, and a 'hammer' approach[129], whereby the communication and musical communication of an individual may be 'translated' into a new context; sometimes congruous as in matching and translation processes, or, in the case of the hammer, incongruous, through the musicians asserting a new energy in order to change overall communication dynamics. In addition, there may be difficulty in finding or agreeing a dominant interpretation of the situation collaboratively, especially when reflexive decisions are made, sometimes leading to what Matthew refers to as *"thwarted intentions"*. As outcomes within the session are not always clear, and individuals may reach divergent interpretations within the same experiences, the project compels people to interpret, reflect, negotiate and reinterpret their own experiences, developing a respect for other's perspectives, and over time, relationships founded on a strong sense of trust.

Space and pace

Interlinked concepts of space and pace underlie many of the communicative approaches adopted by musicians and care staff within the project. It is important to find a pace that enables time for individuals to process, interpret and assign meaning to information transmitted through language. Within a dementia context, it is crucial to find and match the pace of the person with dementia, communicating at a slower pace in which they are able to understand both content and meaning: what is being communicated, and if there are any expectations for a particular response. Opportunities for communication can be maximised through attention to the speed or pace of communication delivery and overall balance of activities. As pacing enables time for someone to process and interpret information, it also enables them to develop a relationship to the information and to the person communicating that information, therefore attention to pacing enables relationships between people to occur.

The concept of pace naturally leads on to space, creating or leaving a space in communication for another to make and enact decisions around how and what they wish to communicate and participate. Space incorporates a willingness to enable another person to speak, to communicate, and to listen openly to what they have to say, collaborating to create a space where spontaneous and truthful dialogue can emerge. It also has a literal meaning, as the physical space can impact upon the social environment, and also in the case of musical silence, or stillness in body language, which may be read as cues of reaching a state of peaceful acceptance.

---

[129] See Chapter 2.3 on 'Applied musical improvisation'.

The impact of physical proximity to an individual, as a way of supporting communication and engagement, is highlighted through these accounts. Looking at the use of space by individuals within the session, a pattern emerges: the location of the musicians within the space, particularly the workshopleader, can serve as a catalyst, stimulating and focusing communication and participation. For instance, in some interactions, the musicians may choose to focus group awareness on an intimate piece built around the communication and participation of an individual within the group. This will often be echoed in their positioning within the room, for example, one to two musicians may sit next to or kneel in front of the person at the centre of the interaction. Similarly, when all individuals are seated within the circle, the physicality seems to suggest a space for active group participation. This can be seen in the following extract from the field notes taken during session three, which highlights the role of proximity in cueing transitions within the musical interactions:

> From the field notes:
>
> Anneliese takes charge and alerts the group to Sarah. Matthew asks her if she'd like to play a piece. Both Anneliese and Matthew are near Sarah. Sarah shakes her ghungharus[130] briefly at Matthew, and a piece starts, with Anneliese imitating the tremolos of the ghungharus, looking at Sarah as she does this. During this interaction, Matthew moves over to Diallo, taking the djembe from Diallo and bringing it over to Anne and Sarah. During this time, Sarah has begun to disengage and has her head in her hands. Matthew kneels in front of Sarah and near Anne, and begins to play the djembe softly, instituting a soft, regular drum beat as Anneliese's harp tremolos transition into a repetitive accompaniment, on which she sings long wordless 'ah's'. Matthew takes Sarah's hand, and transfers the djembe to Anne, who continues the music-making through playing a drum beat on the djembe. Matthew holds Sarah's hand for a while, and then joins in playing tingshas[131], staying near Sarah. After some time, Matthew decides to give the tingshas to Rachel, and another instrument to Diallo before he returns to his seat to sing and play a shaker.[132] The piece begins to grow, becoming louder and more vibrant. Sarah is clearly at the centre of this piece, but others in the circle join in over time. Matthew takes care to thank Sarah after her piece ends.

In this interaction we are introduced to Anne, a nurse and team leader. She is responsible for managing the activities of care assistants within a unit, as well as providing nursing care for residents. Anne is warm, friendly and highly committed and professional in her work, and seems to provide a

---

[130] Also known as Payal, Paayal, Ghungaru, Ghungroo, Ghungur, Nupur, Ghangaroo. An Indian instrument, traditionally worn on the ankles, consisting of a band with two rows of small bells sewn into it. Shaking the instrument produces a high, light sound. See also Appendix V, 'List of musical instruments'.

[131] Small heavy cymbals connected by a leather strap, traditionally used in prayer by Tibetan Buddhist monks. When struck together, the cymbals make a high pitched, resonant sound and are typically made from a bronze alloy. See also Appendix V, 'List of musical instruments'.

[132] *Seed shell shaker or seed shaker*: A collection of natural seed pods connected together by thin rope, and with a loop for holding it in the hand. The sound is produced through shaking the instrument, or using the hand to stroke the pods. See also Appendix V, 'List of musical instruments'.

sense of security for residents through the gentle, patient way she communicates with them.

Additionally, in this interaction the positioning of Matthew, and his proximity to Sarah, is influential in its impact on the growth of the piece from one focused on Sarah to a piece in which the group becomes musically active. Proximity can also be used to send a non-verbal message about the focus of an activity, as Matthew describes: *"If you're sitting back in the group there's a responsibility upon the whole group in a way. In the way that the shaker-piece developed for example, it was kind of open for anyone to be part of the music-making. Whereas if you go to somebody and kneel in front of them then you are making a statement to the rest of the group: this is going to be just us doing this now."*

Proximity within physical space can stimulate communication, and as a result, the development of relationships. Fiona was positioned next to Rosamund, and slowly over time, an enduring relationship began to form: *"I could write so much about each resident, but I really wanted to reflect on one in particular. I often find there is one, or perhaps two residents that I really connect and journey with on a project. Usually these are the people I sit next to (often because I have made a connection with them in the first place). On this project it was Rosamund."*

This use of space can be planned, through careful consideration of seating arrangements, but is more often than not, unplanned and reflexive, and based upon prior learning experiences, captured in Matthew's reflection on his decision making during this particular event in session three: *"I think that when I went over and started that piece today with Sarah, there was this close, tight group, I wasn't thinking, we're going to start a piece with her and then I will back away dadada. You know, the reflexive response, to go over there and make the piece with her and then the kind of thinking starts about what's going on behind me. I would be hard pushed to say whether turning that piece into a whole group piece was a cognitive decision or a reflexive one. I couldn't tell you (...) You know, we've had those sorts of discussions so much in the past that it becomes internalised and becomes a reflexive thing to do."* In addition, if the engagement of an individual in a piece is starting to decrease, musicians may be prompted to re-engage through a change in position, coupled with other aspects of supportive communication, as emphasized in this passage:

From the field notes:

Abigail is given a hand chime in c, so that Abigail, Jessica and Hannah all have a hand chime (making a c major triad). Matthew highlights this in a vocal improvisation, singing their names, connecting Jessica and Abigail. Abigail starts singing along. Harry also highlights this by echoing his words vocally. At one point, when Abigail begins to look a little disengaged, Matthew comes and sits next to Abigail – he explicitly sings to her raising the volume slightly – she appears to reengage, and this prompts her to play her hand chime again. Matthew sings and Abigail imitates it, this goes on when Matthew changes rhythms.

As well as helping to engage and re-engage individuals in the music making, physical proximity can act in a holding way. When accompanied by sensitive body language, such as eye contact and touch, it can help to create a sense of security during transitions, and when an individual appears anxious. Calmness and stillness in the body is important, as emphasized in this passage, describing the arrival of Sarah and Hannah at the beginning of session six:

> Sarah and Hannah are first to arrive at about 10.50 am. Anneliese and Fiona play very softly – there is a nice regularity to what they play – it's undulating and fluttering; Matthew occasionally hums along. It is very still and the musicians take great care to be physically close to and calm with Hannah and Sarah. Anneliese seeks to communicate sensitively with Sarah – Sarah has said "mummy" once; Anneliese leans in close, making eye contact.

Proximity may also create dynamics of reliance. Matthew argues after session three that it is important not to create a situation whereby Sarah becomes reliant on him to be close for support. Similarly, a relationship between Rebecca and Matthew seems to develop where Rebecca seems to draw security from being seated next to Matthew, however, this has an impact when Matthew moves from his position. Rebecca seems highly susceptible to the movement of others within the group, creating a need for others to develop a sense of rootedness and sensitive awareness in order to support her, as Brian observes: *"I think we're learning about Rebecca and where she sits and who she sits beside and how to help her to remain and be calm (...) [When] she's sitting beside somebody who's going to stand up during the sessions, she's also very, very likely to want to stand up. She needs a lot of sensitive support, which she does get."*

However, at the heart of this an ability to respect the personal space of another is fundamental if a strong relationship is to be formed, as emphasised by Fiona, reflecting on her experiences with Rosamund in the first session: *"I felt that I wanted to include two ladies who had seemed a little cut off, so I got up and sat on the floor and played in front of them. At one point I had very strong eye contact with [Rosamund] so moved a little closer but actually it was too close and she broke the eye contact and looked away. I was just reminded of the need to have a highly attuned awareness of people's need for space in this work."* This awareness comes through interpreting the person's responses, understanding if they are endorsing or rejecting this closeness. A closer relationship between Fiona and Rosamund can be seen in the way they physically interact with each other as the project develops, with increasing physical contact such as holding hands, and as described in the final group interview:

Fiona: *...[in the first session] "Rosamund was sitting next to [Gabriella] and so I just got up and knelt in front of them and played for them. And Rosamund kind of looked at me at that point, and as soon as I went a bit nearer, she turned away; didn't want, you know... nothing. So to have kind of come full circle today to have had that shared moment [of creating a piece] with her..."*

Anneliese: *"She actually let you in."*

Matthew: *"Yeah, she let you in."*

Fiona: *"And it's been step by step from her choosing to hold my, she grabbed my hand about four weeks ago, and it's just been tiny steps by steps. So that's been really precious."*

Alongside a very physical realisation of space, space as a concept is equally, if not, more important in terms of creating an environment conducive to enhancing communication and participation. A slow pace is required in order to create space, enabling a person experiencing dementia to interpret other's communication and to act in response. As a mirror of this, space is also required for staff and musicians to interpret the communication of the person with dementia. Pacing in musical communication is therefore highly important from a musician's perspective, as it can be difficult for a musician to process and act upon all of the communication-based information that they register within a session. In order to truly 'tune in' to another person, the pace and degree of development in musical communication needs also to slow down, to become functional, rather than conceptual, and simple, rather than elaborate, drawn reflexively from subconscious awareness. The musicians describe this in conversation:

Anneliese: *"When I play in a Music for Life setting my playing is quite different. It's less complicated, very simple."*

Matthew: *"Because of the other things that are happening."*

Anneliese: *"Yes, there's so many things to think about, apart from, obviously, making music together (...) you're trying to handle lots of things at the same time. Hence, me usually paring things down. Anything complex (...) tends to be a bit much for the brain (...)"*

Fiona: *"I find my intellectual awareness of what I'm doing in a session diminishes. It's almost like I don't always know what I'm playing. I kind of feel like I'm over there, I'm in the other person's space. Because your awareness can't be between the three of us, your awareness is suddenly on the other person. And that's why the default setting, you know, when you have your own default way of playing, sometimes you rely on that in those moments, because you're so needing to tune into the person that you're playing for (...) It's all about your observations about that person, rather than about what you're creating."*

This 'default' mode that Fiona refers to is about accepting that in order for the primary focus to be on interpreting and relating to the other person, concentration on musical exploration and experimentation may by limited, and a more subconscious deployment of musical language is likely to occur. This 'default' mode calls previous learning and experiences to the fore, and therefore makes great demands on the existing skills and musical language of the musicians, as well as an internalised, shared understanding of the effective application of musical language within this context.

Repetition in musical language is a key asset in developing a slower musical pace, enabling musicians the opportunity to interpret and relate to others. A type of 'scaffolding' occurs within activities, in which prior elements are repeated, but then gradually extended through adding another simple developmental step each time the activity is repeated. When paralleled in a musical sense, the development within the music is less focused on linear, 'horizontal' direction, full of contrast, change and development, but on a more static, 'vertical', approach whereby a few key musical motifs or cells are repeated and layered in interaction with each other, and where new elements may be introduced slowly over time to change the direction of the music. This relies intrinsically on the initial development of a strong musical foundation in order to take place.

The most influential musical elements in creating musical motifs or cells are melody and rhythm in close interaction with harmony and pulse; together these create an overall tonal centre, tempo and character underlying the motif or cell. Repetition in these musical elements can support the gradual evolution of a musical piece, whether extemporised, as in the framing piece and welcome song[133], or completely improvised afresh. Repetition gives coherence to the emerging music and a possibility to add further elements over time to develop the form, character and musical elements of the improvisation, whilst keeping it firmly rooted in its own history. Through this repetition, a slower overall pace of development is achieved, enabling each individual to become involved in making meaning from the aural experience. Fiona reflects on how musical repetition can also help to establish an overall sense of continuity and community, after session two: *"The 'welcome song' also was repeated many times, so many that I wondered if we were doing it too many times. It felt very laborious which in retrospect seemed to reflect the energy of the group. However I actually think this was so important in anchoring the group. They needed the repetition to enable them to understand the process and it really helped to establish a sense of group."*

This choice to use musical repetition had been a conscious one, discussed as part of the preparation before session two: *"As last week had felt so unsettled, Anneliese, Matthew and myself spoke before the session about using lots of repetition and very clear musical structures; clear beginnings*

---

[133] See Chapter 2.3 on 'Applied musical improvisation'.

and endings. We gave ourselves permission to keep it simple! I found this really helped me in the session."

Preparation however, does not just entail discussing a concept but exploring it in reality, in a very practical sense, in order to develop a communicative environment for translation into the music session, as Matthew reflects: *"We had a good time together as a team, from ten to eleven, it felt really good. We played the theme together quite a lot, and really grounded it, and bedded it in so that we all felt really comfortable with it, which we hadn't done last week. And I think that helped us to feel more grounded and more connected."*

Attaining a slower pace through musical repetition can be difficult for a musician, although Fiona and Matthew highlight the importance of working in this way. This sentiment is echoed in the following field note extract, in which persistence in repetition within the activity processes, reinforced by modelling and physical repetition in body language, is highlighted as a key element in creating connections within the 'passing instruments' activity[134] in session two:

> From the field notes of the debrief:
>
> Deborah praises the musicians on their "persistence" – in relation to the activity of passing instruments around the circle, "that must have been so tough…it must have been at least ten or fifteen minutes you were doing that… it really paid off…suddenly you sensed there was a group", especially during the singing enabling it to "grow into a sense of group at that moment…you held your nerve" and that "didn't know what was going to happen … the way you tried that, with possibly one of the hardest groups to try that with…it forced people to look from side to side, take it and relinquish it… it helped them to make a connection…"

For the musicians, finding balancing this repetition with a communicative approach of authenticity, structural integrity and spontaneity is an ongoing challenge and area of interest, as Fiona reflects after session two: *"I want to think about how musically I can support the repetition in a creative way. How can I keep a sense of continuity but also a sense of creativity, invention and spontaneity in the music? It is always playing and creating the most simple music well that is the most difficult challenge!"* Through repetition comes this simplicity, and through simplicity, meaning and coherence; there is space to let the music 'breathe' and take shape at a pace in which each new element or contribution, however small, becomes a vital part of the whole. Anneliese describes how the attention to pacing and space within the 'passing instruments' activity, achieved through repetition, began to create a new communication dynamic within the group, one of alertness, dialogue, spontaneity and fun: *"We started handing instruments around (…) we persevered and I felt the exercise paid off. When we finished playing nearly everybody was holding an instrument and there was this intent alert*

---

[134] See Chapter 2.3 on 'Applied musical improvisation'.

silence... for me this was the first real 'Music for Life moment'. Residents were listening and reacting to musicians or other residents; pieces of music were started and sparked off each other; we were having fun."

Through this passage we see that a space to interpret and reflect upon musical language, a literal space of silence, occurs as a natural response within this communication dynamic. This space enables something new and unplanned to take place. This emergence of communicative spontaneity is highlighted in an improvisation initiated by Abigail, Hannah and Jessica, which takes place in session two, directly after this 'Music for Life moment'. The pacing and space created in the passing instruments activity somehow translate into the interactions and conversational nature of the improvisation, creating a sense of a sustained momentum and coherency to the communication:

From the field notes:

The piece then begins to be led by Abigail, Hannah and Jessica. (This is a very interesting and complex series of interactions). Abigail plays a few short taps on the drum which both Fiona and Anneliese copy – this is very obvious in the musical texture. There is space and quiet, until Hannah shakes her caxixi[135] and it is immediately copied by Anneliese. Abigail joins in again with a stronger short motif on the drum – Anneliese copies and Hannah joins, punctuating the texture with her caxixi occasionally. There is a real sense of listening, waiting to take turns and ensemble. Anneliese copies Hannah's shakes with a set of flourishes and Fiona joins in – encouraging Hannah to continue shaking. There is a long pause – Jessica shakes her ghungharus intentionally at Fiona and Fiona responds musically.

---

[135] A woven basket shaker, with a flat bottom usually made from cocoa shell, and filled with seeds or other particles. It is associated with West African and Brazilian music. See also Appendix V, 'List of musical instruments'.

Passing instruments and emerging trio (session 2)

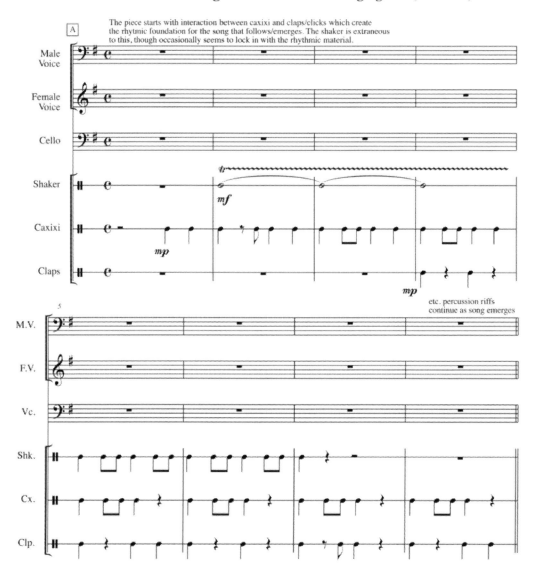

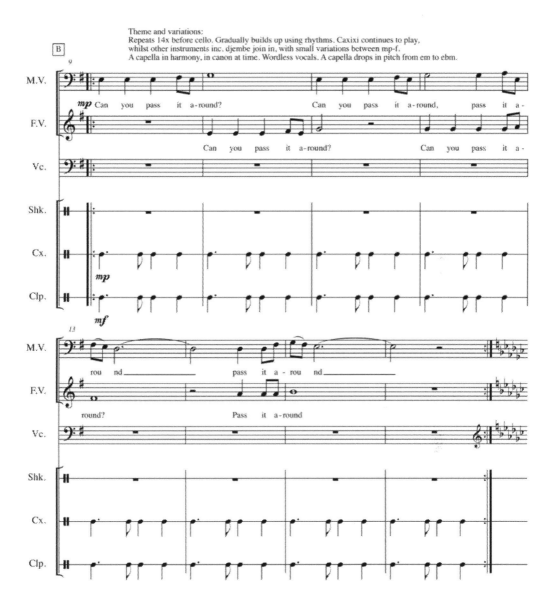

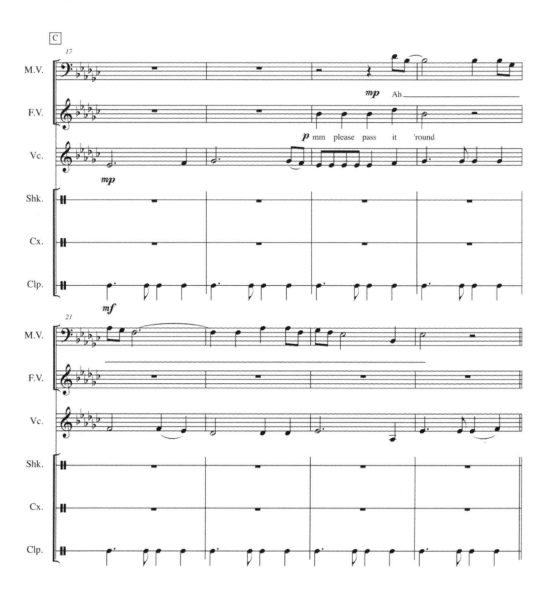

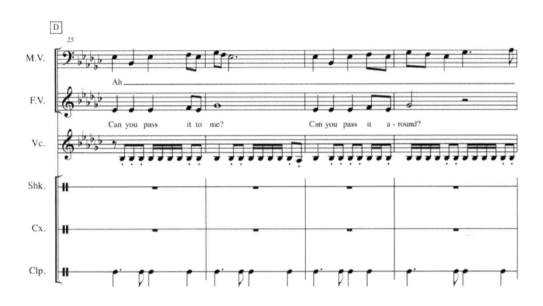

etc. piece continues, then
attacca into passing instruments trio
- bridged by a cello solo

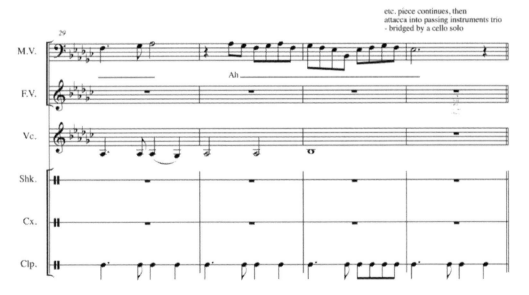

Cello solo linking full group instruments activity into 'trio' of residents. The harp enters and the character begins to change

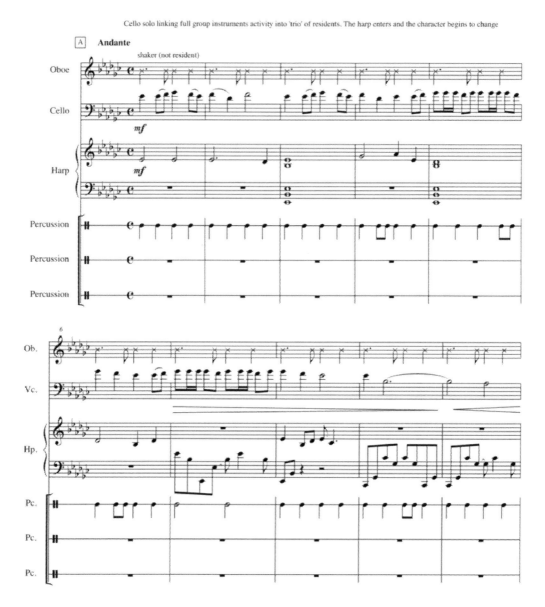

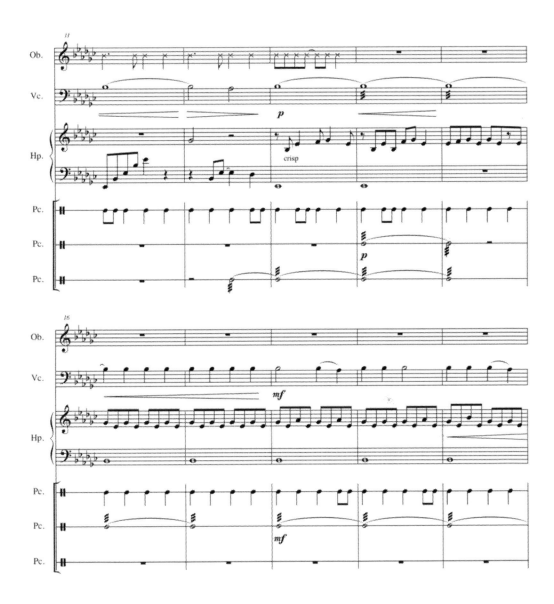

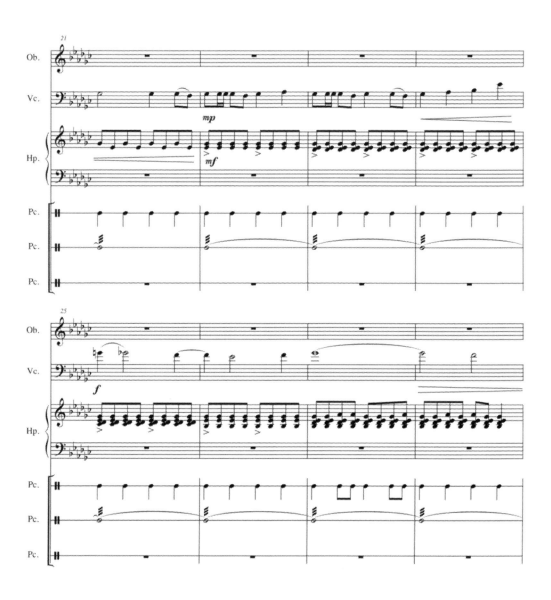

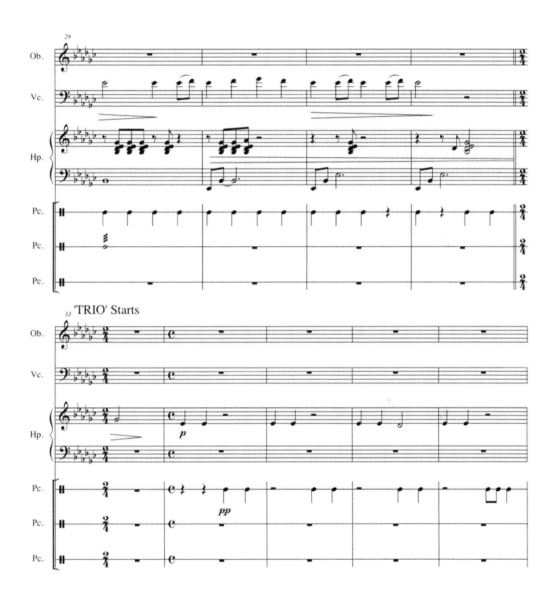

"TRIO" Starts

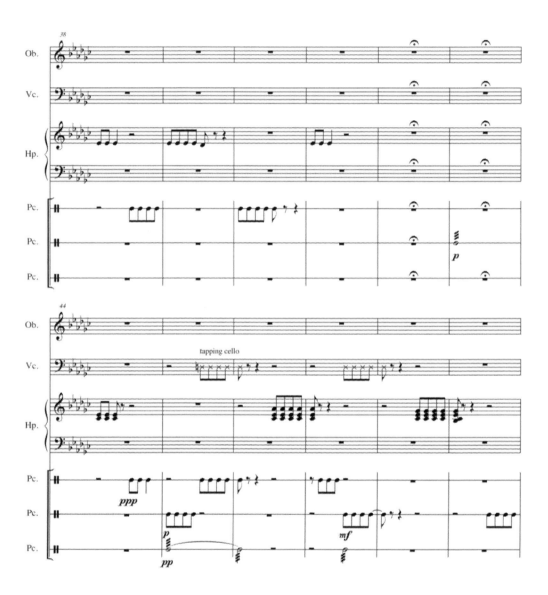

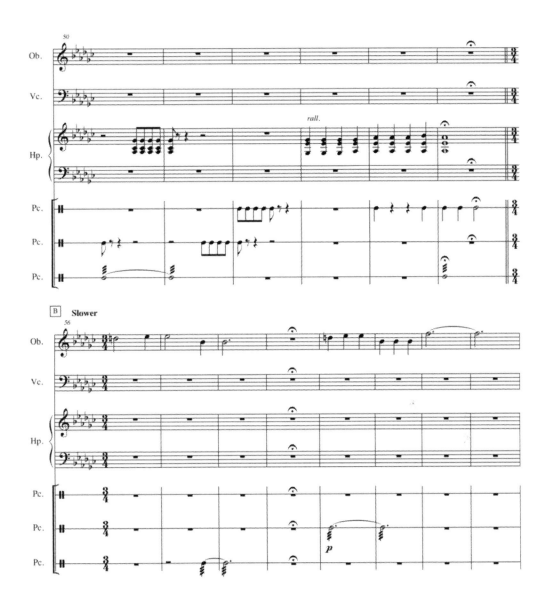

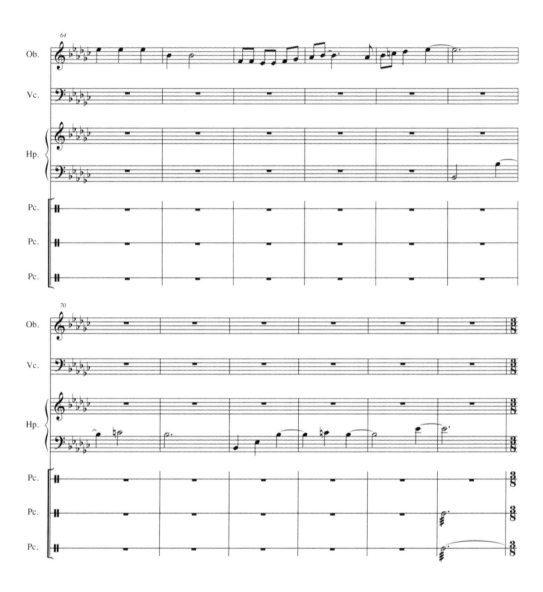

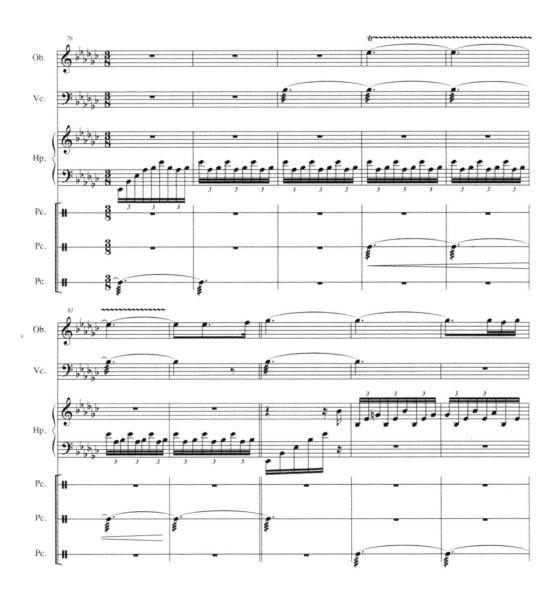

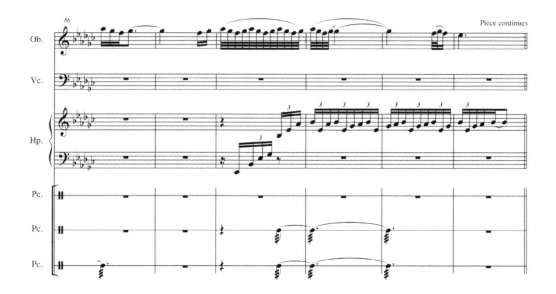

Repetition, in this case through imitation and extension of each other's contributions, has set up the opportunity for a dialogue, and for a larger musical architecture to emerge from the interactions.

Language: quality and form

In relating to a person with dementia, it is important to provide a message of reassurance and validation through communication, that they are accepted and their perception of reality is valid. In recognising the communication challenges that dementia can create, communication needs to be stripped back to its bare essentials, to an essential purity and authenticity where the message being conveyed can be both recognised and responded to. This authenticity in communication can lead to feelings of connectivity, collectivism and communion, a sense of being part of a community.

Authenticity and depth of integrity in musical communication is paramount. Even if the music and interactions within the music may appear to be silly and fun, there is integrity behind the musical communication, and a sense of artistry. Through this artistry and this willingness to find and acknowledge the authentic self of another, comes a sense of a deeper connection through communication:

Fiona: *"You want to bring your best, and have musical integrity, I think, in what you're doing."*

Anneliese: *"But we found again and again that without this musical integrity, you don't get that, you don't get the same depth and connection. I think there really is, there's a real truth there. You can't just go and play something to them, it doesn't work. It doesn't work in the same way, you don't go as deep."*

This 'depth and connection' is achieved through musical integrity of the highest quality, where the music created is coherent and meaningful. Where this coherence in the musical message is absent, it can impact upon the experiences of participants, leading to a sense of anxiety, the message lost in incoherent fragments of music. Matthew: *"For the musicians you can end up feeling like you're playing for the sake of it and you're not making good music. You're just noodling and doodling, making music that you don't feel is very good, I suppose. And I think it can potentially create a feeling of anxiety for the residents as well, if there's no resolution ever. And I wondered whether some of Gabriella's discomfort and her saying: 'Come on, come on, play', I can't remember exactly what her words were, but there was a sense of 'get on with it, do something, come on do it.' And I thought, yeah, we're not playing. We're filling in the background and nothing is happening."*

Authenticity also involves creating music that reflects the uniqueness of the person, and that is relevant within the moment, and therefore indicates a need for spontaneity and adaptability in communication. However, a freshness of approach and language within communication may not always be attained and may sometimes be an ideal, as a result of the vast amount of information a musician is processing and interpreting within the session:

Fiona: *"I think you can always grow in this work (...) to bring my best, and to find other ways [of communicating]. Because you can get into a default mode, can't you, especially when you're aware of all the different things that are going on, you can revert to your safe, oh, 'I'll play this and I can do this kind of thing'."*

Anneliese: *"I do that a lot, sometimes you have to, don't you?"*

Fiona: *"You have to (...) but I want to kind of keep growing that, so that I get a bigger vocabulary, that's the aim."*

Matthew: *"Yes, likewise, likewise. And there is a kind of feeling of achievement, when you've been through a session and you've pushed yourself musically a bit as well, you feel like you've been brave, you know what I mean?"*

Combinations of musical elements, such as pitch, melody, harmony, tonality; pulse, rhythm, tempo; texture, timbre and dynamics interact together in many variations as part of this vocabulary, interacting to form a compelling musical language. The way the musicians apply these elements and how they take form – whether it be an evolving structure or within a musical framework – has a strong impact within this context. As a whole, the qualities of these elements interact together to produce an overall effect, a musical message or mood, which can act to enhance the social environment. At some point Brian reflects on how the musical quality was compelling in creating a secure environment where residents wished to be: *"I personally think it's because the quality of the music was quite calming and relaxing. It led people to a place of calm and still. It was also a lower energy, I think, but in a good way, a relaxed sense of lower energy (…) people were quite relaxed and happy to stay."* This lower energy of the music in turn creates a situation where the quality of the music is causally related to the atmosphere of the social environment.

In another case in session one, we also see a similar relationship between musical communication and social environment, although the impact of the musical communication creates a very different atmosphere:

From the field notes:

The music segues into faster and more turbulent music, beginning with an oboe melodic line with cello accompaniment, and as it develops, a luscious harp accompaniment. Group participation increases during this – Sarah and Rebecca start shaking their maracas, Esther conducts along with her hands and claps along, Hannah's cabasa[136] becomes louder, Jessica and Abigail remain awake and appear alert.

In this example, the sense of direction and full energy, coupled with a fast tempo stimulates alertness and active participation at a group level. However, it is important to understand that this relationship between music and the social environment is symbiotic, and therefore the music making is intrinsically linked to the social environment. Fiona describes in the final post-project group interview how, apart from influencing the social environment, the 'sound world' is a product of the environment in which it is created, fundamentally reflecting the emotional experiences of the group: *"I think it's the physical things like the combination of instruments, that's an obvious one, but I think maybe it's the dynamics of the group. You know, it's been a poignant group with people who were in quite a fragile state, I think. And I think the music has trod that line of kind of holding that fragility and that poignancy, and kind of maybe taking it somewhere safer. It's kind of an emotional soundscape almost."*

The language of music has great potential to act in a number of ways, validating and transforming emotional experiences. One way in which it can do this is to act in a 'holding' capacity, for individuals who may need the music to provide a strong parallel to other more physical forms of reassurance – such as holding, comforting, embracing. This music then

---

[136] Also called 'afuche': cylinder with a handle upon which loops of steel-ball chain are wrapped, adapted from the African Shekere. The Shekere is a hollowed out gourd covered with a net of beads. Both the Cabasa and the Shekere are played through holding the instrument with one hand, whilst the other hand scrapes the beads back and forth over the cylinder or gourd. See also Appendix V, 'List of musical instruments'.

122

becomes a sort of a 'container' for their emotional distress, a safe structure in which they can be comforted and distracted from their sense of turmoil, as Fiona mentions after session three: *"Last week Sarah had been so distressed so this week we decided to bring her in first, and sit her next to Anneliese. This really seemed to help and Anneliese worked wonderfully with her. She was much calmer and although she occasionally called out this was often stopped by a musical distraction. [Sarah] again made a wonderful piece with Matthew, right at the point when she was beginning to cry out (...) It made me reflect on how music can be an anchor, how it can bring people back into the moment and help to stop 'default' behaviour."*

The 'default' behaviour Fiona refers to here is one of a resident's disengagement and distress; a communication mode that Sarah returns to repeatedly when her sense of security begins to erode. In this case, the 'anchoring' quality of the music provides a way for Sarah to communicate in the here and now, to fully engage in a social communicative process and attain a sense of well-being. As described in the 'Identity' analysis, Fiona again reflects on the 'anchoring' potential of music, its crucial role in recognition of identity, as well as the possibility of emotional transformation through musical communication: *"I think the amazing thing about music is that you can be 'held' in the moment, or taken to a new place. You can provide a safe place in music that accepts each person as they are in that moment, or you can help to transfer them out of their current emotional / mental state to a different place, even for a moment."*

Musical elements which influence the pace and quality of musical production, for instance, tonality, tempo, dynamics and tone colour, are particularly important features underlying this anchoring quality of 'holding'.

Through outlining a strong, static tonality within the musical language a sense of reassurance and security can be attained at a social level. Tonality is often emphasised through melody as well as harmony; a static tonal centre is often made more powerful through simple chord progressions, a slow harmonic rhythm and thematic melodies with small contours. A very literal tonal journey can represent a metaphysical emotional journey; a small level of modulation and thematic development can create a sense of change, of hope, and one of acceptance when brought back to the principle tonality. Besides tonality, pacing, repetition, affirmation and decisiveness are again paramount; and when combined with a slow tempo, soft dynamics and instrumental timbre, it has a potent effect.

The following field notes outline two musical interactions, the first in which Rosamund is at the centre of the musical interaction, but during which Sarah begins to become distressed; and then immediately followed by a second interaction where Sarah is called upon to 'help' Matthew by conducting. Within both it is possible to perceive how these elements of tonality, tempo, dynamics and timbre interact, in relation to the social context:

From the field notes:

Anneliese starts a melodic motif in F major in a triple meter; it is quite bright in character, but dynamically soft and at a slow tempo. Fiona joins in the improvisation with her cello – copying Anneliese's melodic motif and developing it, as Anneliese supports it with a simple 'oom-cha-cha' accompaniment. Matthew then joins – taking a melodic role, supported by an antiphonal countermelody on cello and accompaniment on harp; all three occasionally reference the original melodic motif. The piece is gentle in nature, almost lullaby like – at one point it moves harmonically to A minor for a brief period but firmly returns to the F major tonality. During this piece Sarah has begun to shout "mummy" repeatedly and regularly. Diallo is comforting Sarah and holds her hand – this sometimes seems to placate her to a small degree, but she appears to be becoming more and more distressed, with her shouts picking up in frequency and intensity during Rosamund's piece. When it ends they appear to become a little softer.

From the field notes:

Matthew pauses for a moment before heading directly for Sarah. He touches her upper arms and comforts her, saying her name – "mummy" becomes tinged with sadness and is slightly lower in pitch. Matthew asks Sarah: "Can I play a piece of music for you?" to which she replies immediately: "yeah, but it's not easy". There is a pause before Matthew asks: "Can we try?" and she immediately responds with a "Yes". Matthew asks: "Will you help me?" repeating, "will you help me Sarah?" as he passes the baton to her.

In these interactions, as outlined in the analysis on Identity, the role of music in affirming Sarah's identity is crucial; therefore, understanding the musical language from which this sense of 'belonging' arises is important. Matthew starts the piece with an exploratory melody, kneeling in front of Sarah, supported by a spacious and gentle accompaniment from Anneliese and mysterious tremolos from Fiona, which are then echoed by Anneliese. Sarah has good eye contact with Matthew and she rapidly moves the baton, which influences Anneliese's musical response: florid, flowery accelerating and decelerating arpeggiated embellishments on the harp, which permeate the entire improvisation. Fiona's phrases initially are subtle, but grow in intensity throughout the piece; they often act in antiphony to a gentle, sustained and expansive melody by Matthew. The piece transitions from using low and middle registers of the instruments during the initial, calmer part of the piece into the high register, as it develops to a climax at the end of the piece. The improvisation is characterised by lots of dynamic swells, and is in a free, slow tempo. Harmonically, it circulates around one progression alternating between C major and F major, and mostly with Matthew in a melodic role, Fiona in a countermelody role and Anneliese in a harmonic accompaniment role. At times when Sarah appears to disengage, Matthew makes strong eye contact with her, prompting her reengagement. Sarah does not call out during the piece.

Within these extracts, it is possible to perceive how the musicians interact with each other as instrumentalists, to create this sense of anchoring with the improvisations – although both have different stylistic features, they both function in a holding capacity, and elicit strong roles. There is less of a focus on engaging Sarah in the creative decisions of the piece; the musicians appear to 'gift' it to her, their musical language seems to focus less on creative exploration and more on affirmation and simplicity, which is reinforced by the musical roles that they adopt. A three-tier relationship emerges in which each instrumentalist consistently has a clear role, although these occasionally overlap briefly, and in which the qualities of the tone colour of each instrument are used to full advantage. Through adopting clear roles, it also enables the texture of the improvisation to remain clear and simple. Anneliese establishes the role of the harp firmly and consistently as an accompaniment instrument, greatly influencing the harmonic rhythm, progressions and overall form of the improvisations. Through various accompaniment styles, Anneliese influences the style and texture of the improvisations, and acts to provide a beautiful, flowing and uplifting sense of continuity and connectivity to the more sustained tones and melodic explorations of the sensitive and warm articulations of the *arco* cello and the dreamy, floating oboe. Matthew establishes the role of the oboist as providing the main melodic themes within the improvisations, which works well with the oboe's distinct tonal quality and treble register, as it sits well on the bed of sound provided by Anneliese and Fiona. The use of the oboe in this way helps to emphasize the 'grounding' quality of the cello and harp contributions. Fiona assumes a supportive role on the cello throughout, support for both Anneliese and Matthew – acting to reinforce the melodic and harmonic material – sometimes referencing this directly, and at other times, to provide impetus to the development of the melodic line, through antiphonal countermelodies. Employing the low register of the instruments appears to have a calming, grounding effect, and the higher register a more uplifting one.

In addition to the qualities of these instruments, use of the singing voice and elements of the song form have a strong impact during the sessions. Brian identifies an almost 'primitive' quality of Matthew's voice as resonating with Sarah in her times of distress, calling her out of her 'default' behaviour: *"I was trying to understand why, what were the triggers for her calling out and not calling out between sessions? I wondered at one point when Matthew was making, I don't know how to describe it, but he was using his voice. And it felt to me quite, how do you say, almost primitive kind of sounds. And I just wondered whether that would connect with her, a very primeval kind of calling."* In addition, the voice is the key to connecting with Rebecca, according to Matthew, in his account of session seven: *"We began by playing instruments for her and she appeared to be, I don't know if confused was the word, or what, but that kind of tight mouth and the staring eyes was there while we were playing. So instead I sang, I sang to her and that seems to be the key, is to sing for her, to her, whatever it is. And there's just this softness that just suddenly comes. There's a real difference, I gave her my hand to hold and she did do the very tight grip and the patting of the hand, but it was very different. She would pat my hand and then hold it tightly so we got both our hands held together really tightly. And she was smiling whilst that happened, and not the forced smile either, the real genuine smile of, you know, she really was happy."*

The singing voice is a powerful tool; not only can it recognise and call upon the deepest most primeval emotions, it is a source of joy and fun: convivial in the welcome song, and essential in creating a sense of humour through the impact of lyrics. We return to Gabriella, as described earlier, in the analysis on 'Identity', in this extract from session four:

From the field notes:

Harry comes over to Gabriella, and says "Hello Gabriella", she responds: "Hello". Harry comments vibrantly, "that's a fantastic tambourine" to which Gabriella says "Yes it is... it sounds good, doesn't it?" Matthew adds "and Rachel has one too. You can have a tambourine duet, or a trio for tambourines and flute." Rachel and Gabriella start patting the tambourine. Gabriella says "That sounds good!...Yes, yes very good!" There is a brief hiatus in playing, so Harry uses the "sounds good" and evolves into a semi-pitched rhythm for lyrics: "Sounds good." This is used as the basis for 'trading' bars – i.e. flute duet for two bars, followed by "sounds really good, sounds really good." Harry sings and plays, and encourages Gabriella to recite and sing along, and Rachel to tap the pulse. It's very rhythmic and vibrant in F major. At the end Harry says: "Gabriella...that sounded really good." They laugh. Matthew says "Gabriella, how was the music" and she makes a joke "it sounds really good."

126

'Sounds good, sounds really good' (session 4)

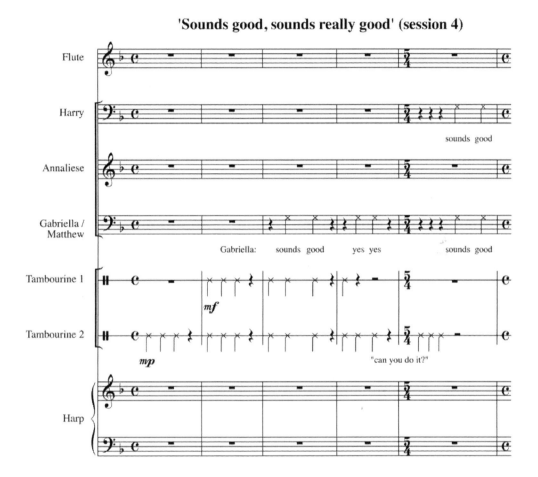

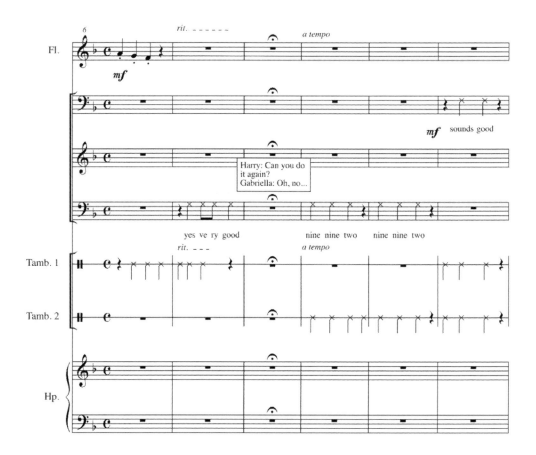

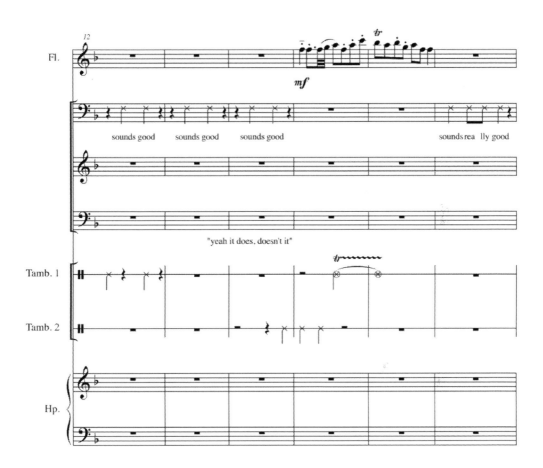

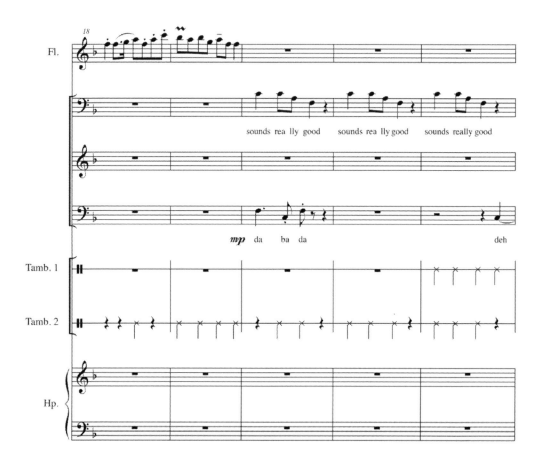

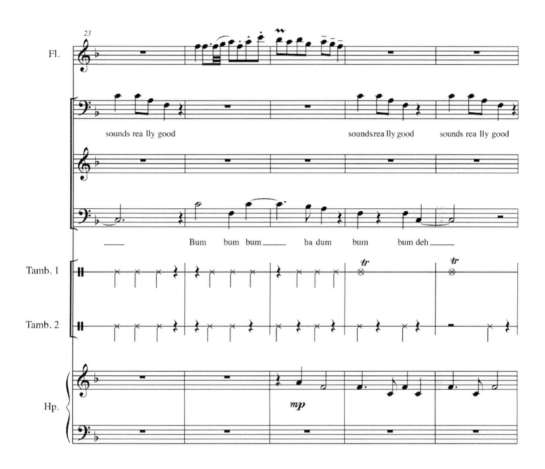

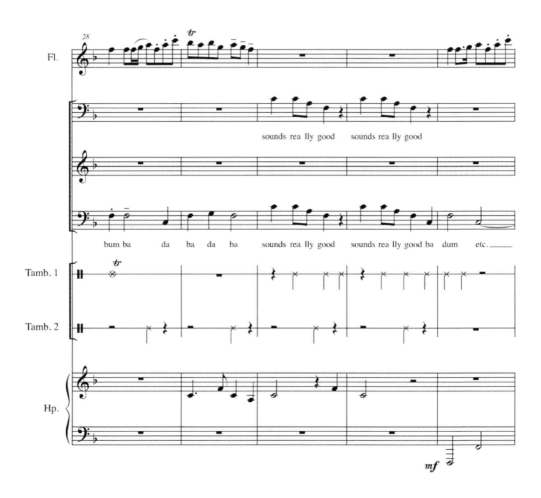

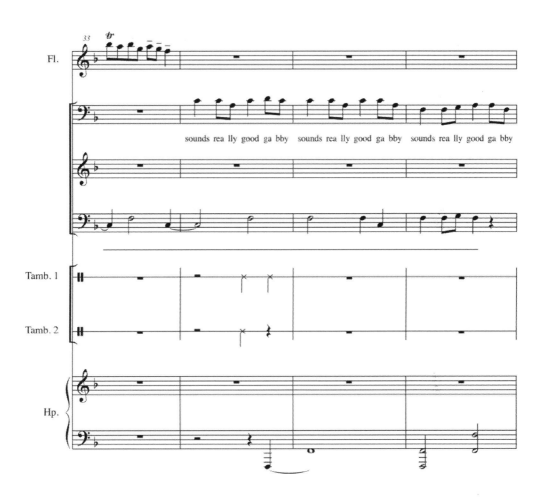

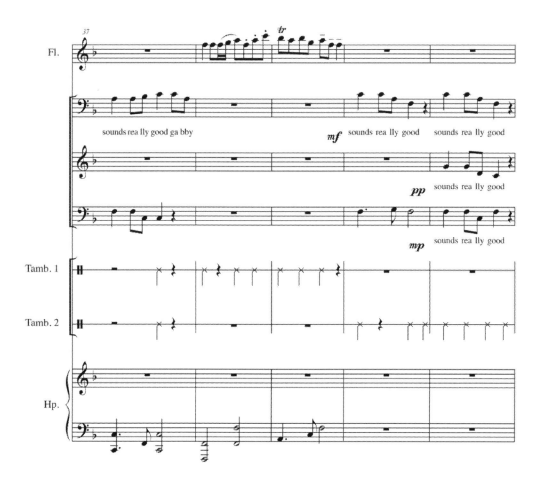

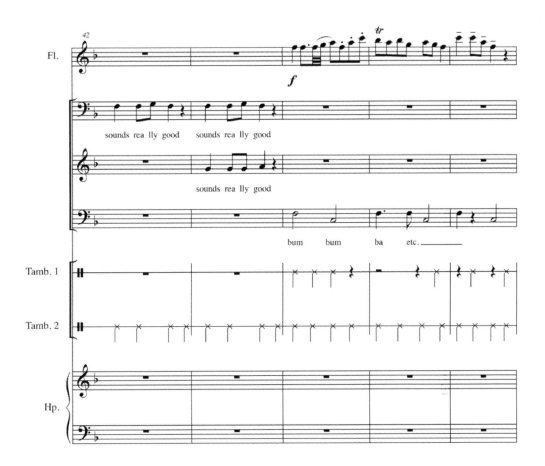

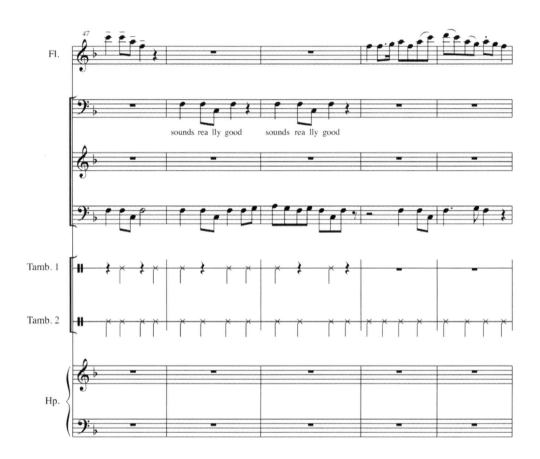

sounds rea lly good   sounds rea lly good

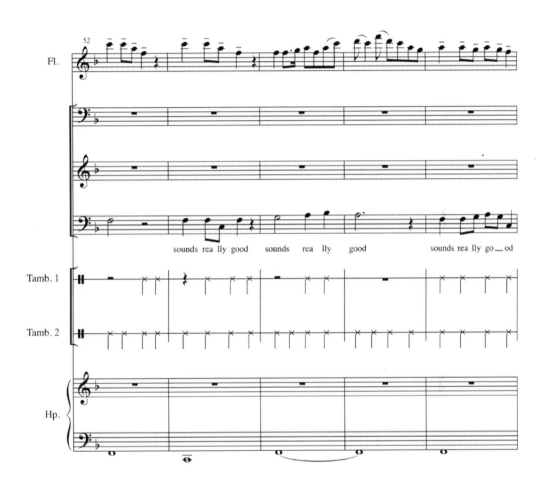

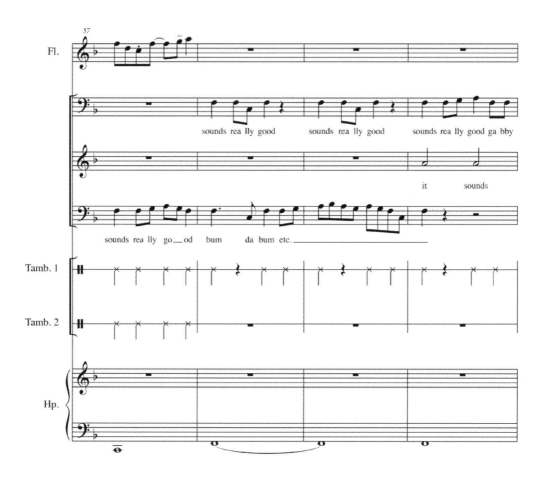

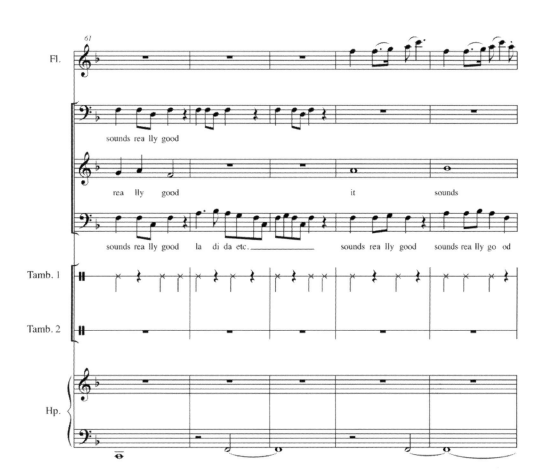

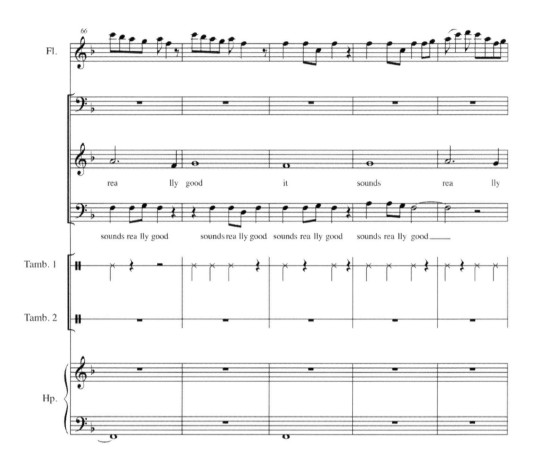

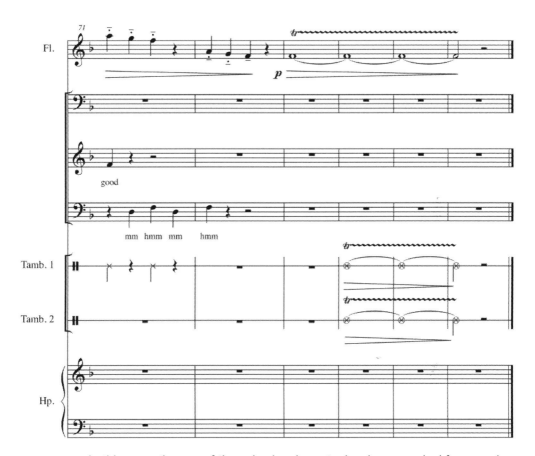

In this case, the use of the voice has been to develop a musical framework in which the musical contribution of Gabriella has been stimulated, incorporated and repeated, becoming a key musical motif within the improvisation. Matthew had reflected after the previous session, session three, the importance of a sense of spontaneity: "*I do really want to let the music 'take off' at some point soon. I think this will be the next stage on bringing the group together, move us all onto the next stage.*" The sense of humour, informality and spontaneity apparent in this interaction is a key sign that this 'next stage' of equality and belonging has arrived.

In other interactions throughout the project, the voice has a strong role in providing means to musical inclusion, for instance: participants singing along in the framing piece and welcome song, especially in the case where

Hannah initiates and concludes the framing song vocally in session five, participants expressing gratitude for the quality of "beautiful singing" such as Abigail and Rosamund, and explicitly 'gifting' music to residents such as in session eight, between Fiona and Rosamund, as explored in the analysis on Identity:

> From the field notes:
>
> Fiona starts to sing to Rosamund. It's beautiful and gentle singing, wordless; a counter-melody to the harp. She uses her whole body in gestures and has a questioning and radiant face as she sings to Rosamund. They hold eye contact with each other, and Fiona gently strokes Rosamund's hand as she sings. Fiona asks at a point: "sing with me?" She continues to sing wordlessly, and then sings once "Rosamund, it's for you". Rosamund immediately responds saying, "it's for you" to which Fiona responds: "No, it's for you!" and laughs, saying "it's for both of us maybe". The piece finishes at this interaction. Rosamund quietly says, "That's lovely", and Fiona responds with "thank you". Fiona then says, a little louder, "thank you for letting me share it with you" and Rosamund responds, "you're very welcome". Rosamund adds: "makes you want to cry" and Fiona responds: "I know, it does make you want to cry, doesn't it?" Matthew affirms to Rosamund: "thank you" and then "thanks Fiona and Anneliese" nodding at them. It's a quiet end to a very gentle interaction.

Through this very intimate, sensitive and powerful use of the voice, Fiona and Rosamund reach a sense of connection deeper than ever reached throughout the preceding eight weeks.

The role of instruments

The choice of instruments used within a session is crucial, with instruments serving as a conduit for self-expression through musical communication. Instruments are carefully selected during preparation prior to the session, keeping in mind prior preferences of and relevance to individuals, and during the session are usually chosen via consultation or coincidentally through the passing instruments activity.

The tactile nature of playing instruments is a sensual act of timalation[137]; each piece of hand percussion elicits a different tactile sensation resulting in a variety of sounds, for instance, exploring the smooth skin of a drum as opposed to the rough uneven texture of seed shakers, or shaking a maraca[138] versus stroking bar chimes. The tactile nature of the instruments creates possibility for those with acute hearing or vision impairment to

---

[137] Kitwood 1997: 90.

[138] Also called chikita of egg shaker: a native instrument of South America, traditionally made of gourd or coconut shells, but also commercially out of wood, plastic and leather, occasionally clay; the shell is usually attached to a handle for ease of playing. The sound is produced when beads or small particles inside the maraca hit the inside of the shell. Chikitas are small plastic versions of the maraca. Egg Shakers work on the same acoustic principles as the Maraca, are handle-less, and the same size and shape as a chicken egg. See also Appendix V, 'List of musical instruments'.

experience music in a different way, for instance, through touching the vibrating skin of drum. Similarly, vibrations produced through using the voice to sing can help to stimulate breathing and may lead to a sense of well being.

At a group level, the interactive possibilities of instruments are important, for instance, sharing a large instrument together, or visually recognising a connection to another person through pairing of the same instrument. At an individual level, the context or sound of some instruments may represent aspects of that person's identity, including their cultural identity, whether this is induced through memories of nationality or spiritual practice. Particular instruments may serve as catalysts for eliciting a different mode of communication than usual. The use of a resonant metal bass bar with Rebecca in session six, as described in the Identity analysis, is such an example; when exploring hand percussion instruments and the baton in previous sessions the fast-paced anxiety underpinning her emotional state was highlighted, drawing attention to the nature of her dementia. However, the resonant quality and gravitas of the bass bar, and the very visual, slow way in which it is struck led to a very different type of communication from Rebecca, one which the musicians could actually match and meet, rather than translating, communication in which there was space for reflection, dialogue and a sense of connection to develop. Anneliese comments in a debrief how she believed the instrument was an excellent conduit for Rebecca's self-expression:

> From the field notes, debrief:
>
> Anneliese says to the group that she was struck by the "gesture... the strength of what Rebecca had to say." She says to Matthew that it was a "good instrument choice – the way it rang... gave it breath" and that it enabled strong contact with Matthew. "She was in charge."

Matthew goes back to this episode from his perspective, in an interview: *"She was hitting it once, which is really different. Normally if she reached for something it would be this slapping or shaking repeated thing that goes on and on until you pull away or something. And she was doing this one strike on the chime bar. I suppose that was the thing that made me think, yes this is good. She's enjoying this (...) this is meaningful for her."* Here, Matthew interprets that the bass bar resonates with some aspect of Rebecca's being, it becomes a communicative device in which she can both create and extract meaning. There are very physical aspects – for instance the resonance of the instrument, the way of producing a sound – but also potentially symbolic aspects underpinning these embodiments. Matthew draws an analogy between the quality of this piece, and a connection with the musical and spiritual language of the Jewish tradition: *"It was a single, very strong beat, like the ringing of a bell (...) And then I was singing very strongly. And I was singing something that was coming out very Jewish sounding. As I was listening to myself I was thinking, 'oh, this is like a cantor', that kind of a*

143

sound. Maybe that will have some resonance for her as well (...) It felt to me like it was almost like a bit of a ceremony. She would ring the bell and then the music would happen again until it died down and it was back to her and she would ring the bell again and initiate the next wave. And it felt very serious, it was very, very serious. And that was what was in her face, as well." Here, within this ceremony, a process of musical 'turn-taking' has been established, leaving space for Rebecca and Matthew to engage in a spiritual dialogue.

Matthew felt an overriding spirituality during the musical communication, a connection between his spirit and the spirit of Rebecca: *"I'm again thinking about Rebecca and singing with Rebecca, I can't think of anything that I've ever done in my life that's anything like it. You know, of kind of losing myself so much in the essence of another person. (...) the musical support is different from the physical reassurance of handholding, it's a real connection with their spirit, I think."*

Brian reflects on the spirituality inherent in music, drawing a direct analogy between the celebratory aspects of liturgy and the communicative rituals experienced within Music for Life sessions: *"Liturgy is often about celebration, celebration of life. You come as you are to give yourself to, whether it is to your community or to a higher power. But you come as you are and you sort of lay yourself open and celebrate with other people. And I think often in liturgies there is a coming together, there's a greeting and then there is something about making something sink a little bit deeper, and then leading into a kind of celebration together, saying 'here we are, this is what we're offering', which is like the music comes up, and usually in liturgy there is a closing down part and a sending forth."*

This sense of celebration, ceremony and spirituality is inherent within the musical communication between Matthew and Rebecca. In this instance with Rebecca, we see a deep connection form with the mode of expression that the bass bar offers. The bass bar seems to suggest a pace of communication and a potential link to spiritual tradition and her sense of spirituality; it also gives her a status as the leader in the interaction. With each instrument comes a status, a combination of the sound the instrument produces coupled with the functional way they are used in musical communication. With this status comes a role, a function; the instrument becomes the visual, physical and symbolic conduit for communication. For instance, the striking of a drum can become a commanding visual and aural presence within a musical improvisation; therefore, as a result, the person playing the drum may take a leadership role in the overall development and character of the music.

Perhaps the instrument with the highest status, and the greatest at symbolizing agency, is that of the baton. Matthew describes in an interview how the baton provided a way for Abigail to 'take charge': *"Her movements were very small and so the baton kind of magnifies that. Gives a focus to it.*

144

So it gives you something to read. There's that very practical reason. Two is, there's the kind of status thing of being given the baton. It's very much about putting this person in charge. And it's by agreeing to take the baton that person is making a choice. About 'yeah, I'll take the baton, I will lead this piece'. And it's a signal to the rest of the group as well. That by taking the baton the person is going to be the focus of the music for the next, however long it takes. And important to have a baton, you know, to have the real thing there. It's an actual conductor's baton and, it's not a compromise, a pencil or a beater turned around or anything. It's the real thing. And everything that it conveys about being a conductor, of being in charge."

Sometimes the taking of musical leadership may occur in a more subtle way. We see this in practice in session seven, when a piece of music evolves in which the majority of participants have an egg shaker or maraca:

> From the field notes:
>
> Jessica explores her maraca, shaking it softly (...) Anne responds to Jessica's shake, and begins a rhythm that catches on quickly. Fiona uses a wooden agogô [139] that slices through the texture and the piece starts to take off. When the piece begins to develop into a song, Fiona adds a repetitive pattern, Anneliese joins in, matching the pattern, acting to embed the pattern into the music.

Within this piece, there is a sense of equality, achieved through individuals possessing the same instrument, however this uniformity can create a limited context for musical development. Through using the agogô, Fiona is able to cut through the uniformity of texture to provide variety from the shakers, enabling the initiation and strengthening of a strong rhythmic motif, which in turn acts as a catalyst for musical development and renewed sense of direction and energy. Matthew reflects on his initial perspective on the challenges that this uniformity created: *"The music was very responsive to people today, but there were some risky moments, actually. You know, the piece that just started off with everybody with shakers. I didn't know what to do, I was thinking 'oh God everybody's got a shaker, how are we going to make a piece out of, with everyone with a shaker'. You know? 'What on earth are we going to do!'"* Matthew reflects further on how situations like this can be confronting as a leader: *"It's like there is an anxiety about what's going to happen next. And it's down to me, as the leader to make sure something happens, and it's got to be the right thing and not the wrong thing. There's a sense of expectation."* However, the desire to communicate musically ensured that a solution was found, according to Matthew, through safeguarding the space for others to interpret the situation and initiate

[139] Agogô Bell, Wooden Agogô, Wooden Double Agogô: Originating from the West African Yoruba and used in samba music, this instrument consists of two metal conical 'bells', struck by a drumstick. The bells are both high pitched, and produce two discrete pitches. The Wooden Agogô imitates the design of the Agogô Bell, and it consists of either one or two bells. Each wooden 'bell' has grooves on it, so that the instrument can either be struck by a wooden beater, producing a semi-pitched sound much like the wood block, or scraped, producing a sound like a guiro. See also Appendix V, 'List of musical instruments'.

communication: *"Wait and see what happens; somebody will signal something, we hope; they always do eventually. Or one of the other musicians can have an idea about what to do next or just begin playing even. I think it's something you can do more as the project is progressing certainly. I think in the beginning, the first few sessions I don't think it's necessarily a useful thing to do. To leave the group feeling they don't know what's happening next. It takes a bit of trust to be built up, that something will happen next."* As Matthew implies, this spontaneity in communication is something that arises from a sense of security and out of relationships built on trust.

Use of 'language'

In addition to, and often alongside the effective use of physical space, space and pacing and a relevant choice of instruments, communication styles and modes have a powerful impact in developing an environment conducive to enhancing communication and participation. This occurs through the type of language and registers within language, in conjunction with the quality of communication. The use of affirming language is an important aspect in communication within the session, in verbal, non-verbal and musical language. Affirming language is gentle yet strong, clear in intent and directed with a warm regard and respect for the dignity and agency of the other person. It enables a sense of invitation and inclusion to occur, as well as reassurance and validation. From this reassurance a sense of security can arise, invoking greater potential for communication and participation.

In session six, Matthew's and Anne's verbal and non-verbal language is critical in welcoming and including Esther, who has characteristically arrived after the session has begun. Matthew also uses vernacular language that resonates with Esther's verbal expressions:

> From the field notes:
>
> Anne and Matthew welcome [Esther] warmly, "would you like to join us? Just come through". They ask if she would like to join in, then Matthew explains that he is finding a chair for her so she can join the circle. Anne waves her tambourine at Esther, enticing her with it. Matthew brings a chair into the circle for Esther, explains what's involved in the session, and says "would that be alright doll?" and then affirmatively "Welcome!" Esther and Anne interact – talking and playing.

During session eight, Esther again enters after the session has begun; this time Fiona welcomes her affirmatively through non-verbal and musical communication:

> From the field notes:
>
> Esther comes in during the welcome song. She quietly observes the circle from the outside and is sat next to Brian (in the outer circle). Esther sings a little, joining in with the rhythm, as Matthew drums and sings – Fiona hears this, turns her body to face Esther, and motions with her hand and sings to Esther, in an inviting and

acknowledging way. Esther gently slaps her bag in a rhythm and happily claps along to the music and it's very musical.

Within the practice, a level of affection and respect is affirmed through verbal and non-verbal language, fostering a sense of inclusion. This affirmation does not occur just between musicians and residents, or between staff and residents, but between all participants within this community, although musicians and staff model it to a high degree, in a multifaceted way; through soothing, reassuring, validating. It happens at a pace that the other person appears to be comfortable with. In this extract from session seven, Fiona's gentle combination of verbal and non-verbal language validates what Rosamund is feeling, and happens at a pace where there is ample space for a response from Rosamund, matching Rosamund's tone, style and pace of expression:

From the field notes:

Fiona speaks to Rosamund softly – she asks how she is today and says "it's really nice to see you again". Fiona asks how her week has been; Rosamund whispers back her answers. Fiona says "you look really lovely, really beautiful", and asks her if she is tired. After speaking to Jessica, Fiona sits with Rosamund and holds her hand. Diallo arrives and helps Rosamund to be transferred into her chair. Fiona asks for a pillow for Rosamund to help her be comfortable, which he brings. Rosamund settles in, and closes her eyes, and looks peaceful.

We see in this example that Fiona interacts sensitively with Rosamund in a variety of ways; she enquires after her well-being, affirms Rosamund's value in her life, compliments her and through enquiring if she is tired, validates Rosamund's potential experience, and validates that she is accepted. She also holds her hand, staying close and just sits with Rosamund, affirming that she is there with her. Attention to the details around Rosamund's physical comfort also enables a greater sense of security to develop for Rosamund, one where she has permission to be as she feels. Another way that the musicians may soothe residents during transitions is through gentle music making, as in this instance:

From the field notes:

Anneliese has returned to her seat and plays her harp softly as Hannah arrives and is transferred into a chair. She also plays to Sarah who is holding her head in her hands. Sarah is clearly distressed and keeps calling out for her mum.

Open facial language and eye contact is also an important tool of affirmation, as within session seven:

From the field notes:

Matthew again is very attentive – he kneels, near to [Abigail] but still with enough space for her. He blinks softly and smiles occasionally, which seems to reassure her. Anneliese also smiles across the circle to Abigail as she plays her harp. Anneliese's eyes are focused on Abigail and the baton, and her facial language, especially around the eyes, is very open and inquisitive.

Similarly, smiling urges the person receiving the contact to also reciprocate the gesture, as with this extract from session eight:

From the field notes:

Rebecca looks happily towards the musicians, appearing utterly relaxed, sitting calmly with her hands folded in her lap. She and Rachel are physically close, in a sort of cuddle. Rebecca smiles broadly and her face comes alive as Matthew plays the drum and sings – she appears to really like this. She also smiles back at Matthew warmly when he smiles at her.

Here we find a new sense of freedom, spontaneity and confidence in Rebecca's communication; previous expressions of pursed lips and intense staring now replaced with smiling lips and soft eyes.

In addition, squeezing and stroking hands, as well as stroking arms and backs, is an important method of non-verbal affirmation within the practice. Holding hands is a literal symbol of not only a physical, but also a social connection between individuals, and it happens often, initiated by staff and musicians. Often, this form of soothing contact can develop into an opportunity to share a musical experience together, through rocking interlinked hands to the underlying musical pulse, as in this case with Samantha and Gabriella from session seven:

From the field notes:

Gabriella's eyes are closed; Samantha gently holds her hand and strokes it for some time. When Gabriella's eyes open, she and Samantha begin to interact in a really lovely way – they wave their hand up and down to Matthew, and Matthew waves back with a slightly larger motion, encouraging her to continue waving. Gabriella's facial expression seems to come alive and she looks well.

Through this extract it is possible to see that this interaction emerges from slowly paced, gentle, non-demanding and affirmative communication initiated by Samantha. Essentially, by holding hands and rocking hands to the pulse, Samantha is, in a sense, mirroring and extending Gabriella's contribution.

Interestingly, as the project develops, we begin to see that residents begin to initiate contact, through holding hands, with musicians and staff. This leadership symbolises a growing sense of inclusion in and ownership felt by residents within the social environment, as emphasised by the following extract from session six:

From the field notes:

Rosamund has been asleep during Jessica's piece. Fiona gently wakes her up at the end of Jessica's piece, and there is an intimate moment between them. Rosamund's hand is on top of Fiona's, and as they hold hands, Rosamund strokes Fiona's hand softly.

The following extract from session eight shows a more complex series of interactions, where both musician and resident feel a natural desire to communicate affection for each other, the product of a strong relationship formed over many weeks of interaction:

From the field notes:

When it is Hannah's turn, Anneliese has leaned in close to her. Hannah senses this and reaches out her hand to find Anneliese's. They clasp hands, interweaving and locking their fingers together. Hannah appears to hold on firmly. A few seconds later Hannah pulls her hand back and stretches her fingers wide. Anneliese then locks her fingers around Hannah's. They start to rock their hands in time with the music and this becomes a bigger gesture. Anneliese is still able to play the harp with her right hand, playing arpeggios as this happens, and they do this for some time.

It is important to note that these interactions take place in a larger group environment. The musicians are adept at affirming individuals within the group as well as simultaneously maintaining a sense of group; they achieve this mainly through non-verbal language, for example, roving eye contact whilst playing, or holding eye contact with an individual whilst gesturing outwards towards the group, directing their awareness to others. Matthew details this approach, when reflecting on the choice to change the nature of a musical interaction focused on Sarah into a group piece with shared ownership in session three: *"I wanted to try to pull her awareness out to the rest of the group (...) I realised there was all this attention on her, with Anneliese on one side on the harp and Anne and me being in front of her; she was very cut off actually from the rest of the group, and my back was to the rest of the group as well. So I guess, yeah, it was a really conscious decision to draw that piece out into the rest of the group. So that she could see everybody, and I guess to, for her to have that experience of her piece being taken on by everybody and as a way of, the focus moving away from just her to the focus being a group focus; that she can be held within that group attention. Because she is part of the group, she has our attention, everyone has our attention without it needing to be so narrowly focused in on one person."* In addition, by drawing her focus into that of a group awareness, Matthew is enabling her to see she has the support of others, that she belongs within a community of peers, all of whom can be called on for support: *"I was also very conscious of not wanting this sort of dependency on my attention being the thing, of needing to demonstrate that she can have the support of other people too. Anneliese was there next to her, Anne is there. You know, it doesn't just have to be my attention."*

Here we can see that leadership decisions, such as changing the focus of an activity or interaction, can help to change the dynamics and awareness within a group, as well as enabling group ownership of the experience. This enhancing of individual awareness of others within the group is a crucial element in helping create a new communicative environment, one that breaks through the barriers of isolation and withdrawal; where the full social nature of our beings can be celebrated:

From the field notes:

When Rosamund's name is being sung, Fiona connects with her and they converse lightly, Rosamund speaking in a whisper. Rosamund smiles at Fiona, and chuckles. She also looks at Matthew as he sings to Fiona and appears curious and engaged. She also begins to look around the circle. She and Fiona share another short conversation and she smiles again at Fiona. Afterwards Rosamund's face seems really relaxed, and almost elated particularly around her eyes, which seem to twinkle.

In this instance from session eight, Rosamund becomes illuminated, a member of a group where she can communicate freely and with joy and regard for others. This is the product of eight weeks of concentrated effort by the musicians and staff; enabling Rosamund, through their communication styles to break barriers and celebrate being part of a group.

Modelling

One of the most important tools for developing a shared language and process, and in enabling opportunities to interpret the musical aptitude, preferences and level of engagement of all participants is through modelling. Modelling is an important factor in musical enablement, as it clearly demonstrates expectations of potential ways to communicate musically, with an inherent invitation to copy and extend an existing action or sequence of actions. Modelling also reduces the risk factor of trying something new by providing a clear example. Modelling creates an opportunity for the musician to assess the initial level of interest when initiating a potential activity, in this instance, introducing the function of a conductor's baton to the group in session one, for the first time. The modelling here takes place at a purely non-verbal level:

From the field notes:

Matthew sits down and then conducts Fiona in a very gestural solo, modelling how the baton works. A soft cello melody evolves. Rebecca becomes interested in what Matthew is doing, and he offers the baton to Rebecca non-verbally.

In this instance Matthew has been able to interpret Rebecca's engagement and transform it into an opportunity for a musical interaction initiated by Rebecca. Matthew's modelling, and the involvement of the musicians in creating a musical example, has formed a bridge – from an activity initiated by the musicians into an activity that Rebecca can initiate and sustain.

These examples involve modelling where it leads to an improvisation initiated by a resident, however, modelling can act more subtly within an existing improvisation. This happens often, and is a way of both supporting, developing and extending the musical communication of an individual, and the resultant musical language and form of a piece, as the following extract from session one demonstrates:

From the field notes:

> Esther has started singing; Matthew picks up on this immediately and copies her. A piece starts to develop. During this piece, Matthew plays a wooden agogô and manages to enable Esther to play one too – initially modelling how to play it to her whilst he continues singing (...) The piece is very vibrant. At the end of the piece Esther converses jubilantly, saying, "I didn't know it was going to come out like that."

Here there is a sense of flow to the interaction, Matthew first of all validates Esther's musical communication by joining in – reflecting her contribution. He is able to extend Esther's musical communication and participation through modelling the use of the agogô; here he naturally models how to use the instrument without compromising the growing energy and development of the improvisation.

Sometimes the musicians may model how to use the baton simultaneously with the person, for instance, in session four, when, after a short improvisation with Hannah conducting, Matthew encourages Hannah to direct again, encouraging her to extend her non-verbal gestures when conducting. Matthew holds Hannah's hand with the baton, helping her to literally feel how she can explore making different, bigger gestures, reinforced by verbal suggestions that she can draw shapes and experiment. Anneliese supports this shared kinesthetic exploration musically, using a musical language that corresponds to Hannah's visual gestures as well the underlying energy and pace of these gestures. When Hannah hears the changes in Anneliese's playing she begins to conceptually and practically understand the musical impact her gestures are creating, developing her musical language.

At the basis of modelling is a developing relationship between people, in which an individual is equipping another individual with the tools to express themselves through communication. For the individual copying, to copy someone means that you are listening, that you are endorsing their action, endorsing their communication; it therefore entails respect for the other person's communication. Modelling also enables leadership; not only does it equip someone with an extended language, but also with a process by which they can communicate this language to another. Throughout the project, we start to see participating staff begin to adopt this way of interacting. Matthew reflects upon the growing sense of confidence in musical communication and leadership by participating care staff after session three: *"Staff did some great playing; very natural playing from Anne and Diallo in particular, very natural. And they judged the level of what they were playing very well, very instinctively, and they didn't play too much, they didn't play too loud, but they played so they could be heard (...) I feel really comfortable about asking Anne to work along in a piece with Rebecca and Anneliese, and kind of being able to start her off and then she's able to continue that. With Diallo as well, I was able to ask him to do things. What I would really like now is for there to be more contact with them throughout the session, more eye*

151

contact and more kind of cueing them, or them looking to me for leads, or checking out, 'shall I do this?'"

Here Matthew indicates the key role of non-verbal communication in reinforcing shared leadership within musical communication. A later example of this increasing ownership of the modelling process is the development of interactions directed by Diallo, with support from the musicians, in the seventh session:

> From the field notes:
>
> Fiona suggests that Diallo and Jessica could start a piece together. Diallo taps his drum and says "alright Jessica!" Diallo takes charge confidently, and asks Jessica: "do you want to start?" Matthew says "who else would you like to play Jessica?" and Diallo suggests: "Abigail, do you want to join us?" "Yeah," she responds. "You give me the start then", Diallo says, and soon after she shakes her ghungharus.

Musical frameworks

The musicians use musical frameworks[140] within the sessions in order to invite and inspire communication and awareness of others at a group level, whilst simultaneously aspiring, at an individual level, towards an inclusive environment in which the pace of communication is personalised for each individual. As described in Chapter 2, the frameworks can be loosely pre-developed or completely spontaneous and emergent, and involve a variety of techniques that seek to connect with the communication of participants. Pre-developed musical frameworks function to provide security, particularly during initial stages of the project, when an understanding of 'what participation involves' is being formulated, and they can act as cornerstones for 'celebration' once this understanding becomes stronger. It takes time for repeated frameworks to become a real shared entity; from it to transition from a constructed activity into one owned and embodied by the group, and in which there is a variety of communication and participation. Over time, an increasing multitude of communication styles and participation, and a growing sense of celebration and community begin to emerge through musical frameworks.

Within the framing piece, which opens and concludes each weekly session, a richness and sophistication of musical language is introduced and explored. The musicians fluidly change musical roles, and transition through a variety of musical elements, partially instilling an atmosphere as well as interpreting the response of the group. Below is an excellent example, from session six, where the fluid nature of these interchanges can be deduced:

---

[140] See also Chapter 2.3 on 'Applied musical improvisation'.

From the field notes:

It's a very gentle start with space at the ends of phrases – Fiona initially plays in the low register, with small punctuations by Anneliese, very much centred in G major. Matthew plays sweetly in the upper register, with echoed phrases by Anneliese, and a pizzicato accompaniment by Fiona. Fiona and Anneliese play the theme together in unison with a countermelody answer by Matthew. They move into E minor very briefly and Anneliese softly hums along. Matthew again plays the melody, whilst Fiona plays an undulating cello line. The group sings, responding to Matthew's lead. The texture thins as Hannah joins in singing the theme. The mood and direction of the piece picks up with a driving drone by Fiona, djembe rhythm accompaniment by Matthew and harmonic outlines by Anneliese. It becomes more rhythmic – Fiona also joins in knocking the wood of her cello. It evolves into a vocal-led theme again, led by Matthew, with the accompaniment of the djembe and the harp.

In this framing piece, a real sense of anticipation and excitement is developed, with enough responsiveness to incorporate resident contributions, such as Hannah's vocal contribution.

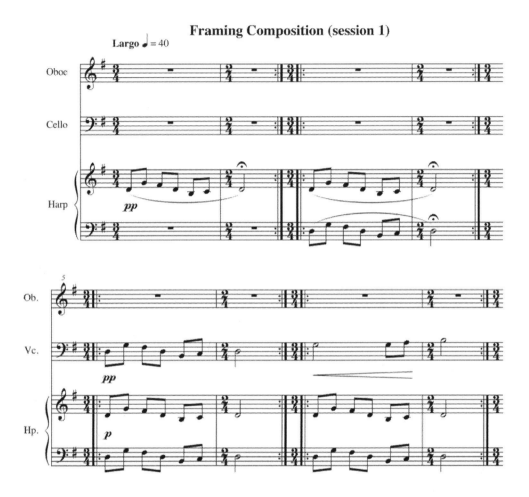

Framing Composition (session 1)

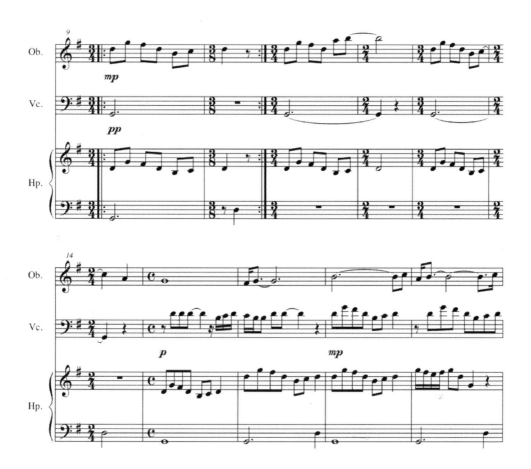

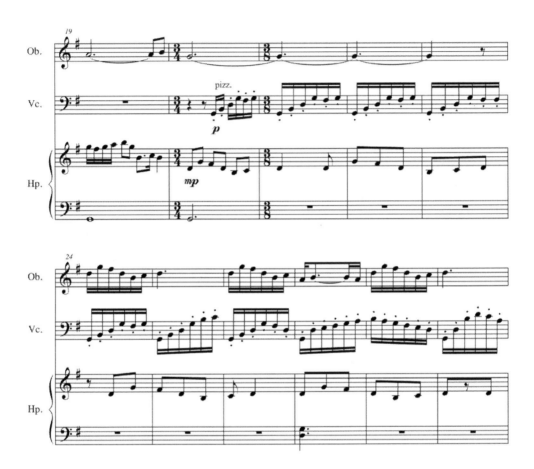

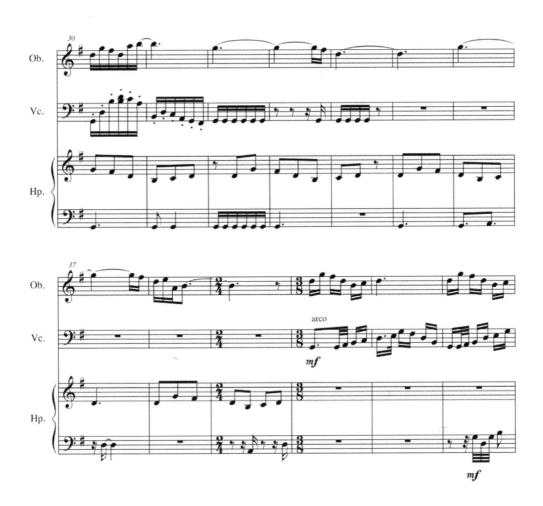

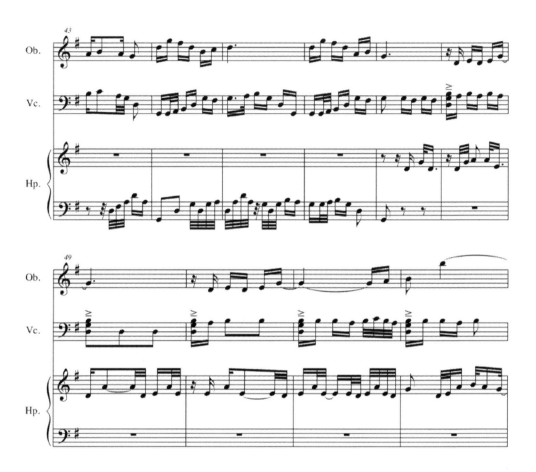

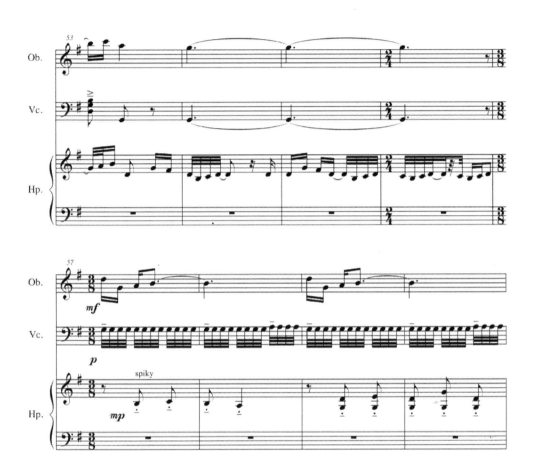

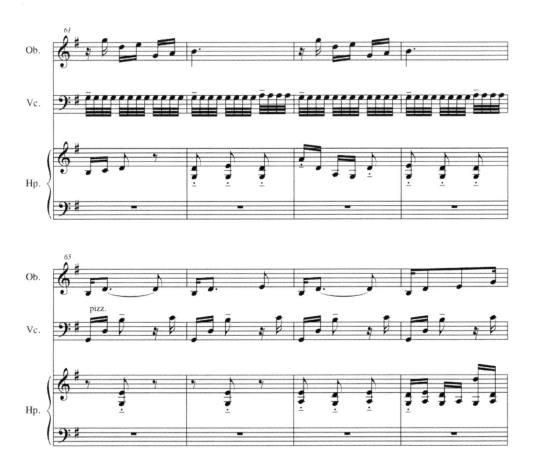

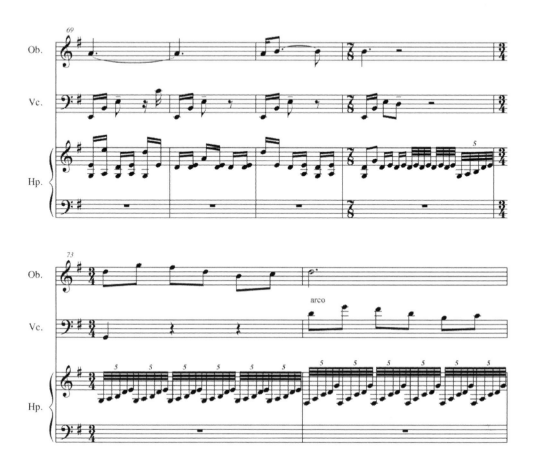

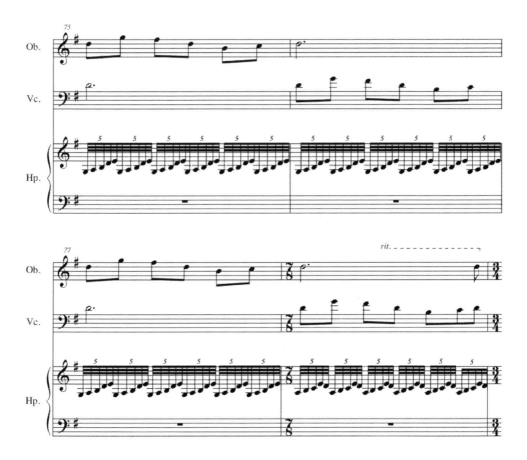

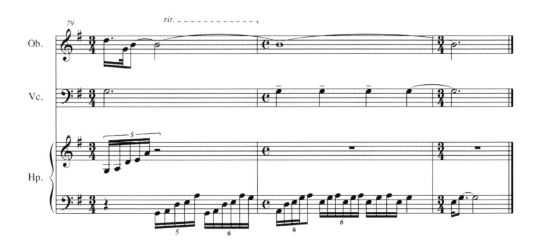

The role of the framing composition is principally to act as a transition from the arrivals and welcoming of residents – principally a social space – into a musical space, where musical and non-verbal communication becomes the norm, and then, at the end of the session, to acknowledge the transition from music-making into everyday routines and traditions of life within the home. The framing piece therefore acts to settle residents, who may feel a variety of emotions during these transitions, and also to create a group experience without any particular participatory demands. The framing piece enables freedom in communication between participants, as emphasized in the following passage from Fiona's reflective journal, detailing the arrival of Esther during session three: *"I sat next to Esther this week. She was brought in just as the framing piece started, which was what we had wanted to try this week. Last week she left before we even began! She seemed to be immersed in the music from the start and at the end of the framing piece there was a lovely moment when we had a moment of real connection. I believe Hannah began singing the musical theme, which sparked a vocal rendition of the theme around the circle. I think I began using a gesture as I sang it to Esther, who often moves her hands in time to the music. Esther is very musical, but can often use very small rhythmic gestures. However at the end of the opening piece we both began to use large sweeping gestures that reflected the motion of the music. This became a real point of connection. I mirrored her hand movements for a good few moments and after a few moments, in the middle of one of our gestures she took my left hand. I just felt it was as if she realised we had been in the music together. She was very affectionate to me from this point on."* Here we can see Fiona first of all modelling an action, and then mirroring Esther's resultant gestures. These gestures have sprung naturally from a shifting relationship of modelling and mirroring into one where a sustained dialogue emerges. Mirroring is a very equalizing, empathic way of 'meeting' someone. It can act to enhance or reinforce a contribution, as well as enabling space for development and dialogue to emerge.

The welcome song follows the framing piece; creating opportunities for moments of individual recognition within a group, as well as encouraging interaction with, and awareness of others. The framework effectively seeks to draw attention to the fact that the music-making takes place in a social group environment, in which each member of the circle plays an important role. The welcome song is characterised by singing; the immediacy and effectiveness of singing is crucial in eliciting responses from individuals within the group, almost as if the voices were calling each person, drawing them out from their dementia, inviting them to communicate and participate. As a sense of group and awareness of others begins to develop, the musicians become more playful with the format of the song – rather than just singing to each individual in turn within the group, very visually around the circle, they begin to pair up individuals adjacent or even opposite each other, through singing and strengthened by accompanying non-verbal language gestures.

The 'passing instruments' activity references the sense of group established in the welcome song through the very visual element of the circle, transforming it into a tactile activity, which calls upon each individual to participate actively in the process. The passing instruments activity enables a sense of security and equality on one level, as it is a repeated activity, in which everyone has a similar sequence of tasks; on another level it allows personalities and individual creativity to be highlighted, as everyone can explore the instruments in their own way. Pacing is very important in the process of passing instruments so that each person has time to understand the sequence of actions, for instance take, explore, pass, and so on. As the tasks begin to be understood, an underlying momentum and consistency of pace begins to develop, and more instruments can be added to sustain and develop the activity, providing a bed of sound for the musicians to improvise over and develop new musical frameworks in response to the communicative environment.

Pre-developed frameworks, whilst useful, also have their pitfalls. Frameworks can serve to invite individuals to participate, but they can also become archaic, antique products that do not necessarily reflect the reality of the communicative situation or process, as Harry suggests, related to the framing piece: *"The framing piece has always been a bone of contention for me. I've always sort of felt that it's a double-edged sword. Sometimes it's a wonderfully settling, calming, unifying thing to have. And people sing it and people go out of the session singing it, and they come into the session singing it. And then there are other times I just think, 'oh we've got to get rid of this horrendous tune, it's just sending everybody to sleep and we just need to shock them out of it.'"*

In addition, it can be risky initiating and delivering a group activity such as the passing instruments activity. For instance, the visual and tactile nature of the activity may inspire and stimulate with individuals to engage within the process, creating a sense of whole group active participation. However, the activity may also act to highlight the presence of dementia, where residents no longer understand the relevance of the object being passed or what is required of them within the process. In addition to this, it can leave a participant in a situation whereby they may feel coerced to participate in a certain way, unable to exercise choice.

Matthew considers, after session two, how this passing instruments activity may not have been a suitable activity for Rosamund at that point in the project: *"She was kind of caught in a pincer movement there, you know what I mean? (...) You either take it when they pass it, or you don't. There was no third option there, which I think is probably a mistake. With some residents it can be the right thing to do, because it gives a sense of clarity about what's happening (...) But for Rosamund that wasn't the case. I think she knew exactly what was being asked of her, but this kind of activity sort of meant accepting she was part of this group and she doesn't accept she's part of the group, I don't think at the moment."* It could be that Matthew is reading into Rosamund's behaviour and ascribing his own meaning to the situation. However, it is important for the musicians to reflect on the nature of frameworks, assessing their effectiveness in creating and stimulating potential opportunities for communication and participation.

Brian also questions the challenges the passing instruments activity may pose to a person experiencing dementia, commenting on Rosamund's engagement within the activity at a later session: *"People did try very hard to engage with Rosamund [during the passing instruments activity] (...) I felt that there was too much focus on Rosamund to achieve something, which was very hard for her to achieve. And I don't think it needs to be about what Rosamund does. It's more about Rosamund being included and being reassured (...) I think there needs to be a level of acceptance of the fact that this person has dementia, which is a complicated condition which involves a number of disabilities (...) Often in these sessions in situations I am also often surprised that the person will actually manage to do more than I would have expected them to do of the physical actual tasks, but my question would be, was it the right thing to do? (...) Because for me there are a number of things going on there: there is understanding what something is, understanding how I use it, understanding language."*

In contrast, Brian reveals a dichotomy regarding the passing instruments activity arguing, after session two, that the activity enables a sense of group to be achieved, and a sense of meaningful activity to take place. These conflicting views are not easily rectified, as the activity can simultaneously have a positive impact on the communicative and participatory environment:

"Today I learnt about the possibilities for creating social interaction between residents. One of the initial exercises in the session involved passing around some instruments from one person to the next. It was very interesting to see how residents managed to do this and to experience a sense of group and togetherness. This made me think about how often residents share the same living space but are not socialising. The importance of finding ways that can create connections was highlighted for me with this simple exercise. I felt that this sense of being together and making connections was well maintained throughout the session."

Similarly, Fiona also highlights the musical consequences; in this case, the passing instruments activity inspired a spontaneous creativity and musical dialogue between participants, as described here: *"Matthew began passing round the instruments and this again was a huge risk with this group. However, the endless repetition really paid off. They really did manage to pass the instruments to each other – it took a little time often but when given that space they achieved this action. We were amazed to see the capabilities of the residents and we had a wonderful moment of a spontaneous piece initiated by three of the residents across the circle, who were each responding to the harp and myself in a call and response like pattern. Suddenly a sense of group had been achieved."*

Additionally, managing transitions within musical frameworks is key. Within this, a clear sense of beginning can be an important tool in bringing closure to interactions and marking a change in focus of an interaction, as Matthew affirms: *"It's important that they know this is their piece, and it's starting now, and then there's a real feeling of it coming to an end. The beginning and endings are important, in order to prevent a continuous sense of suspension, because for them experience needs to be contained (...) They've gone out on a limb, extended themselves to do that, and they made a connection with you, and so if that isn't brought to a proper conclusion they are left exposed and open. It needs to come to an end where they feel that this has been successful, we've made this together, we have the connection."*

Leadership in interpretation

As mentioned previously, the act of interpretation entails risk and requires reflexivity, balanced with an approach informed through reflection. Leadership is about interpreting when there needs to be a change in communication style, or if there are any issues at play within communication. In some cases, it may be difficult to interpret what a person is trying to communicate.

Within the context of the project, Hannah is often an enigma. Her level of dementia, and her ability to hear are often discussed, with great variance in understanding how these factors impact upon her experience of communicating, including her ability to understand others. Anneliese writes after session three: *"Hannah is a bit of a puzzle to me. She seems so coherent and alert. Is there not just a hearing problem? We need to give her more responsibility musically."* Although Hannah often engages readily in musical communication, the musicians feel that they have to find the 'right' way to engage with Hannah, verbally and musically. Matthew often engages in long verbal exchanges with Hannah, trying to find out more about Hannah's history. Hannah appears to cope with verbal exchanges at times, whilst at others she does not understand, although she possesses an awareness of her lack of understanding. This leads to a great deal of experimentation and exploration throughout the project, including giving Hannah the opportunity to play the harp, as Matthew comments: *"We thought we'd had this brainwave of how to connect with Hannah and we had this idea that she would actually play the harp, you know. Playing a real, proper instrument. All instruments are tactile, but a harp particularly is very tactile and that she would be able to feel the vibrations of the sound as well because of the soundboard being so close to you and in such contact. And I think, this is one of these things that we had pictured in a particular way that this was going to be the answer, and Hannah would play the harp amazingly and we would make beautiful music with her."* The musicians endlessly search for different ways of engaging with Hannah at a deeper level, to find the 'right' music for Hannah, music that truly reflects her. In this way they continually reflect on their interpretations of Hannah's communication and participation, in order to develop new interpretations and potential approaches and opportunities for enhancing her communication within the group.

In other cases, interpretation may involve questioning decision-making around the appropriateness of a particular communication style with an individual, for instance, understanding when to employ mirroring as technique. As mirroring involves explicitly and directly copying the verbal, non-verbal, social and musical communication of an individual, it essentially mirrors the emotions driving these actions, enhancing or magnifying the communication of the other person. It therefore entails sensitivity and integrity in approach, in knowing whether it is appropriate or safe to mirror communication, as with this instance between Matthew and Rebecca in session three:

From the field notes:

Matthew has clocked that Rebecca has the baton, and goes and kneels in front of her with his oboe. It isn't clear whether she is smiling or is close to crying. She holds it fairly still, and occasionally shakes the baton vigorously but the musicians don't seem to respond musically in the same way. Matthew decides to go closer to Rebecca's face and sings close to her. He gestures for the baton, which she gives to him, and then he directs Fiona and Anneliese with a very large, fluid arm movement before handing it back to her.

Matthew comments on his own perspectives during this episode, and the rationale behind his approach: *"When she had the baton, she didn't move very much. But what she did, she did this real shaking of the baton, which was like when she grabs your hand and shakes it very hard. It seemed like an expression of her, not frustration, cause I didn't feel she was frustrated at that point. But that was, I mean looking beyond the actual movement that she made, which was this kind of pointing of the baton at somebody and shaking it very fast, was about the kind of recognition or desire to engage or, rather than it being one fast shaky sound, I really don't think that that was what she was wanting. And I think that what she wanted was connection and kind of excitement almost, a desire to connect and it came out as this shaking."*

Here Matthew interprets her non-verbal communication – the shaking of the baton, combined with other aspects of her being – in order to reach a new perspective, one that translates her 'default' shaking from a sign of anxiety and retreat into a call for dialogue. The resultant music is music that does not mirror her movements into music, but instead seeks to translate these movements into a more fluid, connective style of musical communication. Matthew goes on, in the interview, on the nature of mirroring and translation: *"Mirroring is if, well particularly if somebody is doing something that is different. You know, showing a different side of themselves then yes, mirroring is a great thing to do, a great way of reinforcing what they're doing. Translating is when somebody is stuck in a repetitive cycle or it's not useful to further embed them in that repetitive cycle by reinforcing it (...) it's about space, isn't it, I suppose? So if you're mirroring and saying that it's creating space for somebody to be more expressive or to express something new, or whether your mirroring is keeping someone stuck (...) Maybe that's a good way of looking at it, about whether it creates space for people to be more expressive."* Here the approach is dictated by the underlying goal: to enable expressivity in communication. Throughout the project, the musicians and staff continue to reinterpret Rebecca's communication.

Brian reflects on an instance from session five in which Rebecca is invited to conduct, and the possibilities that this presented to the musicians: *"I felt in the debrief there was a nice exploration about whether we should follow her beat and follow her, you know, she gets very intense, that maybe the musical expression of that intensity might happen sometimes; become a loud piece of music, because that's expressed in her intensity, and would that give her a release or not?"* It is perhaps this reading that enables the musicians, particularly Matthew, to feel courageous to explore a different type of dialogue with Rebecca in session six, as detailed earlier in this chapter.[141] In this episode, Rebecca strikes the bass bar, enacting a dialogue in response to Matthew's cantor-like singing; an interaction in which Rebecca's intensity and anger in expression is given a conduit for expression.

In some instances, the musicians may make leadership decisions in which they choose to redefine the communicative situation. According to Fiona, the *"low energy, sadness and pathos you pick up in the circle"* needs *"validating"* as it *"builds trust"* but that sometimes there is a need to *"lift them out of that"*. She speaks in the debrief of their decision in session five to *"really go for it – it's not always easy going against the grain but it has to be at the right time"*. 'Going against the grain' can be challenging to the existing status quo, however this 'right time' was a conscious decision made by the musicians, upon reflection of the previous sessions, and with a feeling that a level of trust had been established in relationships.

In addition, the ability to determine what sort of approach would be appropriate was dictated quite strongly by the nature of the group, according to Fiona: *"We had this phrase about music being this mirror or a hammer: reflecting back what we were feeling and seeing at times, and then at other times trying to cut through and break that. I think we were kind of always somewhere in the middle, steering this very fine tightrope walking, almost, and occasionally dipping one side or the other but you couldn't go too far either way. They weren't able to cope with that, I think, it had to be somewhere in the middle."* Fiona further reflects, writing about the leadership decision to institute a more directed, concentrated energy in session five: *"I think in previous weeks that we have felt so aware of the fragile state of many of the residents and that there was a real need to create music that reflected how the residents themselves were feeling – even to help validate them. I think this has been right and necessary. However the problem in this is that as musicians you can get very trapped in reflecting the atmosphere and creating music that, in a low energy group, has no energy. It is important to, at the right moment, use music that is different and 'breaks the atmosphere', especially when wanting to establish a sense of group. We really tried this in session five and I really felt there was a real breakthrough in the way the group interacted throughout the session. In places I felt that they were carried by our energy and our musical convictions, and that this in many ways created a new sense of life and freedom throughout the group. Also as musicians it is great to have the freedom and confidence at times just to go for it! Often in these sessions one can feel very unsure and as if one is treading on eggshells but to have moments of musical freedom, and clarity as a team really gives you time to regroup and connect."*

[141] See Chapter 4.1 on 'Identity'.

Fiona feels that this communicative approach is releasing for the musicians, reaffirming and reasserting their leadership and artistic creativity. This approach enables the musicians to communicate better together and to re-balance the existing dynamics within relationships, into a context where all participants, including the musicians, really are equal. In this newly emancipated state, the musicians give themselves permission to truly communicate as equals with everyone, embracing their artistic identity and selves, beyond their leadership roles and responsibilities. This changes the communicative environment into one where musicians can be confident to be both responsive and decisive in their leadership, without compromising their own need to communicate within the group.

Occasionally, differences in interpretation can lead to a divergence in practice. This divergence may be based upon different expectations regarding the function and application of music and musical activities, including decision-making around the 'right time' to play in a certain way, use a particular framework, hand out instruments, encourage a focused interaction within the group over an explicit full group interaction, as some examples where divergence may occur. This can result in miscommunication, mostly during the early stages of the project, when the volatility of the 'unknown' combines with an emergent and highly responsive communicative approach where relationships are in a formative stage. Miscommunication can occur between musicians and staff, who are conceptualising what leadership entails within the specific context of the project. For instance, in session three, staff and musicians interpret a situation differently from Matthew, handing out instruments. Matthew describes the consequences of this in interview: *"What I'd intended to happen was for it to continue as just a sung piece, but giving Hannah a role within it. And it was read by the rest of the team, of the care staff, as a signal to hand instruments to everybody. I kind of tried, it had begun to happen before I could do anything about it really, and the one person who was near me who I did ask not to, was Rachel. And it came up in the debrief that she'd felt really dreadful about this. That she'd done the wrong thing and that she didn't understand why she wasn't supposed to give the instruments out, but that Diallo and Anne hadn't been stopped and it was really awkward and difficult."*

Within this episode, Matthew's implicit intentions are unintentionally thwarted, and then his explicit leadership is misinterpreted. However, it leads to a communicative environment in which learning can take place: Rachel raises this issue with Matthew and it enables the group to talk about reflective and reflexive planning, to begin to develop a shared understanding of each other's motivations and vulnerabilities, and in finding ways to ensure clarity of communication in practice.

Additionally, miscommunication can also occur between the musicians, leading to a sense of being at 'cross-purposes' with each other. Matthew explains that this miscommunication was endemic in the first session: "*I felt we were at cross purposes quite a lot and that we confused each other. I don't think we were kind of working against each other in terms of what we were trying to achieve from the session, but just musically we didn't get together as well as we could have done.*" Within the first session, the overall musical communication is described by Matthew as being indecisive, lacking cohesion and 'rambling', as well as lacking clear beginnings and endings and a variety of musical language. As Fiona states: "*The first session of a project is always daunting and full of unknowns and this session was no exception.*" Within this communicative environment, specific instances of miscommunication are apt to occur, such as when Fiona reads a musical cue from Matthew in session one and interprets it as being a cue for the final framing piece, and another instance when Anneliese withdraws musically from a piece, possibly to make 'space', when Matthew interprets the potential for the piece to grow in another way: "*There was a time when a piece we were playing transitioned from being quite a slow, dreamy piece, and then it suddenly it picked up some pace to it, and I said, yes, great, great! So I just got on board there, and I think Anneliese started it by doing something on the harp that had quite a lot of movement to it. And as I started to play, she stopped. And I was like, 'no!' I was about to keep going. So I could ride on top of it and the group would go with it. But she obviously read it as something different. But I was coming in and so she was withdrawing and making space.*"

Over the weeks, as relationships start to develop and grow – musical relationships and social relationships – understanding of interpretations begins to develop into a shared understanding, fostered by group and individual reflection. Although still there are enigmas throughout the project, such as Hannah, and there still may be divergence in the meanings individuals attribute to other's communication, ongoing reflection strengthens the evolving network of relationships that have emerged through mutual engagement in shared experiences. It is through these experiences – reflective and reflexive – that a greater depth of knowledge about each individual's identity, communication and participation styles begins to grow, and a greater convergence of interpretation begins to emerge.

Reinterpretation implies a learning process has taken place, at both an individual and group level. For instance, early in the project, interpretations of Rebecca initially inspired fear and cautiousness in both the musicians and staff; Rebecca is painted as a 'loner', full of 'anger and spite'. However over time, we perceive, through observation and first-hand accounts, a greater sense of connection to Rebecca emerging; reinterpretation of her communication leads to reinterpretation of her participation, and importantly, a greater understanding of, and love for, the woman behind the dementia. The image of Rebecca changes in the minds and hearts of the musicians and staff, and as this image transforms, relationships with her also metamorphose: fear becomes love, caution becomes acceptance, and misunderstanding becomes recognition. As we learn more about others, so too do we learn more about ourselves, about our own fears, misconceptions and our capacity as learners to grow and change.

4.3 Participation

In the analysis on communication, the quality and form of verbal and non-verbal language was explored as a crucial factor in creating an inviting environment for communication. The ability for others to interpret and extract meaning from language was enhanced through the musicians' skillful use of frameworks, space and pacing, and quality of language. Communication was defined as a cycle of dialogue involving interpretation of other's communication, assigning meaning to it and taking a resultant action. This creation of dialogue, in which each person interacts in a group context through a series of communicative actions, can be viewed as participation.

The notion of belonging to a group is the central underlying theme in this subchapter on participation. This sense of belonging can drive the way that we communicate and invariably participate in a social context. To belong, one must feel safe, able to act freely and to explore without judgement, to move beyond risk to an attitude of play. To belong, we must also feel welcomed and respected as a member of the group, with a unique role and a voice; where ownership and leadership is shared. Knowing whether we belong or not to a group is something that we intuitively perceive and feel at an emotive level; we know not only how it feels to belong, but also how important it is to belong for the sake of our own sense of identity and self-worth. In addition, in this analysis on participation, the impact of the social and physical environment upon individual and group participation will be explored.

Participation modes

We are all unique: unique in the way our experiences shape our perceptions of others, our environment and ourselves. Therefore, the mode in which we participate is reflective of our unique and ever-changing selves, the meaning we make from social situations and our sense of what role we might play within these situations. We see a variety of participation modes play out in the researched sessions. Sometimes participants choose to 'actively participate', taking an active and visible role, greatly influencing the resultant actions of people around them. Sometimes they take a more backseat role, actively listening, fully engaged – although it may not be obvious to others around them, to whom they might seem only 'passively aware'. Sometimes participants appear to be completely disengaged, whether this is through a deliberate choice to disengage, placing themselves on the 'periphery', or through disconnection with the present experience, often due to the impact of dementia.

In the analysis on communication, the importance of interpretive skills in understanding a person's communication and participation was raised. These skills involved understanding the different and individual modes of participation that are present during a session, and the fact that staff and musicians can sometimes have divergent views on the significance or depth of resident participation was also explored. Interpreting the significance or participation of a person requires skill, particularly in interpreting the participation of a person with dementia, which may at times seem unclear or fractured. Signs of active participation may be subtle, particularly for residents; these may be attributable to physical health and strength, or reactions to medication residents may be taking.

Matthew reflects on Abigail in session three: *"I can think of Abigail, just with her eyes closed, and just very quietly moving a hand, like this to the beat, which at the time I noticed and I thought, yes! You know, she is not asleep, and she is just connected with what's going on and she is enjoying it."* It is possible to miss noticing the subtlety of Abigail's engagement; she may appear entirely disengaged, or only passively aware. Subtle signs like this could ordinarily be a high level of participation for a person with dementia. Fiona states on the same episode: *"Abigail was asleep for most of the session. There were moments of quiet interaction between Diallo, the staff member, and herself throughout, but actually it felt right to simply let her be. I know some of the staff were worried about her and other quieter residents being excluded but it really felt the right thing."* Here she accepts and values Abigail's level of participation, and also validates the sensitive, subtle, supportive participation of Diallo. Fiona further reflects on how this type of participation seemed meaningful for Abigail: *"At the end of the session [Abigail] simply said: 'I fell asleep...It was the music that did it. It was very soothing. It did me good'."* In enabling residents to 'simply be', music can act as an inclusive platform for drawing out different, valid modes of participation, whether active or passive, peripheral or central.

Curation of space

The motif of 'space' recurs in participation. In the analysis on communication, space was explored conceptually; here it is relevant in a very corporeal sense. The most important aspect in terms of physical space is the creation of a physical environment conducive to enhancing participation; one where safety is paramount. In order to achieve this 'safe space', it requires both an understanding of how a physical environment can influence the social environment, and the development of solutions to mitigate any issues impairing communication and participation. Through consideration of observations, reflections and interview material, we see that the existing physical space can be partially adapted, through enhancing structural aspects of the physical environment, as well as developing altered perspectives on the nature of the environment.

Finding a suitable location for the workshop to take place is a key issue impacting upon the development of a 'safe' participatory environment. Issues may relate to the design, location and sensual aspects of the space; a host of variables all interact together to create a physical environment that may need to be adapted or curated, if it is to achieve its potential as an inviting space for communication and participation. This creates an opportunity for learning and creativity, through assessing and experimenting with variables, as described by Fiona after session two: *"The practical set up of a session is a really important part of this work and this session really helped me to see the difference it can make. It is so important to find as many ways as possible to create this safe space and to find creative ways of achieving that, even when it seems impossible to change the layout of a room/area that you are working in."* Fiona additionally writes about how resolving an issue with extraneous noise, caused by an air conditioning unit, helped to create an environment conducive for communication and participation: *"We experimented with trying to turn the air conditioning off so that the space was quieter. When this worked it made a real difference. The music was the only sound and this really helped to 'draw in' the residents and helped us as a musical team as it was just so much easier to hear across the circle!"* Here, the importance of working from an atmosphere of quiet – which also infers stillness, lack of ancillary vibrations – is highlighted as enhancing communication and opportunities for participation.

Matthew describes how the location of the workshop space, and its traditional use as a thoroughfare, impacted on the coherence of communication between musicians during preparation, thinking of his experience during the preparation hour before session three: *"The room has this office which is sort of part of the room which people keep still coming in and out of and fetching things and coming and going, and I do find that distracting (...) That kind of space doesn't feel secure and safe for us in that first hour, really, and I think that affects the playing. If you're distracted (...) I was trying to listen to what Fiona was playing so I could respond to it. And I could see, where I was sitting there's a mirror which reflects the office behind me, so I can see this sort of to-ing and fro-ing going on in the corner of my eye behind me and people getting files out and stuff. And maybe I just need to sit somewhere different so I can't see that or do something about it, so as not to be wound up by it. But the tiniest things will distract, I think."* These remarks also show that for the musicians it is deeply important to feel focused during the preparation hour, and within this, silence, stillness and safety are important factors.

For Matthew, it seems impossible to communicate on a musical and social level when distracted, although he does refer to it also being a state of mind that can be transcended through altering his own perspective of his experience, continuing on in the same reflection to say: "*It's almost as though those things are a kind of excuse not to engage with the musicians. Maybe we've got too fixated on it, that the room has to be clear and dadada, and people mustn't come in and. So when that does happen we think we can't rehearse properly, while actually we could. But your own frustration kind of gets in the way of being able to connect and to really play.*"

However, in reality, this sense of distractedness can translate into the communication and participation of musicians within the music session. The musicians need to be able to cope with this, moving past frustrations and placing faith in each other's abilities to communicate, as Anneliese writes after session three: "*I did not feel very inspired and free to play before the session. Was I tired? The space (...) does not feel very private. There is no door to close and we never feel on our own. Having said that, I trusted that we would come up with some good ideas in the session. This is a sign of our mutual understanding and knowing that we could play well together.*" Interpreting these various statements, it also seems crucial for the musicians to feel a sense of security themselves, in order to communicate and participate effectively within the session. If they feel uneasy about the physical environment, this will transmit into their own experience of the session, potentially impacting upon their communicative abilities. However, by developing an attitude of trust and letting go of anxieties and frustration they can transcend this.

Beyond the variables inherent in the location and the overall design of a space, the physical layout within a space can create a strong message of invitation. The seating is set-up in a circle, creating an explicit reference to the mandala, a symbol of equality and unity. The musicians emphasise this physicality of the circle through activities within the session, such as the welcome song and passing instruments activity. This circle is set up by the musicians to look and feel inviting; for instance, the use of soft, lounge room chairs with cushions, spaced to be intimate but not crowded, provides a degree of comfort and possibility for physical interaction for residents and staff during the session. The central point of the circle, consists of small, low tables attractively covered in instruments, providing an area of focus, 'drawing' participants into the action. In observations during the preparation hour, it is possible to perceive the great care with which the musicians approach the curation of practical and sensory elements.

From the field notes:

Attention is turned again to the physical set-up. Fiona says: "we need some sort of centre-piece" for the instrument tables. Anneliese moves the instrument tables, so they are more central in the circle, and Matthew checks whether access is possible around the tables to parts of the circle for wheelchairs.

Assessing the sensual aspects of a space can often be key indicators in understanding potential barriers to participation; often this assessment occurs at an intuitive level. The workshop area in the Emanuel Zeffert House was a multi-purpose lounge-kitchen area, which, although very warm and inviting in terms of furnishings, colour, lighting and other elements, was less effective for a context of group music making, as Fiona writes after the first session: *"It felt difficult to know how to use the space. It was a vast, open planned room, which initially looked an amazing space to use, but actually in the midst of the session I was struggling. It was very hard to create 'community' and a sense of group intimacy, and it was also really hard to hear across the circle."* After session two, on the change created through adapting this space, through the use of a folding screen, she states: *"Last week the large open plan space made it very difficult to establish a sense of group and community. It also didn't feel very private and when doing this work we find it is always necessary to create a sense of safety, a calm space in the home for people to come into. The music of course can create this space, but a literal space that leans itself to this is always really helpful. Brian had set up some screens that divided the large space, almost sectioning off a room and this really helped to create a private space. It felt more intimate and was a space into which the residents could literally 'come in to'."* Fiona affirms a holistic view of space; through addressing both physical and sensual aspects, a sense of safety, intimacy and focus was attained.

Seating arrangements

The spatial layout of seating can influence participation, so therefore it stands to reason that the 'social' layout of seating would have an even greater impact upon participation. The musicians craft a seating scenario to stimulate communication, enhancing emerging relationships and helping to develop a sense of belonging within the group. In conversation, Anneliese and Fiona discuss the anchoring quality of seating, where an environment conducive to communication and participation needs to be constructed both literally and metaphorically:

Anneliese: *"There are always new challenges with the seating and trying to get it so that it gels more easily."*

Fiona: *"I just wonder if, this is me wondering out loud, external processing, when of course the home has not been settled in any way, I think that's had a huge impact on the feel and the need to anchor people (...) We're not coming into something that's already established, we had to come in and be that anchorage in every way, in a more present way than maybe we always have to."*

Knowing you have a place in a group can help develop a sense of confidence in your status in a group. Fiona feels that this is important for all participants, including staff, writing after session two: *"I was aware of how important it is for the staff to feel sure. One member wanted to know where to sit and was a little unsure of where to put herself. Normally we label the residents' chairs but not the staff places, just for flexibility. But on this occasion I really felt it would be good to help the staff feel secure and know where they are sitting. This member of staff had never been in the circle before and I sensed real anxiety at this point. It really helps for people to know that there is a place especially for them (and helps us as a musical team to create the best possible circle, regarding the residents behaviour and needs)."* Here, Fiona identifies that a sense of place can help create a sense of safety and belonging for staff, as well as enabling opportunities for staff to support residents in their participation, forming relationships in the process.

Careful observation of the group can lead to discussions on future plans for seating. This discussion between the musicians in the preparation hour in week three of the project highlights some of the rationale underpinning choices behind seating arrangements, guided by their emerging perspectives:

> From the field notes:
>
> At 10.15 am the musicians discuss the residents and where they should be sat in order to maximise their potential and according to preferences. For instance, Sarah should be sat next to a musician, Esther should be sat somewhere where she can get out easily if she wants to leave and flanked on either side by a musician and a staff member, an "optimum chance for her to stay". Gabriella is identified by Fiona as having been "great next to [Matthew]" though he appears slightly reluctant to sit next to her as she "needed a lot of support – it was constant". Rachel is identified as potentially a good source of support for Rebecca and the musicians plan to seat them next to each other. Deborah arrives and the musicians consult with her about some of their thoughts on seating.

This example indicates that individuals who may need a higher degree of communicative support could possibly be sat between both a staff member and a musician, although this needs to be thought through carefully in terms of what impact it may have on the musicians being able to enact their roles within the session. It also acknowledges the impact of musical communication, and proximity to the primary sources of its production – the musicians – as a potential 'holding' strategy. Further, seating arrangements also enable agency: access to the circle for those who may wish to participate on the periphery, in a literal and metaphorical sense, as well as lessening the impact of potential disruptions to those in the core of the action.

Great care is taken to create personalised seating, set up in such a way as to be inviting. However, we see in the project that when the optimal use of physical space is impaired, sometimes through accidental means, it can impact on the continuity of activities. For instance, a vacated seat in the circle can fragment the flow of activities and lead to a sense of incompleteness within the circle. One way in which this manifests is the absence of Esther from the group; Esther usually joins the group for only the very first part of a session, if at all, leaving a tangible sign of her absence, an empty chair. In the following example from session two, Matthew highlights the impact the absence of Esther causes on an already complicated situation: *"There was a mix-up about chairs and the chairs that were intended for the observer got pulled into the circle, so then we had an extra chair and that meant that people weren't balanced around the circle as we planned for them to be; and with Esther leaving there were two seats with a big gap in between Rosamund and Anneliese."* In later weeks, the solution discovered by the musicians was to draw a chair into the circle for Esther when she decided to join the circle, and to remove it when she left. However, in this session, this mix up with the seating leads to a situation where there is a 'breakdown' of participation, as described in the field notes:

> From the field notes:
>
> When the instrument gets to Anneliese, she has to get up to move over to Rosamund. Rosamund has closed her eyes but doesn't appear to be sleeping. Anneliese tries for a while to get Rosamund's attention, by shaking the instrument softly on her lap and saying "I've got a little shaker here", but Rosamund doesn't open her eyes. Anneliese says "would you just mind passing it on for me?" and Matthew echoes her – "would you just mind passing it on to me?"... "Can you take it Rosamund? Can you take it from Anneliese?" and again, more softly, "Can you take it from Anneliese?" In the end, Matthew asks "Can I take it [from Anneliese]?"

Anneliese passes on the shaker to Matthew so the activity can continue. The musicians persist with the activity, as it evolves into a more formalised structure and song. A subtle but very important change in Rosamund's communication and participation begins to emerge, enabled through persistence and gentle persuasion in the communication of Anneliese:

> From the field notes:
>
> Anneliese and Matthew still seem to be finding it difficult to engage Rosamund actively – she still spends most of the time with her eyes closed, though Anneliese repeatedly and sensitively tries to draw her attention out very gently over the long duration of the activity by playing near her, touching her gently and prompting her verbally. Later in the piece, Rosamund stirs and opens her eyes, looking at Matthew for an extended period as he drums. When Anneliese comes and joins Rosamund again, Rosamund looks at Anneliese, though she still chooses not to take an instrument.

Here, we can see that, although Rosamund still chooses not to actively participate in the same way or pace as others might, she does seem to begin to engage in the process. Anneliese writes of the challenge to activity continuity that this physical barrier created, and that proximity, perseverance and repetition in contact was key in influencing Rosamund's participation: *"This was a huge challenge, given the fact there were two empty chairs to bridge (one extra chair ended up in the circle by mistake) and some unwillingness to participate... we persevered and I felt the exercise paid off."*

Instruments

In addition to curating an inclusive environment through attention to the impact of physical space, it is important to consider the resources available in a session. It is also important to consider access to musical instruments that enable opportunities for meaningful musical participation and highlight the abilities of participants. The musicians are regularly involved in wide-ranging discussions, both in debrief and planning, on the suitability of instruments in enabling musical participation. The discussions often assess the physical techniques involved in playing the instrument, as observed during preparation:

> From the field notes:
>
> Deborah and Anneliese try out the hand percussion instruments, meticulously, discussing: what kind of sticks sound best on the gato drum?[142] Does it still work when a resident is seated in a comfortable chair?

Here, we also see that the aural qualities and musical potential inherent in the instruments are fundamental to the musicians; the instruments must sound beautiful and be audible. This type of discussion is echoed and extended in the debrief from session five, with a more specific assessment on the actual reality of playing the instruments for a resident, Jessica:

> From the field notes:
>
> It is agreed between the musicians that the gato drum beaters need to be harder – they were too soft and didn't project the sound, particularly when residents like Jessica tend to hold beaters like a pen, and beaters need gravity to work. It is also agreed that instruments with beaters are not right for Jessica, and that other types of instruments could be explored.

In this example, the musicians are exploring what type of instrument will really give Jessica an audible 'voice', and what she can comfortably play; making shared decisions on what future opportunities could be developed with instruments. In addition, we also see learning about residents' instrument preferences occurring throughout the project; this learning is developed through observation and assessment. Great care is taken to find the 'right' instruments for residents during the session, chosen by and, through consultation, with residents rather than for residents. There is also recognition when an instrument appears to be a strong conduit for expression. In the following musical interaction, Anneliese appears to be searching for the best instrument for Hannah through consultation, modelling and observation:

---

[142] A type of hollow slit drum, crafted from wood into a rectangular shape. Varying widths and lengths of the multiple slits or 'tongues' on the top of the drum produce different pitches when struck by a mallet, wooden beater or heavy rubber beater, with the body of the drum acting as a resonating chamber. See also Appendix V, 'List of musical instruments'.

From the field notes:

> Anneliese explains the egg shaker to Hannah. Later, when Hannah has the African ankle rattle,[143] she shakes it strongly in front of her. Hannah taps her knee whilst Matthew drums. Soon after when everyone has an instrument; Anneliese plays a tambourine[144] gently on Hannah's lap. Hannah tries the tambourine but Anneliese recognises that it looks uncomfortable, commenting to Hannah that it looks quite heavy, and would she like another instrument and replacing it with a caxixi, consulting with Hannah as she does this. Hannah plays along with the pulse. As the piece becomes a bit more free and textural, Hannah shakes strongly in various points where there are spaces for musical interjections, and Anneliese interacts musically with her. Hannah seems to be listening intently. She also responds to Rebecca's drumming on the djembe by echoing it musically with the caxixi.

Sometimes instruments may not be suitable for all participants, for instance the hand chime, which, in order to make a sound, requires a flick of the wrist, which in turn activates an attached beater, striking the chime bar. It can be a strikingly visual and aurally profound instrument when used well, however it can present problems for some residents, according to Brian: *"It's a wrists-thing (...) I think that's quite hard for people to use."* Aside from the very physical barrier to participation it may cause, he also considers the sequence of processes involved in playing the instrument, processes that a person with dementia may find hard to enact: *"The hand chime. I always have a problem with that and I always feel the residents have a problem with that (...) I think it takes quite a bit of learning how to do that, I think you have to know what it's about."* Here, he also acknowledges the cognitive abilities necessary for playing the instrument. He continues, *"I mean there's this thing with dementia, some people can't know what something is. They recognise it but they don't know how to use it (...) and that's because lots of people develop problems in the parietal lobe, which is about knowing how to use something. And I often see that played out."* Through sharing and developing this knowledge of key cognitive issues faced by a person with dementia, Brian demonstrates once more his crucial role in influencing learning and practice around creating participatory opportunities.

Transitions: opening situation

For musicians, the first transition they experience is from that of normal life into a work context, where they must let go of their individual desires and frustrations, and begin to work as a team, personally and professionally. As explored earlier, the physical environment can have an impact on the musician's ability to connect and communicate during the preparation hour,

---

[143] An African instrument, traditionally worn on the ankles, consisting of a band strung with small seedpod shells. Shaking the instrument produces a raspy, rattle sound. See also Appendix V, 'List of musical instruments'.

[144] A ring in which small, thin 'cymbals' are attached to, akin to the frame drum, with or without a skin head. When shaken or struck, the cymbals strike each other to produce a high, rattling sound. Tambourines can often come in an oval or half moon shape, and the ring is commonly made of a light wood or plastic. See also Appendix V, 'List of musical instruments'.

making it a fundamental task to establish strong communication during this transition, beyond any obstacles that may arise:

Anneliese: *"Also when we meet up in the hour before, that's also a chance to connect in that way where we don't have an agenda. Because I feel it's quite a different way of playing, I don't know if you feel it differently."*

Matthew: *"Yeah, it's really different."*

Anneliese: *"But for me it's quite different, and for me it's really important to have that time and sometimes it gets cut short because there are problems and they're not coming in. Somebody's ill, so much time is taken up and you haven't made that connection and that can be quite tricky when you're going straight in because, we also commented on that the last time we met, making that connection is quite crucial, you can be out of practice doing it, you know? If you're doing it all the time it's easier."*

Finding this level of communication where they feel connected and convergent requires a special mindset, with a depth and intensity of connection that can bring a sense of confidence and freedom in communication and participation. In the previous instances, outlined earlier in this analysis, feeling tired and distracted can become obstacles in creating this connection. Through creating this connection, the musicians are able to ground themselves as musicians and bridge the transition into the session, as Matthew reflects after session two: *"We had a good time together as a team, from ten to eleven, it felt really good. We played the theme together quite a lot, and really grounded it, and bedded it in so that we all felt really comfortable with it, which we hadn't done last week, and it think that helped us to feel more grounded and more connected."* In many ways, this musical preparation is like a dress rehearsal for the music workshop session; in the early part of the project, the musicians tend to develop strong musical frameworks, where 'play rules', processes and language are discussed and explored for later application. Later, as the project develops, this exploration turns into a freer musical communication, often echoing a parallel development in session, where a freer sense of overall communication and participation begins to emerge.

In terms of understanding the types of transitions residents may experience prior to a session, it is important to once again reflect upon the nature of dementia, as it shapes the communication and participation of everyone within the community. As explored in the analysis on communication, interpretation for a person living with dementia can become increasingly difficult, often leading to a sense of confusion and anxiety when the meaning of the intended 'message' is no longer received clearly. Sustaining communication with a person with dementia can also become difficult, as they slip in and out of awareness. Transitions are an ordinary part of everyday life, however, for a person living with dementia. In trying to make sense of the environment around them, change, especially abrupt change, can impact directly on their sense of well-being and communication. The reasons for changes around them may not be so apparent and may cause distress, confusion and frustration, all of which can lead to a 'breakdown' of participation, where a previously felt 'connection' may seem lost, fragmented, irretrievable. Brian highlights how the transition from daily routine of breakfast into the session impacts directly on Gabriella's sense of well-being: *"Gabriella is one of those residents who is new to that unit and then she has a disruption. She doesn't have her breakfast immediately as she would do in her own lounge. She's accompanied to another lounge and she has breakfast in that setting. And then she comes back [to her unit for the session]. So I could see that when I met her first, she was quite pleased and happy and in a good space (...) When I went back [to accompany her to the session], just before Music for Life began, it felt like quite an intrusion again into her space, and she found it difficult to be asked to come out of there again, and to come over to the other lounge. And actually being the person who was accompanying her in her wheelchair, I got a sense of how frightening the space can be, being wheeled though these doors and corridors and not really having any control over where you're going, and that's the experience she came with to the group. And obviously I did my best to communicate and reassure Gabriella, but I could tell there were several points along the way where potentially she found it quite difficult, because of the doors, because of other people coming towards us and then the busy environment when we got into the room."*

The arrival of residents is a precarious time, in which confusion and anxiety can reign, as alluded to in the previous example of Brian wheeling Gabriella down the corridor. This is one account, of one person's potential experience, into a space where eight residents and five staff will be arriving. There is potential for a great diversity of experiences and needs of people entering the workshop space, all of which can play out in a number of ways, as Brian suggests: *"Maybe one resident wants to go someplace else and is looking for her daughter, another resident is looking for her mother, another resident needs the toilet just before the project is starting, another staff member gets called away to assist somebody who isn't in the group and can't wait. It's challenging, it's very challenging."* These challenges all add up to create a unique context for participation before the session, which somehow needs to be engaged with in order to bring everyone into an environment conducive for communication and participation. Care staff and musicians need to be able to support residents through these transition issues in a sensitive way; a way that can turn a frightening, almost nightmarish passage, into a peaceful, positive journey. The following observation, from directly before session four, gives a strong flavour of how various residents cope with the transition into the session, and how the musicians and staff interact with them to reduce the impact of this transition, and bridge the transition into the music session:

From the field notes:

Sarah is heard in the corridor and is calling out "mummy", when she is wheeled in, she again shouts "mummy", her hands shaking. Gabriella says, "I feel sick" and begins to count repeatedly. Matthew goes to Sarah once she has transferred from her wheelchair, and spends some time chatting with her, touching the harp as he soothes her. Anneliese sits silently with Jessica, stroking her wrist gently until Hannah arrives. Whilst Hannah is being transferred into a chair, Anneliese returns to her chair and plays her harp softly. She also plays to Sarah who is holding her head in her hands. Sarah is clearly distressed, repeatedly calling "mummy". Deborah and Matthew comment that the colour of Gabriella' blouse is lovely – she responds with a warm open smile and appears pleased. As the other residents and staff are still arriving, Esther says to Harry that she wants to leave. He explains that "we'd love you to stay and listen...we've got a few jobs for you to do" and she takes interest, "Ah, what is it?" She sits again, interested, and appears to immediately settle back into her seat. Harry explains to Esther that she can leave "in about an hour" and engages her in looking at his flute. Esther makes many excuses to Harry on why she has to leave, which he counteracts – cousins visiting, seeing her mum, "to help mum." She asks Harry if he will come with her, but Harry answers that he'll stay here a bit, and asks her why she wouldn't also stay a bit as there are so many jobs to be done. "Well, I gotta go... I gotta help..." Matthew sees this and immediately brings over a set of soprano chime bars for her, and Anneliese begins to play the opening tune which comes out of her gentle playing that has been underpinning the last arrivals.

Here we see that the arrivals of residents is paced to enable gentle interaction with musicians and staff, with ample time for residents to be transferred from wheelchair to armchair as well as comforted; a welcoming period in which participants can adjust to the new social context. The musicians and staff also take time to frame the upcoming experience for residents, announcing that there will be music, referring attention to the instruments and the musicians, and through initiating gentle, soothing musical fragments in the background. Brian acknowledges the efforts of the musicians, reflecting: *"I felt at the start today, when residents began to come in that as always a lot of effort, a lot of thoughtful preparation had been put in place before residents came. I hadn't been listening to the musicians' preparation but it was clear to me that they knew amongst themselves how they wanted to greet people and they had some kind of plan in place for themselves. They were working in a flexible way with that to try and help each person feel secure and welcomed."* Here he recognizes that reflection enabled the musicians to create a flexible, personalized plan for inclusion, in order to help enhance overall participation.

The quality of communication, underpinned by genuine warmth, praise and validation, helps to ease the transition for residents and create a social environment in which the residents belong. In order to achieve this, it is vital that an atmosphere of quiet calm, and attention to the pace of arrivals is achieved. Brian reflects, after session two, that it is not so easy to cultivate this atmosphere, in reality: *"I think it has to do with the feeling of the atmosphere in the group... it all felt so hectic at the beginning (...). So I think we can do our best to manage it but I think it's actually quite hard. In an ideal situation it would be lovely if people could come into a quiet and relaxed atmosphere where music was playing and they could just gently sit down. I think in reality it's not easy to establish that."* Fiona is also able to perceive the difficulty of achieving this, particularly in the context of the new home: *"The arrival time at this home is very chaotic as the residents are coming from different floors and parts of the home. The home has also changed its whole schedule to accommodate the project and this has real repercussions on the staff and residents."* She goes on to reflect: *"Sarah was very distressed in this session. Last week she had been fine throughout, but she had arrived early and had more one to one attention before the session began. We wondered if we tried to do this again if it would help her to feel more secure. However, the logistics of the home may well make these ideas impossible to achieve. The staff are already under huge amounts of pressure."* Here Fiona identifies that a great sense of chaos and unsettledness during the transition into the session has been a fundamental issue impacting upon Sarah's participation within the session, offering a theoretical insight into how this could be approached differently in future practice.

Throughout the project, particularly in the early stages, discussion around the order of arrivals prior to the session, which usually takes place within a window of ten minutes, becomes a recurring element between musicians and staff. Some approaches are identified, such as creating opportunity for those with tendency to walk to come in to an established group where the atmosphere is relatively settled, for individuals such as Rebecca and Esther. Coming in earlier is better for others at an individual and group level, for instance, for those who may need a long period of comforting, such as Sarah, or for those who seem to project a positive social influence, such as Hannah. Over time, a growing sense of efficiency and calmness in arrivals seems to take place, and a corresponding sense of relaxedness and joy begins to emerge during this transitional phase. On a physical level, musicians and staff work collaboratively during this time, taking great care to ensure residents are comfortable. Often this takes on a practical dimension, motivated by a desire to enhance that person's inclusion and engagement in the group, and occurs alongside a variety of sensitive communication. For instance, upon Rosamund's arrival and transfer in session seven, Fiona and Diallo work together in session seven to ensure Rosamund's physical comfort:

From the field notes:

Fiona sits with Rosamund and holds her hand. Diallo arrives and helps Rosamund to be transferred from her wheelchair into her chair. Fiona asks for a pillow for Rosamund to help her be comfortable, which he brings. Rosamund settles in, and closes her eyes, and looks peaceful.

At a musical level, the role of the framing piece acts as a transition from a social space to a musical space, acting to change an environment of unsettledness to calmness, as Fiona reflects: *"In this work I have often found that the time and atmosphere of the arrivals can really dictate the way the session goes, or at least contributes to the general feel of the session. If it is chaotic and rushed or difficult (which it often is!) it really means that as musicians we have to work to create that sense of stillness in the opening piece. We had talked about this before and had aimed for our opening piece to be very grounded – a steady pulse with lots of repetition and broad statements of the theme, which did actually help to settle the atmosphere and residents after a slightly chaotic beginning."*

Breakdown of participation

Sometimes a 'breakdown' in communication and participation can occur, where a sense of 'flow' in the session is disrupted; participation becomes fragmented and communication between participants becomes unclear and difficult. Breakdowns in communication and participation can emanate from a number of situations and factors. The following examples detail a breakdown in communication and participation between the musicians during musical interactions. The impact is two-fold; the musicians become divergent in their leadership and actions, and there is a sense that neither resident's contributions are at the centre of the interaction:

> From the field notes:

> Whilst Gabriella's 'calm and gentle' piece is being played, Gabriella has passed the baton on to Rachel who has then passed the baton on to Rebecca. Rebecca smiles and points it towards Fiona, who responds to her intense waving of the stick. She also points it towards Anneliese who also responds, however Matthew hasn't picked up that Rebecca has the baton as he is very gently singing to Gabriella at this point. There is a tension with two clear activities going on at once. The musicians appear to choose to continue directly with Gabriella' piece, but Rebecca appears to be confused by this interaction. At times she appears frustrated and angry in her facial expressions.

In this instance, the passing of the baton to Rebecca – the conductor's baton, a directive instrument with authoritative status – has created a situation where the piece potentially has two directors, and two directions. Anneliese and Fiona at this point are torn, unable to honour the authority of Rebecca's direction in this instance. Upon reflection, Anneliese reveals she could have sung to Matthew to direct his attention to Rebecca, thus finding a way to integrate the two directions into one. Another incident occurs where Fiona misreads the musical signals of Matthew, leading to a breakdown of communication, as briefly detailed in the analysis on identity. For Fiona, the 'struggle' of reading the group's communication and participation had resulted in fatigue for her; and her skills at reading the musical and non-verbal communication of Matthew momentarily lapsed: *"I found the session so uncomfortable that at one point I prematurely introduced the closing piece as it felt time to end! In fact we had another twenty minutes to go, but somehow to me it had felt like it had been such a struggle and had gone on for so long that it felt time to end – I was convinced that it was 12:00 pm already and that Matthew was signaling the end with his G major improvisation!! I've never mis-read that before!"*

In the analysis on communication, the notion that the communication and participation of a resident in distress can disturb the participation of others was explored, with Brian reflecting on the potential impact of Sarah's distress and calling out on others, as well as the example of Rebecca's susceptibility towards changes in the environment, mostly in response to physical cues. Earlier within this analysis the example of a breakdown in the participation of Rosamund was visited, which was augmented by a physical factor – in this case, the seating arrangement. However, another instance in a later session highlights that this may not be the only factor leading towards a breakdown in participation for Rosamund during the passing instruments activity:

> From the field notes:
>
> Matthew tells the group it's time to pass instruments around the circle (...) Anneliese shakes the egg shaker briefly before passing it to Sarah, who in turn passes it freely to Samantha. "Samantha's got something she'd like to give to you". When Samantha shows Rosamund the egg shaker, Rosamund says: "Yes, I think that's pretty." Harry confirms: "beautiful." The process of passing the shaker appears difficult for Rosamund; there is a long exchange as Rosamund tries to pass the egg shaker to Harry. She drops her tissue in the meantime and Harry and Samantha are careful to give her tissue back. When the focus has been on Rosamund for some time – about twenty seconds – and she still hasn't passed the egg shaker, Matthew introduces another instrument, the hand chime, into the circle, which seems to change the overall dynamics of the activity, detracting focus from Rosamund. Rosamund eventually passes on the shaker to Harry.

This focus on Rosamund leads to a tricky moment for everyone involved; the activity seems to be exposing Rosamund's understanding of the task involved. The passing instruments activity can create an awareness of being within a group, and promote positive interactions between group members; however, in this instance it seems to be highlighting Rosamund's difficulty in understanding the processes involved in the task. Brian reflects on the potential impact of dementia on Rosamund's cognition: *"I think there needs to be a level of acceptance of the fact that this person has dementia, which is a complicated condition which involves a number of disabilities. And I think we need to explore a little bit more about what that really means for Rosamund (...) For me there are a number of things going on there: there is understanding what something is, understanding how I use it, understanding language, and disinhibition as well."*

For the musicians, Hannah seems to be an enigma at times. She readily participates in the music making, however, the musicians aspire for a deeper level of participation, a deeper level of musical and social connection beyond the relationships they have built with her. As revealed in the analysis on identity, questions over the nature – and even presence – of Hannah's dementia are raised by musicians and staff during the project; such is the complex and inconsistent way in which it presents to others. Sometimes Hannah even comments on her ability not to understand specific questions directed to her, an awareness that may not always be so acute for someone lost in their dementia. In addition, Hannah is visually impaired; she seems to have problems with some aspects of her hearing, aspects that present in an inconsistent way. Sometimes she can hear and respond to the subtlest details of music, at other times she can't seem to hear speech directed to her in close proximity.

One poignant example of a breakdown of participation happens when Matthew attempts to engage Hannah in directing the creation of a musical piece. Here, the breakdown of participation arises from extensive verbal communication. During the interaction, Hannah seems confused at times, asking him to repeat his requests, stating "you're too far away, I can't hear you" and "I don't understand you". Matthew tries to find out what kind of music she likes, searching for a way to create music that will reach her and resonate with her identity, however, the way he asks her questions seems to be too difficult for her at times:

From the field notes:

Matthew: "Hannah?"
Hannah: "Yes."
Matthew: "I wondered if we could make a piece for you?"
Hannah: "Pardon?" Hannah's hearing appears to be not so good.
Matthew: "I wondered if we could make a piece of music for you?"
Hannah: "Yes."
Matthew: "I wondered whether you had a favourite composer... or a kind of music that you enjoy listening to? Do you have a composer that you like... of classical music... or jazz... or a favourite kind?"
Hannah: "I don't understand you."
Matthew: "...That's fine... I wondered if you enjoy listening to music?"
Hannah: "I enjoy all music."
Matthew: "Have you been to concerts?"
Hannah: "Yes."
Matthew: "What kind of concerts?"
Hannah: "Classical concerts."
Matthew: "...and did you have a favourite... favourite kind of classical music?"
Hannah: "A favourite? Yes, I had, but it's a form that I can't remember."
Matthew: "Could we play a piece for you?"
Hannah: "hmmm?"
Matthew: "Can we play a piece for you?"
Hannah: "Yes."

Matthew then asks her if she would be willing to conduct the musicians, to which Hannah agrees. Matthew verbally points out the musicians to her – telling her where they are sitting, what they play, and then asking them to play for her;
Matthew: "Could I, can I if give you a baton, a conductors baton, and I wondered if you would conduct us?"
Hannah: "Yes." Hannah takes the baton.
Matthew: "So we have... Harry is over across the other side of the circle from you."
Harry: "I'm right over here, Hannah."
Matthew: "You can hear his voice, and he plays the flute, can we just hear that?"
Harry plays the flute – something bright. "So we have Harry there. And just next to you is Anneliese with the harp." Anneliese plays. "I'm going to go sit on the other side of you on your right, and I play the oboe."
Matthew tries to explain to Hannah that he would like her to start and finish the piece and that the musicians will follow.
Matthew: "So, Hannah...?"
Hannah: "Yes?"
Matthew: "If we make a piece with you, would you be able to show us when it's time to start and also when you feel the piece has reached a time to finish?"
Hannah: "You're too far away, I can't hear you."
Matthew: "Sorry, I'm sorry, I'm sorry... so would be able to show us when it's time for the piece to start and when you think the piece has reached an ending – then you can show us it's time to finish."
Hannah: "I still can't understand you."
This seems too difficult for her to absorb, so Matthew tries to explain in an easier way:
Matthew: "So when you... if you conduct for us, then you're in charge, so we will start when you start and we will finish when you finish. Is that ok?"
Hannah: "Yes."
Matthew: "Okay then, we're ready."
The musicians then improvise a short 'crisp' piece in F minor. Hannah puts the baton down after a minute or so and the piece finishes.
Matthew: "How was that Hannah?..."
Hannah: "mmm..."
Matthew: "How was that, how was the music...was it okay?"
Hannah: "I can't understand you."
Matthew: "Was the music okay?"
Hannah: "Yes."
Matthew: "Would you like some more?"
Hannah: "Yes"
Matthew: "Okay, then you need to keep conducting...will you keep conducting?"
Hannah: "Yes."
Matthew: "...and maybe if we draw, if we imagine drawing some shapes as well like this..."
He holds her hand with the baton letting her feel how she can make bigger gestures.
"...You get some different sounds like this, ok? ...you can experiment."
Matthew holds her hand with the baton letting her feel how she can make bigger gestures, as the musicians join in; Hannah appears to understand. She really starts to conduct, and with a variety of different motions from before. At the end, Matthew says, "Thanks Hannah – how was it that time? Did you enjoy it?"
Hannah: "Yes."
Matthew: "Was that the music that you wanted to hear?"

Hannah: "Yes, but it's not quite the music I wanted."

Matthew: "It's not quite what it is... are you able to tell us what it is that you want to hear?"

Hannah: "Well, I don't know what it's called what I wanted."

Matthew: "Where did you hear it... where were you when you heard it?"

Hannah: "Mmm?"

Matthew: "Can you remember where you heard it... or when...? Where were you living?"

Hannah: "I don't know."

Matthew: "In Germany?" She appears to give an indication of a yes.

Matthew confirms: "In Germany."

Hannah: "Yes, I m sure I heard it in Germany, but not only there".

Matthew: "So, it's a famous piece... How does it make you feel, your piece? Is it a happy piece... or a sad piece? ... Or a thoughtful piece?"

Hannah: "I don't know where you are but you're too far away."

Matthew replies: "Okay, I'm sorry... Maybe we'll try it another time, should we try it another time?"

Hannah: "Yes."

Matthew: "Thanks Hannah... I did enjoy the music that you made anyway.
I thought it was nice anyway, and we can try again another time... yeah?" – she nods – "Great, thank you very much."

During this interaction, it becomes clear that this exchange leaves both Hannah and Matthew quite vulnerable and exposed at times, the group an audience to their long, awkward and sometimes fragmented interaction. There is a sense that as Matthew strives to find out more about Hannah and the identity of the music that is important to her, he is thrown off guard by her responses. He becomes further embroiled in a verbal dialogue with her, trying to find a multitude of ways to rephrase his questions. At times, Matthew's method of questioning elicits a closed response of 'yes' from Hannah, or challenges her to recount facts and knowledge, which may be beyond her. However, the breakdown is averted through the music making. Matthew's joint conducting with Hannah, where he models the use of the baton in a very tactile, non-verbal sense, proves to be an effective way of engaging with her through the music making, a way in which they can both express their intentions with full understanding.

Breakdown of participation: musician perceptions

Fiona points out that the project is about 'being in the moment' and that a breakdown of participation is naturally part of the reality of working in this context, and that there are "no neat endings". However, for the musicians, situations where this breakdown of participation occurs can be very disorienting. The musicians describe a metaphor of being lost at sea, representing a perceived lack of focus and safety, where they are less in control of the situation, and trying to process a vast deal of information. In the initial group interview, Anneliese reveals how, in these moments, it is possible to lose touch of your rational abilities, saying *"you can't even think straight anymore."* The workshopleader can be particularly vulnerable to these feelings; expectations of the group may weigh heavily upon their shoulders, due to the visibility of this leadership role, even if all of the leadership responsibilities do not actually reside in the workshopleader's hands. Whilst the workshopleader has the ultimate responsibility for initiating, developing and sustaining frameworks within the planning and music session, everyone involved has a shared responsibility to support, develop and sustain the frameworks. Within this responsibility, the leader may move between a variety of roles: vision setting, coordinating, management, coaching, enabling, modelling and 'filling in the gaps'. Leadership decisions and communication in this role can be a stressful responsibility, placing the workshopleader in a vulnerable position, especially when others may have different viewpoints, and when there are breakdowns in communication and participation.

Matthew reflects how, even though in some instances silence in the group can signify a sense of acceptance, peace and togetherness, in other instances it can also be a cue that there are communication issues. He describes silence that is a result of a breakdown of communication as being a sort of "tumbleweed silence". He reflects on his feelings when these moments occur: *"There's panic, then there's the need of making a decision about what's gonna happen next. It feels like there's not a comfortable flow, from one piece or one activity into the next one. The session has lost momentum, I suppose, if you have that tumbleweed silence, which is kind of like stuck, I think."* Here, Matthew sees his role as vital in both the creation and solution to this problem of tumbleweed silence, perceiving this as a sign of failure in his responsibility to direct and shape a session: *"It usually comes from, I think, a kind of imbalance in the relationship between the leader and the other two musicians and with the staff; me, as the leader, not having created a good working relationship with the two musicians. They don't feel... because for there actually to be moments where nobody has got an idea of what should happen next in a group of three musicians is a pretty, it shouldn't happen... that there isn't somebody that's got an idea or spotted something or has an idea for something, there must therefore be a lack of confidence in expressing that. So for that thing to be happening, where nobody is initiating or having an idea must be a sign of dysfunction in the team, I think. Must be. Must be. People don't feel able to express something."*

Sometimes a sense of frustration can be felt, where a breakdown of participation has occurred due to the actions of a resident affecting another resident's participation. Matthew describes a moment in a session where Esther's participation dominates that of Rebecca's: *"At the time in my mind I'm just thinking: shut up! Shut up! You know, it was really frustrating. Rebecca's really making an effort here. Something was happening and part of you is really frustrated by it. Obviously. And you have to, you know, the other part of your brain is totally in a place of compassion for Esther. So yes, balancing those two things; and the frustration is not with her, it's with the situation."* In this situation, the actions of Esther have disrupted a significant moment of interaction with Rebecca, with whom connections can be fleeting; in the observed situation Matthew skillfully manages this breakdown very well, validating Esther and valuing Rebecca's contributions, despite his internal monologue. Here, this monologue shows how although Matthew was frustrated in the moment, he is able to develop an attitude of compassion beyond his aspirations for Rebecca.

It is in these sorts of moments, and the moments where the musicians are most challenged to create a sense of continuity in breakdown, that salvation is needed. In order to cope with breakdown of participation – whether it is between just the musicians, or between musicians and the other participants, the musicians need to find a way to reclaim a sense of focus and safety. Music forms the basis of this practice, and it is through the language of music that the musicians can connect and sustain participation through the session. Through musical means, by creating pre-developed musical frameworks or 'musical islands', they can again begin to focus as musicians, artists and people. The musicians refer to musical islands as a formal concept; in the past, when the practice was in its infancy, musical islands consisted of prepared extemporised pieces that they could play as a way of regrouping as musicians. Within this project, musical islands were also present: returns to familiar musical frameworks, as well as unprepared, more inwardly focused improvisations with simple 'default' musical language, with the character of a 'gifted' piece. In these islands, there is a sense that the musicians' awareness in communication becomes more centred and focused on their own small trio and less influenced by the participation of others, meditative in nature.

In the initial group interview, the musicians reflect on what musical islands mean to them; a chance for rescue from the turbulence of being lost at sea:

Anneliese: *"Musical islands, it was just when situations got really bad, it was like: 'what can we do?' You know, you can't even think straight anymore. And then we would just try and have some musical ideas ready, they were our islands, so that you could sort of default. It's the same idea, so that you could go back and sort of climb back on land again. Because, very often when things get sticky, if there is music, even if it's default music, that can be much easier than if there isn't any. And you try and communicate by a language or there is silence, you know. There are different types of silences. And we used them an awful lot, because we were all out there, going: 'what do we do now? Let's get on the island'."*

Matthew: *"Climb back on an island."*

Fiona: *"There's the lifeboat."*

Anneliese: *"But it's a default thing. And it was that sort of thing and as a group maybe we would agree a default thing. And it wasn't maybe the introduction and the ending piece, it was something else that we could just all know, that we all sort of had up our sleeves. And even sometimes you didn't need to use it, but you knew it was there and that was good enough to make you feel a bit less vulnerable."*

Here, the reassurance of 'climbing onto the island' is gained through returning to familiar musical material and limiting the level of development in musical language. Here, by creating musical islands, the musicians can come together, to find their voices again in order to send 'lifeboats' to those who may need them the most.

Risk taking

In the analysis on identity and communication, risk taking was introduced as an integral part of the project. At an individual level risk taking involved being authentic, surrendering to the moment. Risk taking is an integral part of communication, in relation to the musician's leadership, where the risk is having the courage to act upon one's interpretation, an understanding of a situation that may not have any clear or 'right' answers. As Matthew phrases it, taking action in this context is risky; it is like "*stepping into the unknown*" and into a mode of exploration and reflexivity. Fiona details how "*you always feel unsure*", and that there are "*always questions*" around decision-making.

This act of risk taking does not just apply to the musicians; risk taking is a fundamental aspect of leadership and creativity, and is therefore experienced by all participating in the project. Risk taking involves embracing a spirit of exploration and curiosity, freedom and spontaneity. Everyone, for different reasons, is out of their comfort zone, being called to bring their authentic selves to the group. The musicians are the proficient experts in music, the prime language of the music session, whereas interaction through musical communication is potentially a new and risky experience for staff and residents, who may be less certain about the underlying 'play rules'. Even for the musicians, music – the prime medium for communication in the project – can be a risky and elusive art form. Additionally, the musicians are also visitors, coming in to an established community where different play rules may apply. All of these elements can impact upon the ability to feel safe for those involved in the project. In order to take risks, one must feel safe, and therefore the concept of safety is again important; with safety also comes a sense of belonging.

The aim to promote a safe, inclusive environment for all participants appears to underpin the ethos of Music for Life and this project, influencing the way that people communicate and participate in the sessions. It is incumbent on everyone involved to promote this ethos if a sense of belonging is to be reached for all. Matthew recognises the need for this shared vision and collaboration: "*Everyone is trying things all the time and is moving out of their comfort zone and trying new things, you know, and being brave and being courageous and we recognise that in each other. And that's why it's nurturing, because it's an environment where we're all doing that, and there's an understanding of it, and a support therefore as well."* Here he reflects that recognising risk-taking and vulnerability in all other participants, in a non-judgmental and safe environment, is crucial. Through this understanding, trust and a sense of belonging can emerge. In order to achieve this environment of understanding and support, it is important to communicate, to find a shared vision and language working towards a shared leadership model. However, this is not always so easy, as everyone involved has different, unique perspectives, values, experiences and vulnerabilities.

Earlier, in the introduction of this analysis on participation, we explored the possibility that different interpretations of other's participation – in this case, resident participation – could emerge. Through the project, divergent expectations for a particular type of participation from others in the group play out, particularly in regards to resident participation. These expectations can lead to a culture where the act of participation can feel unsafe. High expectations of resident participation can mean that there may be coercion for active and visible participation. As explored in the analysis on identity, there can be a sense of disappointment at a personal and professional level if expectations of resident participation are not attained, as Matthew phrased it, *"the desire for them to play an instrument can be very much tied up with our own feelings of success".* Often some of the most poignant, beautiful and meaningful moments are when there is a focused interaction on a resident within the group; where there is a sense that authentic selves are meeting and merging, that the person with dementia has 'come out from the darkness'. Matthew describes how these sort of moments can emerge from a place of complete emancipation for a resident, *"where somebody kind of just forgets themselves and they forget the context of where they are and they become so engrossed in the music making with one of the musicians that a solo or a duet piece emerges."* However, moments of this type are rare and fleeting, made all the more poignant for that very reason.

Matthew recognises the intense level of risk taking in the leadership of residents that this sort of interaction requires, and that he, as a leader, needs to step back from imposing his own aspirations, in order to create a safe environment: *"It's very exposing for people to do that. It is very exposing to put themselves on the line and play a piece just with one of the musicians, or something; very, very exposing. And just allowing for those things to emerge at the right pace and the right speed, rather than to push too hard for it and to just let them come."* In his role as a leader, Matthew, alongside the musicians and care staff, needs to interpret and recognise exactly when someone feels ready to take that risk, reflecting on the importance of respecting the person with dementia's right to participate on their own terms, writing: *"Really important not to thrust people into the spotlight before they are ready. But there is a pressure/expectation from the musicians and care staff for 'something to happen'. Staff in particular need to have some 'evidence' in order to really get behind the project."*

Positive experiences and tales from previous Music for Life projects can fuel expectations, particularly those of the care staff, according to Matthew. He points out that this pressure can be present from the very start of a project, when everything is new and unknown: *"The first session feels like a challenge, there is anxiety, feeling of pressure and the unknown. Staff may expect big things from residents."* One can sense that this feeling of pressure can seem inescapable for the musicians, for the workshopleader, as Matthew details further: *"And of that issue: that's there all the time, of how much do we want the residents to perform for us, so that we feel we've done a good job, so that the staff see what the project is about and that the staff get something out of it, and that they see the transformative possibility of it. You know, we want the staff to see these big moments and we want them for ourselves, to feel good. And just making sure that we keep it with what the residents want, whilst pushing them and whilst challenging them as well, and giving them the opportunity to move out of the place that they're in to really, really find balance."* For Matthew, this balance is about safety, about respecting that person's right to participate at a pace that feels safe for them, to create opportunities but not 'thrust' them towards taking risks until they give signs that they are ready to take a participatory risk.

Membership

Throughout the project, strong stories emerge that shape the musicians' views on what constitutes meaningful participation for residents. Interactions with each person, as they find their way in the group, create uniquely new situations and issues, enriching, challenging and re-shaping past learning from previous experiences and perspectives. Through meeting Esther, the musicians learn that it is possible to perceive that someone can belong to, and meaningfully participate in a group, even if it is only sporadically. Esther is a clear example of an individual who belongs to the group yet sits on the periphery. This often happens in a very explicit and physical way, for instance, when she chooses not to sit within the circle of residents, musicians and staff, sitting physically on the outside, with observers of the project. It also happens symbolically; she sometimes actively participates in the group, whether inside or outside the circle, and she also chooses when she wants to be with the group, or leave the group. This leads to a sense for musicians and staff that, as she only occasionally interacts with and within the group, she does not fully belong within the core of the group, she is on the fringe.

Esther expressively and effortlessly claps and sings along to the music, engaging in banter, most often with the musicians and those outside the circle, showing occasional aggression towards other residents, such as Rebecca, as well as a tendency to elaborately verbalise her reasons for leaving the group. Matthew details how this unfolds in session three: *"What she kept saying was, 'oh I got to get to work', or something like that. But there was a sense then that almost she wanted to stay, but she was feeling this obligation to be somewhere else. That was so much of an excuse for her, as happened the week before, 'oh, I've got to go and meet my mother'. It was like she was giving us a reason why she wanted to leave, and actually she just wanted to leave. Whereas this week it was like something was keeping her there a little bit, but she felt that she had to go because she had some obligation to be somewhere else and do something (...) she went on good terms and it was fine."* This reflection of Matthew's is interesting for a number of reasons. One can sense that Esther, despite leaving the group, feels enough a part of the group to want to verbalise her reasons for leaving to others; in some way, at some level, she feels that she does belong to the group. It also shows the importance of respecting Esther's right to participate in which way she chooses, even if that involves leaving the group.

Despite enabling a culture where Esther has permission to join in at her own pace, this dilemma of Esther leaving the group is one that the musicians constantly return to. The musicians and staff even discuss at times whether she is a suitable candidate for being involved in the project, as Fiona comments: *"There has been some discussion amongst us as a team as to whether Esther has really been a suitable resident for the project. It has been very difficult to engage her fully and I think she has only stayed for one complete session. Her normal behaviour is to say she has to go and to leave the group after maybe five or ten minutes."* Although they can rationalise Esther's behaviour, they also aspire for Esther to become part of the group in the same way as the other participants, as Matthew surmises: *"It'd be really interesting to see how that plays out for the course of the rest of the project, actually, to see whether she can just relax, and be there and allow herself to enjoy the music. That would be what I really hope for her; that this happens, that she finds a role for herself within the group, where she's useful and enjoys being there and wants to stay and doesn't feel pulled away to do something 'proper', you know?"* It is a natural and necessary aspiration to hold, if the musicians are to continue to strive to build an inclusive and engaging environment for participation. However, through interpreting these statements, it becomes clear that Esther is perceived as not belonging in the same way as other participants; she is not deemed a full member of the group from the current way that she chooses to participate.

Nevertheless, we can see that being involved in the project has had a positive resonance with Esther, in its own special way, and in the moment. Fiona reflects on an interaction with Esther before the seventh session: *"This week I saw a very vulnerable side to her. She walked through as we were rehearsing and said she didn't feel well, and would we mind if she sat down. She was obviously very confused and couldn't remember where her room was. We were warming up at the time and she simply listened for a while. She kept saying how lovely it was, especially Anneliese's beautiful harp, and her whole expression changed. At the end she gave me a hug and said that she would 'remember it forever'. It was actually a very special moment. I then took her to her room where she was again very confused."* This interaction shows that Esther is indeed attracted by the music, the musicians, the space, and feels she does belong there with them, even if she is present for only a short time. Esther is lost in her dementia, yet in those precious moments she has been found.

Respect for an individual's personal space, and accepting and valuing the right to participate freely and uniquely within the group, is integral to the story of Rosamund. The musicians learn that an attitude of inclusivity towards residents does not translate directly or immediately into a sense of belonging for residents. Throughout the project, brief moments elucidate Rosamund's experience of dementia, one in which she appears isolated from others. As detailed earlier in the analysis, during session one Fiona kneels in front of Rosamund and Gabriella during the creation of a group piece. She makes strong eye contact with Rosamund, to which Rosamund responds by holding her hand to her head, hiding from Fiona's gaze. In this case, Fiona is too physically close to Rosamund. In the other highlighted case, the opposite occurs – Matthew and Anneliese are seated too far away from Rosamund to be able to strengthen her participation. Here, the issue of physical space is very different from the interaction involving Fiona, however, as before, the need for personal space is again crucial, as Matthew observes: *"When we were passing the instruments round, she wouldn't, she didn't take part in that, she would absolutely not engage with that. She wouldn't even say 'no', she just totally absented herself from that process. I'm very keen that she doesn't feel coerced or pressured, or, because I think when we push her she will get uncomfortable, she will be angry about that. So there is a challenge there."*

In the same quote, Matthew explores his own thoughts on the reasons why Rosamund may feel disconnected from the group, and the organic way he needs to work with her to help her feel a sense of belonging: *"Rosamund, I feel really unsure of where to go with that because I think she senses very much about whether I, I think she will feel coerced, I think there's an awareness there. I feel she's more aware of where she is and that she is in a circle of people with dementia. And my instinct is that she holds back because she's fearful of accepting her illness perhaps."* Fiona is able to somewhat confirm Matthew's interpretation, sharing the details of a conversation she had with Rosamund after session three. After starting to develop the tentative beginnings of a relationship with Rosamund, Fiona is able to take a risk with her, in this case, seeking to understand Rosamund's perception of her social environment and validating it. Fiona writes: *"After the session I had an amazing conversation with her. I felt that we had formed this sense of connection and decided to ask her how she found the home. I discovered that she didn't know anyone and in her own words: 'didn't want to know anyone' as 'they are all old fossils.' I simply said that I understood and she asked me if I felt the same."*

Through sharing reflections and insights into Rosamund's communication and participation, the musicians and staff begin to develop a richer understanding of her and the factors influencing her participation. Fiona recognises the potential of the project in creating the opportunity to move past this isolation, reflecting: *"I would love the project to continue to provide a safe space for her, where she feels respected and empowered, and to help integrate her more into the life of the home."* She sees the opportunity for this 'integration' happening through participation in the musical experience; through acknowledging aspects that Rosamund finds beauty and meaning in, aspects that she identifies with.

Fiona's sensitive communication with Rosamund creates an opportunity for Rosamund to feel a sense of belonging. Fiona shares a drum with Rosamund, in session three, modelling how to use it but also leaving space for Rosamund to develop her own relationship with the drum. Here, the modelling is not only in a musical context, it is also social, with Fiona offering a way for Rosamund to belong in the group, to begin to communicate at a social level:

> From the field notes:
>
> Fiona gently taps the bodhran[145] sharing it with Rosamund – it is rested on Rosamund's knee. Rosamund smiles at Fiona and appears interested in the drum and occasionally tries touching and playing it. Rosamund appears to engage differently throughout this song, particularly when Matthew sings "Hey Oh". There is a period in the music where there is a breakdown to harp and drum stops where Fiona plays a jaunty loud short break on the bodhran – sharing this with Rosamund, who laughs.

Matthew reflects, after session five, on the sustained change in Rosamund's participation that he sees emerging, subtly from week to week: *"Today in the session there was, what I observed was a real sense that she was enjoying being there and did want to belong. And reaching out to hold hands with Fiona and, you know, if that's not a sign of wanting to be somewhere, I don't know what is. She actually wanted the physical contact, which is a kind of reaching out, a need to feel safe and wanting to belong, which I hadn't seen in her before. And something then very subtly must have changed for her to open up and show that vulnerability."* Fiona perceives that the music has had a great impact in creating this environment in which Rosamund can express herself and express her love for others. She reflects, after session

---

[145] A frame drum with a goatskin head originating from Ireland, usually around 35 cm to 45 cm in diameter. A sound is traditionally made by using a special wooden beater (called a cipin or tipper) or by hand. The drum is struck with the dominant hand, and the non-dominant hand is used against the underside of the drum to control the pitch and tension of the drum. See also Appendix V, 'List of musical instruments'.

seven, on how: *"Rosamund was very frail this week and more confused than I have seen her but it was still wonderful to have her as a part of the group. I was just thinking that although she has not been seen to actively participate that she has in fact made huge progress just in terms of being part of the group (...) I really feel she has just needed to be there, to be part of the music which she has often said she has enjoyed and to be affirmed simply for being her and being with 'us'. There was a real sense of 'us'– 'us' as a whole group this week."*

Throughout the weeks, Rosamund's way of participating is not necessarily about doing, but being, as Brian phrases it: *"It is more about presence than what somebody does"*. It is about social participation; developing warm relationships with those around her, and expressing love for them are important signs of her feeling a sense of belonging, and are just as valid a form of participation as that involved in initiating, creating, and developing musical contributions. Acceptance of Rosamund, the qualities she brings to the group, is fundamental to creating an inclusive environment for her to belong, one where she is perceived as a valuable member of the community. Slowly, over time, Rosamund begins to feel that she is part of this community, and starts to express her own feelings. This growth within this particular community continues into the final session, where Rosamund accepts the gift of a piece, dedicated to her. Matthew reflects on this moment from his perspective, as an observer of this intimacy: *"what I think did happen and was there today, that Rosamund did for a moment at least, accept being part of the group and enjoyed it. She enjoyed a feeling of connection with the group. She allowed the music to touch her and to move her. And she was happy to say so as well. She said, 'it makes me want to cry'. To open yourself up that much, you know and to admit to emotions like that is a really significant difference from how she was at the very beginning of the project, when she was extremely closed and very guarded. And there was not showing any emotion at all. So then to actually vocalise how she felt, and to admit to something like that."* With acceptance of Rosamund comes the possibility of sharing experiences with her, experiences where she is not only giving but also receiving love. Music provides the space for her to be deeply rooted in this group; as she receives the music, she also receives love and affirmation.

Rosamund's Song (session 8)

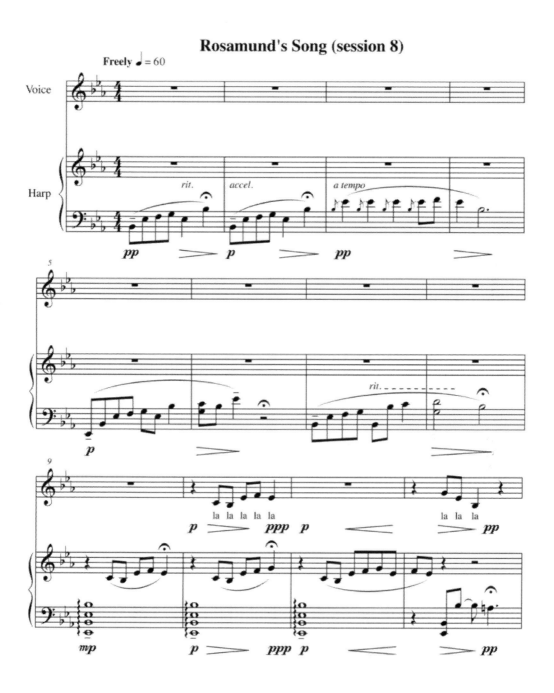

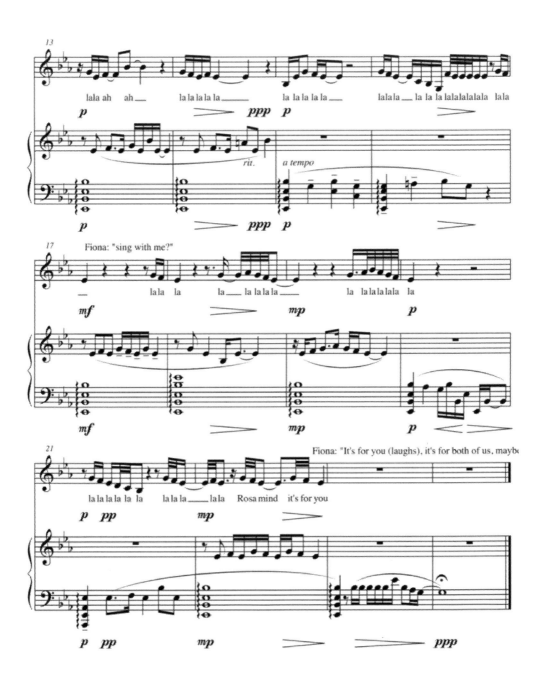

Both Esther and Rosamund's stories reaffirm the importance of acceptance of a variety of participation modes from participants in the group. This acceptance requires patience; patience in creating the space and opportunities for a person to interact freely in the group – whether that be on the periphery or at the very core – and a consistent attitude of love and care in every interaction, every note played or sung. This same sense of love is present in interactions with Sarah. Brian reflects on her participation in session six. Here he highlights the key role of Anneliese and Samantha, whose relationships with Sarah seem to anchor her to the group, to call her to the 'present'. These relationships provide a space where she can tolerate being part of a group, where she has no need to call out and express her anxiety, as the anxiety is not present: *"I think Sarah was very, very intensely present throughout today; she led pieces, she took the baton. Even when the attention wasn't focused on her, there were times when I saw her looking around, really enjoying using the large shaker. She used that quite a bit in one of the sessions. She was really on time, and her looking, I could see her engaging very well with Anneliese and Samantha beside her and yeah, her engaging with those people. And with a smile on her face as well. You know, her not needing to call in those hours. We haven't really, apart from the first two sessions it feels like, had so much of that calling out. Which I think is saying: 'in this space I feel looked after, I feel care, I feel involved, I feel comforted. I don't feel insecure'."*

Brian reflects on how the balance of individual expression and social togetherness begins to emerge, midway through the project: *"I feel that the project is well established now with the residents and each person is responding in their own individual ways. It is clear for about four of the participants that they have retained a sense of the group and they have learned how to participate within it (...) It feels like a group now and not just a collection of individuals."*

Feeling involved, cared for and comforted is also important for Rebecca. Like Esther, Rebecca appears more comfortable in the periphery of the group at times, whether it be for whole sessions, when she chooses to leave the group, and even in sessions, where she may either sit on the fringes, or seems to oscillate dramatically in varying states of comfort and distress. As relationships build however, there is a sense that she is able, like Sarah, to tolerate being part of a group, and to even find her voice, metaphorically and literally, through membership of the community. As Rebecca finds her voice, she is also able to find a meaningful role within the community, which translates even outside of the sessions, as in this example from the field notes:

From the field notes:

Rebecca is standing in the reception area of the home, looking at visitors in a friendly way. When Deborah comes in, Rebecca turns to her with a big smile. Deborah asks Rebecca to help with bringing the instruments. Rebecca seems confused at this at first but repeats after Deborah "instruments for music". Rebecca helps Deborah by carrying a few small items. There are still more to bring to the workshop venue; Deborah asks Rebecca if they will continue to get the instruments. Rebecca looks at her, not understanding the question. Then Deborah says: "for making the music". Rebecca beams all over and repeats: "for making the music!" She hits Deborah's hand, not angrily, but enthusiastically. They leave to do their job.

This observation of Rebecca is very different from the anxious woman we have met during this analysis, a woman prone to pacing the corridors relentlessly, staring wordlessly, in apparent fright and confusion.

Shared leadership

As explored earlier in the analysis, risk taking comes in many forms for the musicians. One risk is developing and using skills beyond the usual experiences and practice required in other professional music contexts, in, as Matthew observes: *"an environment where everyone recognises we're out of our depth, out of our comfort zone."* The musicians need to be brave pioneers, confident in their artistry and professionalism; moving past their own perceived vulnerabilities is crucial, as the musicians discuss in interview:

Matthew: *"Improvisation is not my strongest skill. And I don't think of lots of different chord structures or you know; the music I feel like playing is not particularly sophisticated when I'm playing."*

Anneliese: *"You've got so many things to handle at the same time (...)."*

Fiona: *(...) "But I want to kind of keep growing that, so that I get a bigger vocabulary, that's the aim."*

Matthew: *"Yes, likewise, likewise. And there is a kind of feeling of achievement, when you've been through a session and you've pushed yourself musically a bit as well, you feel like you've been brave, you know what I mean?"*

In this context, to be brave is to take risks, and taking risks can lead to vulnerability. In order to be brave, the musicians need to develop an attitude of collaboration, in which they can trust and support each other, as Matthew comments: *"Yeah, you need that kind of, a little bit of looking after a bit, because we're about to do something that is quite brave, you know. You open yourself up and you feel very vulnerable to do that, and you need that bit of reassurance."* Through trusting each other, the musicians feel able to push themselves further in a social and musical context: *"You know, when you feel that somebody is there and support is there musically. You can push yourself both musically and to the degree which you allow yourself to connect, actually."*

This sense that they are supporting each other seems to be based upon a feeling, an instinct, validated through non-verbal means. Reflecting on a piece that emerged during session two, Matthew describes the intense feeling of validation that this musical support can provide: *"There was a moment where I consciously thought, yes, we're going in this direction where the piece had really developed its own momentum by that point. And Fiona and Anneliese were sensitive to that as well and supportive and Anneliese was playing a lot on the harp (...) Which is just fantastic, when she really kind of digs in deep and this big sound comes out, it's just phenomenal. It's such a powerful thing, such a powerful thing, that sound, I think. So that then supports you to go further because you get the reassurance from the other musicians, that yes, we're with you and you're on the right track. It's like an acknowledgement from the other two musicians that, yes you're going the right way with this. And that encourages you to keep going in that direction, I suppose."* This support enables Matthew to push himself further, to be brave, to take risks.

Shared leadership is particularly important in creating a sense of safety, enabling the ability to venture into new, risky territory. Through this collaboration, Matthew is able to sense, in session six, that there is finally an opportunity to engage with Rebecca in an authentic way. This has been the result of weeks of reflection and discussion between musicians and staff, exploring different ways of helping Rebecca to feel included. However, in the context of the session, Matthew makes a spontaneous decision to take the risk, initiating a piece with Rebecca using a metal bass bar. He looks to the musicians for support in this risk and is validated by Anneliese, who endorses his leadership decision: *"The very first time I did this big bash on the bar and I sang back at her really strong and gave a quick glance at Anneliese and she was looking at me and nodding like, yes, yes yes! That's it, let's go for it! And I could see that she was there, and yes, let's try this. And I knew I wasn't going to be high and dry, I wasn't going to be stranded with taking on something bigger than I could manage on my own. The support was going to be there for it."* For Matthew, this support is particularly relevant at this moment. When he recalls this episode, he is able to confide just how risky his decision to interact with Rebecca was, how vulnerable this authentic and intimate connection made him feel. He even gives this criticism a voice, the 'Snark', as revealed in the analysis on identity. However, having the support of Anneliese and Fiona gives him a real sense of safety, urging him to 'go on' past his own internal, destructive critical voice: *"Sometimes when I can be brave, ignore the Snark, and manage to forge that connection, I'm sure that's when the best music happens. Having a great team who recognise what is happening, and are there with solid, affirming playing really makes this possible – almost as though they are the safety net, or the people "watching your back". They feel the moment, and aren't afraid of the intimacy. "Yes", their playing says, "go on, go on."*

Here, this 'safety net' can again be likened to the concept explored earlier, of being lost at sea; the safety net a metaphor for being rescued from a turbulent, potentially dangerous environment. This ability to act as a safety net for each other has been built up over a series of shared experiences, experiences of the 'heart': intuitive, beautiful moments of non-verbal connection in sessions, and of the 'head'; sharing reflections, hopes, values, fears and vulnerabilities.

For Fiona this sense of team is important, as she reflects, in discussion with Matthew and Anneliese, on the shared values held within the wider team of Music for Life, and the support that this offers her:

Fiona: *"I was just thinking about, like, the sense of team is really important for me; I mean, I really love our training days. I've come to really look forward to them, because I go just knowing that I will see a group of really lovely people, and it feels like a real kind of understanding. We're all really different, but there's a core kind of value amongst people in the Music for Life team that I don't find necessarily in other places that I work. And I think that comes from a shared…"*

Anneliese: *"…experience."*

Fiona: *"Experience, yeah, and to a certain extent a kind of shared heart. In different ways, people express it in different ways, but there's a similar kind of vision, I guess, isn't there?"*

Matthew equates this 'shared experience' and 'shared heart' as being as emotively powerful as spirituality and family experiences, and ultimately engendering a sense of belonging: *"you've shared these experiences which you can't explain to anybody else, so you feel understood by each other."*

However, developing this level of trust, mutual respect and collaboration is not always a straightforward journey. For Matthew, he becomes more critically aware of his own attitudes towards leadership, as explored in the analysis on identity. He relates this to his own biography, with experiences in his early childhood contributing to his need to feel in control. He reflects how this need to feel in control permeates his leadership style, observing his tendency to act authoritatively, to be in charge: *"The temptation is that I drive the session, I just drive the session. Not necessarily allowing enough space and opportunity for the other two musicians to work. It's something that I need to remain aware of, it's a tendency I have, to lead, lead, lead. And then I can feel a frustration that the other two musicians are not…'where are you, where are you?', you know, to me. But I'm not allowing them any space to do that. And so I'm relieved to notice that in myself right now."* He identifies a solution, that his leadership could be less about taking an authoritative stance, and more about enabling others: *"I need to allow the other two musicians space to work. My habitual and reflex mode of working is to take control. To truly lead means allowing EVERY person to give of their best, to take risks, express themselves. This includes the other musicians, who are both extremely skilled."* This awareness starts to lead to a sea change for Matthew, as his own understanding of leadership and shared leadership begins to broaden. He begins to reflect not only on the values underpinning shared leadership, but to find new ways of achieving this, not only within the team of musicians, but also when working alongside care staff.

During the project, an important area of learning for Matthew is the understanding that convergence in communication between the musicians can be attained in many ways other than playing music in preparation. He first of all describes, after session two, about how this convergence comes through a spirit of collaboration in which the three musicians are involved in planning all aspects of the project at an equal level: *"I really opened up the prep hour to Anneliese and Fiona, who had done a lot of thinking between sessions about the seating, good instruments for specific people etc. This practical stuff, and talking about it together is a great way for the team to connect, and a way to 'come together' that isn't about playing. We have always placed such a great emphasis on playing together as the way the team 'connects', but I wonder whether this very practical stuff isn't as equally important, and a way to connect that can do some of the same things – listening, letting go of one's own pre-conceptions about what is going to happen, taking on and working with the ideas of each other, supporting each other, negotiating over something as simple as which beater is best for which instrument."*

He further reflects that this collaboration on practical aspects can actually be a crucial precursor for creating musical connections: *"The way these simple, almost banal things are handled can have an impact on how the team feels about being together. If a team member chooses a beater for an instrument that another team member feels is inappropriate, this has to be worked through with openness, consultation and above all respect for each other. By the time the team sits down to play together, many of the little niggles can have been worked through already. A way of being with each other has already been worked through."* For Matthew, these initial thoughts about collaboration become an ongoing area for reflection and learning. He begins to understand that a collaborative connection is formed through negotiation, through taking the time to listen to each other and sharing ownership and responsibilities in the planning process: *"You know, you're making these really important decisions together. And it's negotiated all the time and done with respect for each other, and awareness of each other and… so yeah, I've really enjoyed it, I've really enjoyed the way that Anneliese and Fiona have kind of really come forward and taken a lot of responsibility."*

For Matthew, attaining this state of shared leadership is important, a state that enables people to grow, to develop and find their own voices within the project: *"It was something I was very keen for it to happen on this project, because, for myself, the idea of being able to not be the one person who carries all the responsibility (…) I think it's really important that they have the space to be able to try out their ideas and to feel confident, and to make those decisions and to share the leadership."*

This new level of communication and shared leadership with the other musicians creates for Matthew a sense of convergence, that they are able to intuitively understand each other, and reach a shared consensus on decision-making: *"The connection with Fiona and Anneliese feels good. And it feels like there's a good communication between those two, they played very well together. It feels like we've come together very strongly as a team. And that the music is…, that we're on the same wave length."*

Beyond this relationship of shared leadership amongst musicians, Matthew begins to perceive the role and value of his leadership in a way that creates more space for everyone involved in the project to take initiative, and to find their voice. Negotiation, listening, enabling and supporting each other, all hallmarks of the relationships between the musicians, are crucial leadership elements underpinning all interactions and all relationships within the project: *"It's something that I would certainly consider on all projects: thinking about how much of the leadership can be shared with the intention of leading in that way, of allowing as much as possible for everybody to input and to feel they are leading the work. And as an idea it goes beyond the musician team; you want everybody in the group to feel that, the care staff, everybody (…) So it's an interesting thing, leadership is, as I'm really becoming more and more aware of, it's not about telling people what to do. Really not; if you really are truly leading it's about everybody fulfilling what is possible for them to do."* Here, we can sense that the shared leadership Matthew is talking about is one that promotes egalitarianism; that recognises abilities as well as potential, and where everyone can feel a sense of agency, ownership and belonging.

Achieving this state of shared leadership with care staff and residents was a difficult journey, and the changing relationship between the musicians and staff is a key narrative within the project. Both staff and musicians are experts: musicians in the language of music and the practice of the project; staff in their relationships to individuals and the setting, and in developing pathways for sustaining the legacy of relationships that emerge from the project. The musicians adopt a strong leadership role in both an artistic and generic sense, responsible for enabling and shaping the activities and musical voices explored during the music session. Empowering staff to take initiative and share leadership and ownership is a fundamental value of the project, yet, for a musician it can be a tricky process: trying to find the right balance in shaping the sessions and allowing space for others to shape events.

Attaining a model of shared leadership takes time, as care staff and musicians gradually learn to understand and trust each other through mutual engagement in the music sessions and reflective debriefs. In order to truly collaborate with each other, they must first go through a period of negotiation, where values and expectations are explored and tested. With a threatened professional identity, staff may feel disempowered, unable to care for residents or work with colleagues in ways their role traditionally calls for; it may feel risky participating in an environment where play rules are less formalised, unclear or inconsistent. In addition, disempowerment may result in frustration for staff, a sense that the leadership of the session is out of their hands. Brian reflects on the views of staff, discussed in the debrief of session three, when the rules of engagement are clearly being explored: *"That was the big theme, that was going on regarding staff. You know, what is their ownership and what is the musician's ownership of what's happening in the space? (...) How do I work in this place, what do I do? Do I have power or do I not have power? Is all the power theirs or do I also have some power? Is all the responsibility theirs or do I also have responsibility? And there was quite a lot of uncertainty around that (...) It was also about 'when do I take initiative and when is it somebody else's responsibility to take initiative? And how do I negotiate that? What happens if I try to negotiate it and I get it wrong? And is it ok to get it wrong?'"*

These questions have to do with leadership, with responsibility and permission as key issues underlying interactions. After the project, Matthew mentions the 'natural' dynamics that might typically occur in projects between musicians and staff. He reveals his own expectations of the type of roles staff may adopt in their participation, in relation to their roles and personalities, and how this may affect the participation of others: *"Intrinsically within the team you're working with a sense of hierarchy, and we were trying to establish a position where everybody is equal, the musicians, the daily carers; we were striving to have an equality there. And not naturally, but probably habitually, people in the management, or in management roles would feel themselves to have more equality with the musicians and it's more of a natural relationship. And I think there's also something about social status in there as well. That the jobs that the care workers are doing are low grade, low paid jobs, and that affects the self-esteem and the confidence to connect with the perceived experts and professionals coming in. And I do think that that is an issue."* Matthew hopes for equal participation from staff, and, however valid his perception is, he detects that the existing dynamics of relationships in the home may need to change in order to achieve a real equality of participation.

Both the musicians and staff have a responsibility towards creating opportunities for residents' well-being, although they may naturally approach this in different ways. This may lead to conflict at times, in the music sessions and debriefs, potentially leading to perceptions that critical judgment has been made. For instance, the musicians may feel at times that staff are making a critique on the quality of the musical outputs or approaches within the session; musicians may seem critical of staff relationships with residents and other staff, or musical consequences of staff actions during the session. Brian feels it is important for both sides to be able to understand the challenges inherent in their roles, and in their work. He expresses that the reality of the situation is that working in a care environment is challenging, requiring an immense level of teamwork between staff and understanding by the musicians: *"I think the thing I would want the musicians to build up over time would be a sensitivity to what a care environment is, and that care is challenging. And that, how would I say? Not to be critical, not to be judgmental of care situations (...) In particular situations it's just really important that musicians are able to identify with the experiences of staff groups working with limited infrastructure, and limited conditions and limited time, and what that must be like."*

One key aspect that was raised during the project was the equal access to opportunities for sustained, intimate interaction with residents. Musicians felt that they were drawing out residents until they were ready to participate as individuals within a group context, yet some staff perceived that some residents could be given more individual attention. This dilemma is highlighted in a joint debrief discussion between musicians and staff from session three. Afterwards, Anneliese reflects on the different perspectives, writing: *"There was a lot of participation by the clients. On the other hand two of them seemed rather sleepy. I still felt they were with us though. (Staff felt very differently about that!)."* For Matthew, he initially feels sensitive, angry, judged in this instance: *"So there was a very direct comment, which almost felt like a bit of a telling off. About, you know, there were some people who didn't get the attention."* However, the issue is more complex than this; perhaps, as Brian states, it is endemic of a feeling of professional responsibility of the staff in their relationships to residents: *"A lot of that then, there was quite a bit of discussion which centred around some residents participating and other residents not participating at all. And there seemed to be a sense of responsibility on behalf of the staff that there were some residents that didn't participate, and they felt quite responsible, but they didn't know how they could do it differently. Because they didn't feel they had the power to intervene. They didn't really feel at this stage that they could do that, so they were agreed and that was a question to bring back to the debrief with the musicians, which we did do. And I thought it was a very good and mature discussion around that."*

For staff, the reality was that they did not feel enabled to, in Matthew's words, *"input and to feel they are leading the work"*. Matthew acknowledges that creating a space where staff feel involved in decision making, engaged as full participants is fundamental, and that this can only happen when staff feel safe and confident. He recognises that creating this space is a responsibility of the workshopleader. Matthew describes after session two the sort of relationship he would like to have with staff, and his aspirations for their participation: *"I guess at this point of the project my focus is still so much on the residents that I feel like I don't put enough into those relationships with the staff, about building those relationships and building their confidence. And they are kind of an add-on a little bit. And if I can include them in pieces, then that's good, but I could do more to incorporate them into the team, and how the team is functioning."* Brian reveals his own aspirations for staff participation, acknowledging after session four that the issues of permission and ownership are still very present: *"I would have liked if, for the staff, there was more of a connection in the sense of staff being able to feel that they can follow through on musical pieces, and that they can take on instruments for themselves and actually join in. And I still feel that they don't feel that, even if this was talked about last week, about their participation and I don't feel that they feel permission yet to do that. (...) I felt today that it still felt the only people who can lead Music for Life are the three musicians."*

However, this narrative begins to change, as both staff and musicians begin to articulate their perspectives with increasing clarity. Finding ways to negotiate and collaborate are a natural part of any collaborative process, as Brian suggests: *"I think every working relationship has to work out how to communicate. And that's what people are doing. In order to work with somebody you have to clarify what your role is. And I think that's what people are saying: what is my role? And how do I communicate with you? And actually, do I have power in this situation? And are my opinions important? That's just what people are articulating."* In addition, to acknowledge vulnerabilities and areas of conflict can entail risk; however, this level of risk is needed in order for a truly authentic collaboration. Brian details the courage of a staff member who was able to express her own vulnerabilities and therefore grow personally and professionally in the process, acknowledging that not all staff have the courage to address these sorts of issues: *"And this team has decided to address it. I noticed the last couple of weeks they've asked questions and they've articulated those questions much more clearly this week. And one person had the courage to actually say that they felt very uncomfortable with an interaction with a musician, a direct interaction between her and a musician. Which I think takes courage to say, so it's about being able to have that, yeah, being able to say, or reflecting on what's happening and they are reflecting on what's happening to them. Not just with the residents. And I think the fact that they're doing that, and not focusing it totally on the residents, is where they will build their strengths. There's a parallel development that's happening alongside of what's happening with the residents."* This point is particularly important; Brian views the project as a uniquely transformative opportunity, one that they can invest in personally at great depth, beyond the responsibilities of their jobs.

This is a view that he holds strongly; in the pre-project interview, he details the growth of staff from other Music for Life projects: *"It feels a bit contrary to the culture they're always working in, and to be able to tune in a little bit into the feelings and to talk about their feelings. What I've noticed is quite a lot of staff don't need a lot of encouragement to do that; that they actually are able to do it. And it affirms my belief that if we give people the opportunities, they will, they will share. A lot of people have those skills (...)*

209

So I think in this forum, people realise and think, oh yeah! This is all it's about, I can do this." It may be initially difficult to share vulnerabilities and perspectives, but where there is a safe and honoured space to share these feelings and thoughts, a community can start to emerge.

Brian describes how this process of belonging begins to emerge for staff and the impact that this has on residents, an awakening inspired by the participation of staff. Staff are clearly becoming more confident and comfortable in expressing themselves through the language of music: *"I was really, really pleased with the fact that from the beginning the three staff were encouraged to have their own instruments and to be part of making the music. I think that helped and that created a sense of group and I think the residents were able to pick up on that, because there were more people beside them playing. So they got a greater sense of what was happening."* Staff now lead and share ownership of the process alongside the musicians, each with their own role to play.

Fiona reflects on the dynamics of this new relationship after session seven, acknowledging the impact that project has made on the staff at a personal level: *"I really feel that the staff have also grown so much. They seemed very comfortable this week. They worked so sensitively with the residents and took the initiative in many moments. They also seemed to enjoy the sessions and really enjoy the connections they had made with the residents."* Fiona detects a greater sense of freedom in staff; they belong, they feel confident, comfortable, and able to enjoy expressing themselves within the group, beyond their roles. Matthew feels this too, reflecting on how this translated into musical connections during the same session: *"We had this crazy shaker piece that started and I don't know how it..., I think I started to make a piece with Gabriella with the shaker and she shied away from being put on the spot. Didn't want to do it publicly. And so Anneliese suggested that Samantha also took a shaker and then somehow we ended up with trying to give everybody shakers and everyone was just sitting there shaking their shakers, waiting for something to happen. And little connections just sparking off around the circle, people caught each other's eye and little conversations going and, I don't know whether Fiona started to play, I think, I'm not quite sure how it happened. And Jessica sitting really upright with a shaker in each hand and really having fun with it. And said, 'who's getting who', I think is what she said. I think she'd really picked up on the sense that nobody was leading and what the fun of that was. That everybody was waiting for something to happen and she said, 'who's getting who'. And Anne then sang it to her. And I sang it back and we had this really, really fun piece. Which was great, great to see Jessica really having a lot of fun with that, I think."*

Here, Matthew details the link between staff taking initiative in their communication and participation, and the impact it has upon residents' participation, in this case, Jessica's participation. It becomes obvious that there is a complex set of relationships at play; everyone is leading and owning the process. It is a process that is uncertain, but in which uncertainty and spontaneity is celebrated, and each voice brings a new dynamic of 'fun' to the improvisation. Furthermore, the ability to engage in such an uncertain, potentially risky creative situation demonstrates a new sense of belonging for everyone, where trust, freedom and respect are key, and shared leadership is essential. Matthew recognises that it takes time for this to happen: *"We know each other and it's okay to have these moments where we just have a moment of nothing happening. It isn't the end of the world. So, it's definitely something you can do when the group has reached that kind of feeling towards the end of a project or something like that, really."*

Matthew sums up the legacy he perceives of the project; learning through the project that he, as a leader, can have a broader view of leadership, and that he is not solely responsible for change, although he is a key figure. Leadership is not just in the realm of the musicians, everyone involved has a part to play, and is a valid member of the group. The legacy the musicians leave behind is not one of music, but one of relationships: relationships of equality, of shared ownership and leadership, of belonging: *"Everyone is part of the team (...) The needs of EVERYONE need to be considered, ALL OF THE TIME. The web of interconnected relationships and needs is so complex. It's not easy to negotiate it, trying to address someone's needs while advocating on behalf of another, and not completely losing sight of some of the main aims of the project, let alone one's own needs. Maybe this is the very crux of the project – it's all about relationships, and not about music at all. Music is just the way in."*

4.4 Development

After an extensive analysis of the categories of 'Identity', 'Communication' and 'Participation' and following the very interesting learning processes that we were able to observe, there remains the question of the actual *result* of the process that we have been able to study: can we discover any developmental progress in the participants? Has a new characteristic of mutual engagement emerged?

What does 'development' actually mean in this context? Is it a continuous learning process drawing upon new experiences, or a qualitative leap in the intelligence and behaviour of all concerned? The question is by no means a trivial one. It addresses the fundamental philosophical problem of how development is to be understood: in the sense of Leibniz, that nature never makes any sudden leaps (*'natura non facit saltus'*)[146], i.e. that there is a continuous process of development, or in the sense of the much older *Menon's Paradox*, in which Plato's protagonist, Menon, in dialogue with his

[146] Leibniz 1704/1756.Vorrede.

mentor Socrates, comes to the conclusion that man is not actually able to learn anything new;[147] "He cannot search for what he knows – since he knows it – or for what he does not know; (...) for he does not know what to look for."[148] The Socratic solution, that he 'remembers' what he already knew at the time of his birth, without any foreknowledge, seems to be an unsatisfactory explanation for our modern way of thinking. The solution must lie somewhere between a continuous accumulation of knowledge and a qualitative new level of intelligence. Hegel, who also advanced the level of developmental thinking during his time, insists on a kind of "leap in quality".[149] For him, the actual 'goal' is important, and it is this goal that should have a different, or a new, knowledge characteristic.

However, is development truly a question of 'goals'? Must our goals always be predetermined? Is not the unexpected interim result sometimes more fascinating than the final result? Are we not surprised by those who achieve stages of development that were considered impossible when we predefined the scope for them? Perhaps, development is therefore not applicable to an individual as such, but rather also pertains to her environment, her sense of integration, and it also applies to the cooperation and support of others.

Indeed, are such preliminary considerations appropriate for the topic of *Music and Dementia*? Can we actually speak about *development* when considering the cooperation with those who live with dementia? Does it not appear to be exactly the opposite to the independent observer: that there is no development at all, and that a possible loss of development prospects must be considered? The previous chapters have certainly shown that the interaction between musicians, residents and care staff, requires a kind of identity formation, through which new forms of communication are created, and participation and a sense of belonging can emerge. But does this not happen in an isolated and situational way? Can that be considered 'development'?

Perhaps, the answers to these questions also depend on empirical examples. A look at the empirical data used will probably be more beneficial than preliminary theoretical considerations. We have been able to identify five distinct dimensions that make the phenomenon of 'development' in the Music for Life project particularly demonstrative to us: the level of *ratification*, whereby the participants become aware that they are part of a developmental process; the dimension of the *improved quality of the team*, which not only enhances the experiences of the musicians, but shows a new quality of cooperation; the insight into the *sustainability* of the collaborative learning process, that admittedly remains fragile; a new kind of learning, that can be described as *transitional learning*; and lastly, the intuitive experience

---

[147] Platon 1988: 37ff.
[148] Ibid: 38.
[149] Hegel 1955: 150.

of belonging to a *community of practice* and the understanding what this means for one's own professional practice.

Ratification

Preceding the project Brian answers a question from the head researcher about how members of staff were chosen for inclusion in the particular project:

"Well, that's again, it's not very formalised, it's not very..., I don't think anything about Music for Life is very fixed, I mean there is a fixed formula, but I think a lot of it are more informal discussions, talking about it. Some of it is about the practicalities. Like, who will be available? Who can make a commitment over eight weeks? (...) After that, it is about a mixture of strength. You need to have some people who are going to go with it, who are really going to be able to support residents, that's a big factor. Because the primary reason why you have staff in the project, regardless of staff development, is that residents are supported. So that's number one. We need to make sure that residents will be supported within the project. And after that it's about ... maybe we can take some educated risks, so you may say. Maybe this person, I think this person really... they have something. I think this will develop them and I think they will be able to go, I hope they will be able to go and take it forward. And there might be other people who maybe... maybe there's something there, and maybe there's simply an opportunity, like a new worker or something, yeah, I do quite like to have some people who are new. On this project we have a new volunteer. So I think it's about... at the start of her career to have a chance to see something which can influence your whole career, about the way you work, your perceptions about people with dementia, your perceptions about how we work, the importance of being able to talk and share, so I think that's good. And then if we feel secure enough, maybe we can take some risks with the fourth or fifth member of the team (...) And maybe this Music for Life project can make a breakthrough, and maybe it won't, but let's take a risk here and let's see. So it's all those factors."

Brian makes it clear at the beginning of the project that 'development' should at least be one of the central options available to the staff. However, development is not something that can be guaranteed by a technical process (e.g. 'staff development') or by rigidly defined goals. Instead, Brian sets two dimensions as prerequisites for the developmental process: the first condition – *"that's number one"* – is the security that the residents will be supported. Changes are unthinkable without this general framework. In practise, this means that he needs to make experienced members of staff available. These staff members are trusted by the residents and are familiar with their particular idiosyncrasies. The second prerequisite is a certain degree of openness to possible learning processes – especially with the new team members: *"like a new worker"*, *"we have a new volunteer ... at the start of her career"*. Development cannot be guaranteed, but the possibility remains: *"maybe this Music for Life project can make a breakthrough."* That is not without an element of risk – *"maybe it won't"* – but the risk is worth it: *"let's take a risk here and let's see."*

As far as Brian is concerned, 'development' has belonged to the Music for Life project from the beginning; a kind of development in terms of qualitative leaps – *"breakthrough[s]"* – is conceivable at the very least. This openness to embrace new ideas, however, is not a particularly risky game. It is based on the assurance that the residents have a sense of security in all circumstances. A risk that would affect them directly would not stand a chance. Brian considers carefully: *"And then if we feel secure enough, maybe we can take some risks with the fourth or fifth member of the team."* Three of four staff members guarantee security in any event. Only when this fundamental condition is met, can the opportunity for new experiences be created for other team members.

For the staff, development is an important professional option, but it is only feasible if security is initially guaranteed for the residents. A foundation of reliability and trust may then be expanded through unplanned developmental processes. Brian does not specify how this would work. He foresees the potential for failure – *"maybe it won't"* –, however he considers the prerequisites of security and openness to learning as factors stimulating development.

This unconventional tension between security and openness is well known amongst the musicians. We will go back to their deliberations as we saw a few of them already in the part on Participation:

Fiona: *"It's really lovely when you (...) can have the scope to express the parts of your instrument in different ways. So for me it was a real treat whenever we met every, when was it, Thursday. Because Anneliese and I, we can kind of share that role, more in support of each other which is really lovely. I like not being responsible for all the harmonic progressions, I always get really nervous about that. So, yes that can have an impact. It sounds really simple, but actually the instrumentation, it's like a chamber ensemble, I guess. What is your role, what is your voice? And until you've worked together I don't think you learn what your voice is. And it felt really nice, actually. Lots of listening, it felt a really sensitive group in terms of everyone was really listening. I love that when it feels there's space."*

Matthew: *"Yeah, there was space. There wasn't somebody just playing and playing and playing. Which can happen."*

Fiona's description shows a feeling of freedom on one hand, and a sense of well-being – *"treat"* – when she ponders on a specific musical experience, namely with Anneliese: *"we can kind of share that role, more in support of each other which is really lovely"*. There is also an aspect of mutual help in the passage. Simultaneously, however, there is an apparent insecurity as well, almost a type of performance stress: *"it's like a chamber ensemble, I guess. What is your role, what is your voice? "*. A solution, when considering development, can only be found when the musicians, together through continuous musical experience – *"lots of listening"* –, can develop a feeling which creates a kind of *"space"*, in which it is possible to move freely with their instruments: *"I love that when it feels there's space"*[150]. The spontaneous reaction from the workshopleader, Matthew, –*"Yeah, there was space"*– supports this feeling.

'Development' is therefore also not merely an educational process for the musicians, where a specific goal is taken for granted, but rather a fragile approach somewhere between anxiously feeling one's way forward and having a certain feeling of security gained through a shared experience. Undoubtedly interesting is the fact that this feeling is directly connected to the metaphor of 'space'.[151] Of course this does not simply refer to a physical space, but rather, as it were, a mutual 'playing space', created to guarantee each participating musician the opportunity to unfold. As in Brian's example, 'development' is therefore established as opportunity and possibility.

The ratification and, likewise, the fragility of the notion of development again becomes very clear in a passage from Fiona's reflective journal that was also processed in the part on Communication[152]: *"I think in previous weeks that we have felt so aware of the fragile state of many of the residents and that there was a real need to create music that reflected how the residents themselves were feeling – even to help validate them. I think this has been right and necessary. However the problem in this is that as musicians you can get very trapped in reflecting the atmosphere and creating music that in a low energy group has no energy. It is important to, at the right moment, use music that is different and 'breaks the atmosphere', especially when wanting to establish a sense of group. We really tried this in session five, and I really felt there was a real breakthrough in the way the group interacted throughout the session. In places I felt that they were carried by our energy and our musical convictions, and that this in many ways created a new sense of life and freedom throughout the group."*

Fiona's thoughts are based on great insecurity: *"we have felt so aware of the fragile state of many of the residents"*, and the danger of feeling trapped in the reflection of the low energy of the residents. But exactly this awareness provides the insight that an alternative is required: music has to be *"different and 'breaks the atmosphere'"*, it can change the ambiance. And that is exactly what happens in this session: *"I really felt there was a real breakthrough in the way the group interacted throughout the session. "*

[150] See also Chapter 4.2 on Communication, under 'Shared leadership'.
[151] See also Chapter 4.2 on Communication.
[152] See Chapter 4.2 on Communication, under 'Leadership in interaction'.

Exactly what caused this 'breakthrough' is not specified. There are no 'recipes' available that guarantee such a breakthrough. Only subtle indications are present which, through the 'drifts' and 'tensions', indicate a kind of developmental process that affects not only the musicians but also the residents and care staff.

This awareness is significant. What Fiona describes is representative of the development idea of the Music for Life project: it is not about a process that is to some extent 'do-able', or which can be manufactured 'instrumentally' so to speak. In fact, it is that process which the logician of pragmatism, Charles Sanders Peirce, described as 'abductive'[153], as a result that could not be previously anticipated. And yet, there are certain requirements for this type of 'breakthrough'. Fiona never refers to the musicians in the singular, always in the plural form ("*as musicians*"). It therefore has to do with a *cooperative* process. Her reflections are not focused solely on the performance of the musicians, but also on that of the residents and care staff. It is the collaboration of the entire group that makes the breakthrough possible: "*the way the group interacted throughout the session.*" That means that the development that is ratified here stems from a collective occurrence, an occurrence that is not guaranteed. There do seem to be certain underlying conditions which facilitate such development, including a high level of sensibility, the ability to pay attention and to react to each other, and the sovereignty to accept the 'otherness' of the fellow participants. This results in a sense of freedom and trust when interacting with each other: "*a new sense of life and freedom throughout the group.*"

During one of the interviews, Brian makes the need for cooperation even clearer, specifically the collaboration between the musicians and the care staff:
"I think the thing I would want the musicians to build up over time would be a sensitivity to what a care environment is and that care is challenging. And, how would I say, not to be critical, not to be judgemental of care situations (...) Because I think it's easy for anybody to come into a care environment and say: 'why don't they do this?' and 'why don't they do that?' 'Why isn't this like this or like that?' That would be easy to do. But if you're to work in care you have to come in and be part of it. What I'm trying to say is, the reality is in dementia, we don't have the resources we would like to have. And we haven't reached where we would like to be. So we need people to be with us, helping and supporting us as we are and not making judgements about us. Hopefully staff working in care environments can be helped to grow, and to move to the next step. We really need Music for Life because we need to grow."

Brian talks about the urgency of the cooperation from the care workers' perspective, and emphasises that the dependence on the understanding of

---

[153] See here again Chapter 3.2.

the musicians is almost 'existential': "*So we need people to be with us, helping and supporting us.*" Overcoming the daily problems is not a special aspect of the care that is provided, but rather the dementia itself, which overwhelms all concerned – especially the care staff involved: "*the reality is in dementia, we don't have the resources we would like to have.*" There are no routines in place to deal with dementia: "*we haven't reached where we would like to be.*" There is only the common endeavour for further development, and to this end, a level of external support is needed: "*Hopefully staff working in care environments can be helped to grow, and to move to the next step.*"

Brian's hopes lie with the musicians: "*We really need Music for Life because we need to grow.*" The provision of care, indispensable such as it is, does not guarantee 'development'. External stimuli are needed, as well as recognition and a sense of purpose, which will give the notion of care a new level of significance. The music is able to make the care staff support the residents, visibly, provided that the music is able to take up this challenge. If so, it will give a lot of purpose to the heavy task of care.

Brian's reflections again make it clear that the way that society deals with dementia is not only a question of professionalism, it also depends on new and creative forms of cooperation. Music for Life is a magnificent opportunity, as Brian considers in one of the interviews: "*Well, I think for me it's about having arrived at a place where there is a group, and that includes musicians, staff and residents. And I think people know one another. But in terms of the work of Music for Life it is very much that being able to believe that it is making a difference. And I think up until now there was a lot of questioning. And my hope for the last sessions has been that people rather accept that this is a powerful interaction that people are benefiting from and enjoy that experience with the residents. And not to worry about it. Cause I feel for musicians that in the initial sessions they're exploring a lot and trying to find a way forward, and trying to find the connections. And I think actually in this group they have been very successful. I've been involved in quite a number of Music for Life projects, and I would rate this a very successful one, if you were to compare projects, in terms of connections being made.*"

It is Brian, the staff development practitioner, who makes the clearest connection between the project's development and the cooperation of the three groups of players, namely the musicians, the care staff and the residents. He also sees the difference between when the project began and its current status: "*up until now there was a lot of questioning (...) actually in this group they have been very successful.*" He therefore discerns the presence of development, and recognises the depth of connections emerging in this particular project. Indeed, the developmental process does not mark itself out by superb musical performances or a visible increase in the professionalism of the care staff, but rather it distinguishes itself by "*the connections being made.*"

Such relationships are also addressed by Matthew in an interview: "*I think, for the people without dementia there's a security in being able to pin things down and understand them and make sense of them for themselves. 'Oh, this piece is about that' (...) We're making a piece about this, that's what we want. And we feel that we've succeeded if we can do that. And just the being there in the uncertainty and allowing that kind of shared discovery with the person with dementia and for the meaning of it to develop, or to become clearer, or clear, is a different process, ... it includes the person with dementia in finding what the piece is or what the relationship ... the piece is about the relationship between the people. In a way, by withholding from imposing meaning on the piece, you're also allowing the relationship to be... you know, what is the relationship between the musician and the person with dementia, and leaving that a bit more open and more equal. This person who comes in from outside on Monday morning from this time to this time, it keeps it clearer and easier to deal with if you define yourself more by deciding what pieces are about and all of that kind of thinking. It's a lot less certain and a bit messier to leave that kind of thing open.*"

The relationship between the musicians and people living with dementia also extends to the music itself, ideally, which is created collectively, it: "*includes the person with dementia in finding what the piece is.*" It is a searching process, trying to find a "*piece*" which is the result of such cooperation. This process requires a certain sense of openness, and activities that work on an equal footing – "*leaving that a bit more open and more equal.*" A significant aspect is that Matthew takes the perspective of the residents – "*This person who comes in from outside on Monday morning from this time to this time*"– and indicates that, in order to reach a higher level of openness in all participants, a raised level of insecurity is necessary for the musicians: "*It's a lot less certain and a bit messier to leave that kind of thing open.*" However, as discussed in the analysis on Communication, frameworks that can provide a sense of security for everyone also play a key role in the sessions; this can seem contradictory to Matthew's statement above. People with dementia may need a lot of repetition, 'pieces', that have already been 'agreed' with the musicians, as with the repeated welcome songs which feature the names of the residents, which have already been extensively elaborated upon in the above.[154]

A central finding in the research conducted by Kitwood[155] is that such 'celebrations' are of great significance for people with dementia, as these provide them with security and protection. It is also an important insight in the experience of the Music for Life project itself, as Brian writes in his

[154] See Chapter 4.1.
[155] See Kitwood 1997: 90.

reflective journal: *"For me, celebration is important. Music for Life is planting a seed of belief in our ability to celebrate and enjoy life with residents ... I felt a great sense of joy in the active participation of the group this week (...) At this stage of the project, I feel that the appropriate questions for staff and musicians are about how to allow the experience to fully enrich our lives, in strong belief that it is enriching the lives of the residents. If we can move on from the project knowing what the experience has given us as individuals, perhaps this is the greatest compliment that we can give to the residents."* Here Brian gives in his reflective journal a wonderful interpretation: the mutual celebration of a song or a piece of music can bring immense joy to everyone involved, and for staff and musicians, experiencing and 'gifting' this joy is a crucial factor in enhancing opportunities for residents' well-being.

Once again, development is not a randomly manufactured state in the Music for Life project, but rather a result that is shared by all participants: the musicians, staff and residents. A particular scene taken from the field notes at the end of the project convincingly illustrates the feeling of community:

> From the field notes:
>
> Matthew continues: "It's been lovely spending time with you and getting to know you, and you getting to know us a little bit too ... and thank you for your music making, and for making music with us, and allowing us to make music with you ... it's been an honour and a privilege, thank you, thank you."The musicians start to thank the group. Gabriella beams and raises her hand to the musicians, waving over the circle to Matthew and then Gabriella says "you're welcome" to Fiona's "thank you." Fiona thanks Rosamund.

The pleasure, the gratitude, and the acknowledgment are all reciprocal. The end result is not simply having met an educational objective, i.e. the pure result of goal-driven processes, but the profound experience of having gained something from being with one another. Musicians, staff and residents have given each other a gift.

In his reflective journal, Brian has a very fitting summary of the special quality of this gift and, at the same time, the characteristics of the 'development' associated with it: *"In the wake of the last session of the project, and feeling the stark reality that people with dementia cannot recall their participation, I feel consolation that if a moment is to be no sooner lived than forgotten, at least, it was a cherished moment and was worth living for its own sake. The musicians are masters of improvisation in the domain of music. However, for me they live on in my memory as masters of the technique of cherishing moments. For them, no effort is too great to achieve a connection. They express it through music and above all they cherish that moment and celebrate it, then and there. Never mind about tomorrow's challenges or yesterday's memories, let's know how to live in the here and now!"*

It is all about the appreciation of the moment, or the moments, in which a feeling of community was present – communality between the musicians and residents, as well as with the staff that also took part in these moments. People living with dementia may have no opportunities to recreate such situations themselves at will. Attempts may be made to find similar moments again, but there are no promises for any success. In this way, instances of this kind of experience are important, as they themselves have intrinsic value for their own sake, 'a cherished moment worth living for its own sake'. Moreover, even if these moments are significant, 'for their own sake', that does not mean that they occur 'by themselves'. They are the result of consistent artistic effort: "*The musicians are masters of improvisation in the domain of music.*" This mastery is, to some extent, a prerequisite for another type of mastery, as Brian explains: "*for me they live on in my memory as masters of the technique of cherishing moments.*" Each of these moments needs a background, needs 'development', needs the growth of its specific sensibility. The project would not be conceivable without this kind of development.

Improved quality of the team

Working in a team during eight sessions was in the first place a task for the musicians. Teamwork, even for experienced groups, can sometimes still be a challenge – especially when their task involves making contact through their music with people with dementia. However, their increasing experience leads to more insights and an increasing sense of security amongst the musicians.

It is interesting to note that, at the beginning of the reflective journal entries, i.e. those concerning the team's cohesion, the focus is not on the artistic quality while playing music together. Matthew emphasises other aspects ("*practical stuff*") such as the seating arrangements and the distribution of the instruments to the residents as a "*great way for the team to connect*". Matthew's reflections are denoted by a remarkable humility. He realises that there are many other important aspects impacting on the sessions beyond purely musical excellence. Indeed, that does not mean that the artistic challenge is less in any way. On the contrary, completely new challenges are created, that particularly concern the team of musicians as a group: "*... there were times when I was sort of going out on a limb, making the pieces with Jessica and with Sarah and they were just really there. I really felt the musical support, they knew what to play at the right time. There were times when I was playing, I took a while to settle on the tonality, or several times, I think, I was kind of exploring and they didn't seem particularly fazed by that. They were kind of groping their way behind me, but found me and so yeah, that was great. Just that support that means that you can push yourself a bit more, I think. You know, when you feel that somebody is there and support, is there musically. You can push yourself both musically and to the degree which you allow yourself to connect, actually.*"

The beginning of Matthew's reflection is a feeling of relative despair: "*I was sort of going out on a limb.*" The attempt to make contact with two of the residents is endangered. His fellow musicians are present at exactly the right moment – "*and they were just really there.*" They help him: "*I really felt the musical support*"; they give him security and self-confidence:"*you can push yourself a bit more*", and facilitate his contact with the residents: "*to the degree which you allow yourself to connect, actually.*"

The 'performance' that results from this process is not actually an artistic matter, but really a *social product*: without Anneliese's and Fiona's musical sensibility, their ability to play along and give him musical security, it would have been impossible for Matthew to establish contact with Jessica and Sarah. In her reflective journal Fiona also confirms Matthew's impression: "*I felt we really came together as a team this week and the music we created felt very supported and coherent. I particularly remember Sarah's piece. It was very much led by Matthew and yet I felt like all three of us were in tune with the situation and the music. We were all on the same page. I felt that throughout the session we were grounded as a team and this helped to anchor some of the rocky and difficult moments.*" Not only does Fiona confirm Matthew's feeling: "*I felt we really came together as a team*", but she also puts the team development back into the greater context of the project: "*I particularly remember Sarah's piece.*" She remembers the musical experience as well as Sarah's 'piece'. Interpreting Sarah's communication was challenging for others and there were, particularly in the beginning, problems in engaging with her: "*some of the rocky and difficult moments*". However, there is obvious success in the musical and social interaction, which not only touches the team of musicians, but also the residents – including Sarah.

Again it is Brian who in his reflective journal explicitly elaborates on the social dimension of the music: "*I found the music very moving and I felt it was generated by the musicians but from the residents. This is a very amazing process. The musicians allow themselves to become the medium of communication for the feelings in the room. It is equally amazing, that even the seemingly least engaged residents are actively communicating and this is translated into music. For example, when some residents were sleeping, I felt that this was reflected in the pace and quality of the music.*" The expression "*generated by the musicians but from the residents*" is characteristic of Brian's sensibility in also seeing the shared development process from the residents' perspective. They actively share in the successful musical improvisation. Even when apparently asleep, they give the music a sense of quiescence and colour. Nevertheless, Brian also shows the highest appreciation to the musicians when he characterises them as the "*medium of communication for the feelings in the room*", turning the active communication of the residents into music: "*even the seemingly least engaged residents are actively communicating and this is translated into music.*" Brian has the gift of putting the different layers of aesthetic, social and ethical development found in the Music for Life project into words and images, and with it he finds convincing forms that express the complex developmental occurrences.

The members of the care staff also take an active part in the learning process:

From the field notes (debrief):

They speak about how Diallo brought the baton to Abigail, and whether this was the right action – although she was "copying rather than leading with the baton" it was seen as a positive action. Deborah says that Diallo was "brave...natural...part of the team today" and just how brilliant he was at "interpreting what Abigail was doing" and judged instinctively during Fiona's piece "just the right time to take the gato drum" from Anneliese. It is also noted that Anne and Diallo kept the rhythm going steadily and appropriately during the 1-2-3-4 section of the instrument activity.

This short scene shows how the 'spark' can jump from one group to another; that the music does not remain with the musicians, but also involves the staff and residents. It is certainly true that this is made possible through the atmosphere that must first be created by the musicians, emerging from their successful collaboration. But it was exactly this sense of security that continued during the actual session, as Matthew observes in the interview afterwards: *"It feels like we've come together very strongly as a team. And that the music is... that we're on the same wave length. We read each other well, and there's very little miscommunication, actually. For all that sort of talk about, 'oh, that happened and it's messy', or dadada, or we try things and they don't work. It actually doesn't feel that way with Fiona and Anneliese. It actually feels like we're very tuned in and we do go in the same direction most of the time. That's good. I don't know what that comes down to. I think it's a happy coincidence, you know, the kind of instinctive thing that we like to work in the same way. They're the same things we're thinking about, we're not pulling in different directions."*

The conviction, or even better, the strong emotion of belonging in a team, one that communicates almost "*instinctively*" is, without a doubt, the result of long and shared experience – "*we've come together very strongly as a team*"–, yet this has to be proven anew for each subsequent project. Matthew succinctly describes the effect of this emotion on all those present and it does not necessarily have to be the final point of the developmental process: "*I don't know what that comes down to.*" The team's development, as high as the level of mutual musicianship may be – "*we're very tuned in*"–, remains open in a sympathetic way.

Sustainability

The emphasis on these 'moments', in which not only a musical, but also a kind of social contact is established between the musicians, the staff and residents, leads to a shared experience which in turn provokes questions of what happens following these 'moments'; what remains of the shared experience? How can the experiences of the eight sessions have a sustainable effect? How can these 'moments' be preserved?

From the field notes (debrief)

Brian raises the concept of legacy and what might happen after sessions. Diallo talks about how they will keep the group together and will meet next Monday. Helena says that they will probably use some very simple piano music, and will include a couple more residents and staff. It is acknowledged that it is important for those residents involved in the project to have some sense of continuity, and that one of the important factors is keeping the group together, whether that be through music or other types of activities.

Symptomatic of their need, the staff members, especially Brian, Diallo and Helena, are interested in preserving the positive experiences attained during the music sessions. They work with the residents – every single day. The danger of 'forgetting' those experiences, and reverting to the normal daily routine, is considerable and is strongly exacerbated by the dementia itself.

However, Brian in an interview correctly points out that the typical misconception that people with dementia are not able to take in or retain an experience which is felt during the positive 'moments' of the sessions, is incorrect: *"I really think if I see these eight weeks what difference it has made for Rebecca and what difference it has made for Sarah ... I think Music for Life is a big factor in Rebecca's change over the last eight weeks. I don't think I need to say more about that, it's just a fact. And I think that will spur the staff on to do something as well. I think that's a big thing."*

Genuine development can incidentally be observed in the individual residents. An example is that Rebecca starts to speak again, after not having said a single word for a long period of time.[156] Other residents reveal new activities, awoken from their states of lethargy. The Music for Life project experience definitely has sustainable effects. Life with dementia is not a state of total 'non-development'; the 'person behind the dementia' becomes more and more visible over time, as Brian goes on: *"I think I will always remember Rebecca in this project and how much she's achieving. And the fact that she's now beginning to say words, and say things. I'm sure it's not just down to Music for Life, I'm sure she's getting more of a sense of belonging in this house and maybe feels a bit more secure. But she's getting some of her voice, her articulation back. She was, often people talk about dementia being just this constant degeneration, there can sometimes be a little bit of regeneration. I think that's happening with Rebecca, it's lovely."*

Brian's idea that Music for Life triggers a process that gets back something which seems lost – in this case it is Rebecca's 'voice' – is provocative and encouraging at the same time. The shared 'moments' described above do have sustainable effects. It would be tempting to fall into the trap of thinking

---

[156] See the following quotation from Brian's interview.

of this regeneration of Rebecca as something that could continue endlessly, that Rebecca could be 'found', never to be lost again. Similarly, Rosamund's and Sarah's journeys can also be perceived in this light, with both individuals expressing themselves in ways that reflect their growing sense of belonging in the group. However, this is a journey that belongs to this community; for the residents, some sense of well-being and learning may be sustained for longer than a moment, through the session and potentially in the hours beyond. However, the reality is that it may not continue in this trajectory. Nevertheless, through consistent attentiveness to the present moment, and an attitude of love and patience, a legacy of positive relationships can form, which can create a deep-rooted sense of belonging. These relationships lead to confidence and familiarity for everyone involved, and with that a sense of belonging to a community where everyone can both form and play their own unique part and where they can express themselves freely and authentically.

"While the music lasts", drawn from T.S. Eliot's poem, finds real meaning in the encounter with people living with dementia. Fiona writes: *"Jessica has made some wonderful pieces over the course of the project but today was a real highlight. There were two pieces that she was very key in: a nonsense-rhyme shaker-piece, 'Who's getting who?', and a wonderful duet with Diallo across the circle. There was a real spark, energy and groove about Jessica this week and it was wonderful to see this! I really loved the obvious relationship that she had with Diallo and in my memory I really saw them as equals. Once again it felt like the 'legacy of relationships' that we hope to leave behind."* Fiona views the proceedings of the project with a perspective of great empathy: she looks at Jessica, who astonishingly becomes an equal partner with Diallo while they are playing music: *"a wonderful duet with Diallo ... in my memory I really saw them as equals."* The scene seems to be a 'legacy' of what could remain, following the intensive eight weeks of the Music for Life project: *"it felt like the 'legacy of relationships'."*

The question of what remains after the project also motivates Harry, the flautist, as he observes in the group interview after the fourth session: *"It goes back to that question that Deborah always used to fire: 'What do we leave behind?' And if we only work with residents, if we only focus on residents, and the staff continue to treat them in exactly the same way as they always have done, the effect will be, we will not really leave anything behind but momentary feelings of well-being. Which can then probably be lost fairly quickly. Whereas if we can show in some way the staff different approaches to dealing with the people that they're dealing with all day, all week; you know, we're only with them for an hour. And if we're able in that hour to get a different response, and maybe a more positive response from residents than they might usually get, then we are leaving something very positive behind."*

Deborah, the project manager is always interested in the pressing question: *"What do we leave behind?"* When talking about the musicians' relationships with the residents, Harry's answer, that the musicians have to create experiences that inspire the staff to develop their own approaches of care, is certainly appropriate, yet it is somewhat general. The observations during a debrief session a few weeks later show a differentiation and, at the same time, a colourful picture:

From the field notes (debrief)

Deborah asks the group, "how do we close session eight ... how do we withdraw carefully?" Helena comments that she feels that "the residents have come together and feel included" and highlights, "Rebecca is so settled in that group." Deborah says that she wants to revisit Matthew's point about changing perceptions. She asks if "the legacy of the project will affect any change after the project's gone, are there any perceptions that might last longer?" Helena says that she feels she knows the group really well now and that it has been a blessing for her in the early stages of working with new staff and residents at Emanuel Zeffert House. She talks about how the project has aided communication and for residents like Sarah and Rebecca that "they feel they are part of something." Jessica and Abigail had remembered that there would be a music session and were looking forward to it during the week. Anneliese says, "we should have prepared them more" for the ending. In the morning of the session, Abigail had said, "Ah, it's the music, isn't it, who is coming?" It is decided that during the week, it should be made clear that next week is the last session of Music for Life. It is also discussed that we should bring cameras next week so we can take pictures of each resident with the musicians for their memory boxes. Matthew talks about how "the legacy has to be in the relationships." He speaks of the relationship between Diallo and Jessica, how it is full of "humour" and "sensitivity" ... "hope it remains." Anneliese says, "I hope it will spread ... go beyond the group." She refers to Samantha's comments of having such a good time with Gabriella, so much fun, and Matthew says, "when would you ever expect that from care staff?" Deborah tells the musicians: "you're role models. Not only the music is inspiring but also the way you communicate ... the way you show your care." Deborah also speaks briefly about the impact they are having on other staff in the home. She says, "it shows in funny ways like 'here's the milk and biscuits'" but that this contact with the other staff "is really important". She also says that she feels the project has been "quite cut off" from the other staff groups, more so than in other projects.

The situation of the last debriefing session convincingly documents to what extent all the participants, the musicians, the care staff, staff development practitioner and the project manager, apply themselves to the project. They define its after-effects, assess the complex influences on the residents, they acknowledge and appreciate the impact beyond the immediate circle of participants. But also, if necessary, they criticise the strict isolation: "*the project has been 'quite cut off' from the other staff groups, more so than in other projects.*"

This discussion is living documentation of the sustainability of the experiences that have left none of the groups without a strong impression: not the musicians, nor the staff members, and certainly not the residents.

Nevertheless, when thinking about real limitations, there remains – as Brian reminisces in his final interview – an element of thoughtfulness, even grief: *"There is such potential that so much can be achieved for people and I do feel the pain and the fact that there's so little, it feels like we're giving so little in comparison. And for me Music for Life highlights that given the circumstances and given the right attention that people with dementia can actually achieve a lot and can communicate a lot. But in our day-to-day working I just feel we have so much to do, we have so much to achieve. I still feel in this home we have an awful long way to go and it's quite, sometimes when I get in touch with those feelings, it's quite a harsh thing to face. And I think staff involved in the project feel that also. They say, 'well that's all well and good, that was Music for Life but our real life is very different from this little snippet'. There are feelings there for all of us to work through as to how we can take what's best from Music for Life and bring good from it that we continue on. And it is very special and the reality is that, you know, it's not possible to provide that all of the time, it's not possible. I still feel a little bit... I'm going to terms with that, really. I know up here, intellectually, but emotionally I feel quite sad. I'd like to be able to produce this for all the residents at least once a week or, you know, regularly (...) I don't really feel that the staff gave very much about how it touched them, how Music for Life touched them in that last debrief. But that's something that will take time. For people to move from the head to the heart level, it's a challenge. I think probably it takes more than one Music for Life project for some people to get there."*

The difference between the two 'worlds' – the Music for Life project on one hand, and the normal constraints of the daily care routine on the other – is a sobering one. Brian even describes a great sense of grief: "*emotionally I feel quite sad* ". Despite a complete willingness to ensure a sustainable effect: "*there is such potential that so much can be achieved for people*", there remains the insight into the disillusionment of the reality: "*I do feel the pain and the fact that there's so little, it feels like we're giving so little in comparison*". The utopia of offering the project to all residents, possibly on a regular basis, and not just for eight weeks with a selected group of participants, is so far removed from reality that the only thing remaining is to capture the undisputed small successes of the project: Brian is certain that the staff members are touched in a completely sustainable way by their experiences with the musicians, even if it takes time to comprehend that this has occurred: "*But that's something that will take time.*" Most likely, he realistically sums up, "*it takes more than one Music for Life project for some people to get there.*"

Interestingly, Brian uses a metaphor in this context, which seems to be typical for the sustainable learning processes in the Music for Life project: "*to move from the head to the heart level.*" A type of development is indicated, that will be discussed in more detail below, a development from 'head' to 'heart', from intellect to emotion. During his interview, another of

Brian's reflections is helpful in illustrating this, and it also refers to the care staff: *"And their own question was: 'what happens now? What happens after Music for Life?' So that's what they're asking. Within that I asked them to look at two separate things, really. One is as a group (...) what they can do and will do with residents. What are they taking away? But the other is about themselves as individuals, is their own personal responsibility, really, is what they as individuals are taking away. How it has impacted on them. What it has said to them about their work, what it has said, what difference has it made to them as a person (...) And that only they, only each individual can take forward in their own way, because I believe it has touched each of them."*

Brian does not doubt that every care staff member is affected by the project experience: *"I believe it has touched each of them."* It interests him that the staff learn to differentiate this impression: *"Within that I asked them to look at two separate things, really "* by asking the question: 'What have I gained professionally from the experience – for my job with the residents?' And at the same time: 'How has the experience affected me personally, my development as an individual?' This differentiation is connected to the difference between 'head' and 'heart', the central message of the citation above. On one hand, there is the career and the professional skills that may be gained, and on the other, there is one's own self and the biographical development as a person.

Brian touches upon an important insight of new scientific learning theory[157]: all strong experiences of staff members that are shared with others, the learning processes that emerge, the development that is triggered; all of these aspects are experienced on their own terms as a unique individual. This does not only apply to the care staff who participate in the project, but also equally to the musicians, and the residents. Sustainable development requires active individuality, which provides the skill needed to be responsible for oneself and others, and also facilitates cooperation – with others and for the benefit of all.

It is without a doubt that the Music for Life project continues beyond the previously mentioned impressive 'moments'. The reflections of the musicians, the staff, the project management and – indirectly – even some of the residents, are all a convincing testimony to the fact that a process of sustainable development has been set in motion. Significantly, Brian, in his role as staff development practitioner, repeatedly indicates the fragility of the development, and that it is particularly endangered by the reality of the daily routine in the care home.

[157] See here in summary Alheit 2009.

Transitional learning

And yet, the notion of learning that is described in the above example, seems to be intriguing – albeit in an unconventionally provocative sense, as Brian comments in one of the interviews: *"But we're not doing enough for people to see what you get back for working in this kind of environment. And Music for Life does that. Music for Life allows people to see how they as people are growing. And it can give people creative ways of growing that they can use in all of their life skills. Which is very, very fulfilling. So that I think is the passion. That bit that people can learn and say, 'this is fantastic'."*

The project Music for Life, according to Brian's conviction, requires 'holistic' learning opportunities: *"it can give people creative ways of growing that they can use in all of their life skills."* The special aspect is that the participants are able to observe, as it were, the way that they themselves change: *"Music for Life allows people to see how they as people are growing."* The project creates the prerequisite of reflexivity, which affects one's whole life. *"Growing"* means more than simply understanding. It includes the entire being: intellect and emotion, 'head' and 'heart'. Brian classifies this learning process as *"fulfilling"*, as *"passion"*, and *"fantastic"*. Such euphemisms naturally lead to scepticism. They require extensive empirical data, as drawn from the pre-project group discussion:

Fiona: *"You're constantly challenged and you connect with the people you're working with, and you also connect with more of yourself, I think. Because you're constantly looking at yourself as a musician and as a person. So it's a very rich kind of place of work, I think. If that makes any sense."*

Matthew: *"Yeah, absolutely, it makes sense. The thing that you said about ... that is one of the personal challenges. It does challenge you to connect with yourself, and to be honest with yourself."*

Fiona: *"Totally."*

This is the challenge – first and foremost as a musician, but then also as an individual – as alluded to by Fiona. She obviously refers to the encounter with people living with dementia. To be confronted by them does not merely mean finding the right music, the right 'piece', i.e. a successful collaboration with other musicians and the residents, but also to find a new regard for oneself: *"you connect with the people you're working with, and you also connect with more of yourself"*, or, as Matthew puts it, *"to be honest with yourself."*

Thinking back to the moment where Rosamund had to be hoisted from her wheel chair into an arm chair[158], Matthew and Fiona comment:

---

[158] See also Chapter 4.1 on Identity.

Matthew: *"That was a very important moment."*

Fiona: *"Yeah, for me too, really influential in how I will think about the work. And what are you trying to create, and how. Because you can sometimes want to create this bubble, but actually that bubble needs to be grounded in reality. And that means that everyone coming in with their baggage, so to speak, 'cause we bring our own in. And you know, it's like, 'how do you create this safe space, where it's okay to be exactly as you are in that moment?'"*

The repeated realisation that the indignity, which Matthew and Fiona feel when they see the hoist being used for Rosamund, does not diminish Rosamund's dignity, but rather starts a process which in turn gives her a new level of dignity in their eyes, really seems to provide a new characteristic of the musicians' insight when dealing with people with dementia. This realisation changes the creative approach used by them to some extent; it places it on a new foundation: *"you can sometimes want to create this bubble, but actually that bubble needs to be grounded in reality."* This is the 'safe space' that gives the musicians the authority and opportunity to completely be themselves.

This 'transitional learning' is an irrefutable fact. Fiona elaborates on this idea in her journal: *" 'Permission to be real' needs to be a core aim for us as individuals and as a team. Integrity is a core value in Music for Life – integrity as a musician, as a person, as a team and in what we are wanting the residents and staff to experience. We need to give permission to people to be just as they are – whether that is using a hoist or feeling free to express an emotion like anger or joy. Music is a really safe and inclusive medium to enable this to happen."* The chance to be 'real', the integrity to be able to express and live one's own 'self' is a privilege, it is a prerequisite of the learning process; to let others be as they are, to allow them to recognise their own 'otherness' – as is the case with Rosamund. Music helps with this recognition, because integrity, as Fiona describes, belongs to the very core of values but, at the same time, music is not a guarantee that such recognition is successful. It is a *"medium to enable this to happen"*. The prerequisite is that it is always a learning process for the participants, a strategy that creates a new characteristic, but which also contains risks.

Matthew says in an interview, relating to playing with Rebecca: *"It's like releasing something. It's interesting. It's like that thing of almost, like I said, that I was able to tell Anneliese how moving I felt her playing was. It's like a similar thing, the kind of release of doing the thing that you're slightly afraid of doing, maybe. Or the thing that for some reason you hold back from doing. Because it's gonna be too intense. That you're afraid of the intensity and it breaks through the etiquette in a way, and it's going to expose yourself. Yeah, exposing for the resident as well to have all that focus on you and for it to be really very intense in the way it was. It's very exposing."*

The musical communication with Rebecca creates "playing spaces" that also open new dimensions for Matthew and Anneliese: Matthew is affected by Anneliese's playing, and her music touches and challenges him to open up in turn. He is quite apprehensive –"the thing that you're slightly afraid of doing"–, the music could become too intense or the focus upon him could become too great, and therefore it could lead to unexpected outcomes: "That you're afraid of the intensity and it breaks through the etiquette in a way, and it's going to expose yourself."

However, the foundation is not merely playing music, but the (aesthetic) communication with Rebecca. The new characteristic – intensity that produces anxiety – can be a natural part of communicating with people living with dementia. Matthew's attempt to cope with his own anxiety, with the justification that the focus on the residents could become too great, is not particularly convincing. Perhaps the real reason was, as Matthew stated in the group interview, to "create this safe space, where it's okay to be exactly as you are in that moment." It is exactly this aspect that is also applicable to the residents. Matthew's sensibility, his honesty in speaking about his subtle anxieties show the ambivalence, and to some extent, the risk that the project carries. On the one hand there is an opportunity to go beyond the limit, for example in the incident with Rosamund, namely the discovery of a new dimension of 'dignity', and on the other hand the vulnerabilities and anxieties that are connected with these transitional learning processes. Both aspects are also made clear in Matthew's reflections at the end of the project: "And so the time to end the project arrives. As usual, it feels as though it has come too quickly, too abruptly for everyone. It feels as though we are just starting to really get to know the staff, they are opening up, letting us see more of themselves, their sense of humour, their musicianship. As a musician team we have become very close on this project – closer than usual. We have all been moved hugely by this project, by each other's work, by the courage and effort that has been made by the participants. And for the residents, it feels as though we are abandoning them, just when they had begun to trust us. But we know that it is important to leave, and the fact that it feels as though it is too soon, that we can't lose what we have worked so hard to achieve, means that we know it has been deeply valued, and that something will remain. The staff have decided to keep the group together, meeting on Monday mornings to have some musical activity, but mostly to explore communication, and to preserve the sense of group that has been established, and this is great. From this, hopefully, things can ripple out to the rest of the staff and residents."

Matthew talks about the different dimensions of the learning process; first, it seems that all participants feel quite sure that something very important has occurred, despite the fact that the Music for Life project has finished much too early – "we have all been moved hugely by this project"– and that it has a sustainable effect: "that something will remain." Second, he feels that the learning process has not only affected and changed each individual, but also the entire team – the musicians: "*As a musician team we have become very close on this project – closer than usual*"; the care staff – "*they are opening up*"– and also the residents: "*The staff have decided to keep the group together (...) to explore communication, and to preserve the sense of group.*" Lastly, the described process does not conclude with the end of the project, but continues, with different conditions. In some ways it is actually just at the beginning: "*It feels as though we are just starting.*" The project is therefore a milestone, a transition to another reality: between the musicians and the people with dementia, between the musicians and the care staff, and between the care staff and the residents.

Anneliese writes in her journal: "*Looking back from here to session one, I do feel we have all been on a long journey together. What a difference in understanding and trust amongst all of us! And although I am leaving this group behind with a heavy heart I know and trust we have made sufficient impact on staff for the 'seed we have sown to grow'.*" Anneliese confirms the certainty that something will remain and unfold later: "*the 'seed we have sown to grow'*".

Fiona discovers an additional aspect: "*It has been a wonderful, intense, challenging, emotional and rich experience and has felt like we have really worked at a real depth throughout the project. It feels like it has had a real emotional weight to it, and I'm not sure if this is due to the research element that has made us reflect even more on our work and carried the residents through the whole eight weeks or simply just that it has been one of 'those' projects.*" She considers whether or not the "research element" of the whole project has influenced the intense emotional process of reflection, perhaps has even provoked it, in that it constitutes its very nature. She leaves this question open. Perhaps, so she writes, it was only one of those exceptional projects that exist, but that do not represent the norm. In any case, she is also convinced that something extraordinary has happened during the eight weeks.

Brian's summary sounds somewhat more contemplative: "*I've been into the home a few times since Monday and I've met some of the residents who took part in the project. I am very conscious that [for them] the project has come to an end and I feel a sense of loss on their behalf. However, as far as I can tell, they are unaware of this loss. They were part of something beautiful and it was now consigned to the past. For me, I can relive moments of the past from my memory. I feel very conscious of how special that is. I remember the faces, the sounds, the gestures and, most of all, the emotions in the Music for Life sessions. I remember the emotions evoked in me and the emotions that I saw in others. I find myself thinking about it and reliving it. However, for the primary protagonists of Music for Life, this reliving of the experience through memory seems to be denied to them through the condition of dementia. I am struck by the enormity of this loss. I can hardly imagine what life could be like without being able to recall pleasant and fulfilling events, emotions, encounters and thoughts that have made up my day."*

Brian's conclusion seems to be somewhat disillusioning: from the residents' perspective, the project is over. Despite the fact that they may have taken away some of the good and significant experiences or emotions in the 'moments', actual memories of these do not remain. Compared to Brian's own associations, which are essential to him: "*I can hardly imagine what life could be like without being able to recall pleasant and fulfilling events, emotions, encounters and thoughts that have made up my day*", he is somewhat aggrieved by this insight: "*I am struck by the enormity of this loss.*" However, the very fact that Brian has been affected so deeply by this sense of loss, means that a legacy can emerge; his empathy in understanding residents' sense of loss can be carried into the way he interacts more generally with people living with dementia.

It is precisely the challenging relationship, between *moment* and *duration*, between *situational experiences* and *sustainable learning* that makes the Music for Life project so worthwhile. It shows that dealing with dementia cannot be reduced to more or less effective techniques when managing the condition, but that it represents a challenge for all participants, one which forces both musicians and care staff members alike to engage in developmental processes that extend their limits. Perhaps it is not even excessive to say that it is society as a whole that is challenged by dementia, and that it is not merely a matter of creating a new process, but also a *new set of ethics* when dealing with a social group that is continually growing. The Music for Life project gives us an indication of how both a humane and creative process could be applied when dealing with people who have, until now, been out of our society's focus, but who will surely shift to the centre of social and healthcare policies in the next decades.

Community of practice

Finally, we want to re-examine this conclusion on a theoretical level that makes the notion of development in the researched project somewhat clearer: the emergence of a *community of practice*.[159] We will see that we are not dealing with pure theory, but with a concept that is closely linked to a pragmatic process, supported by real data.

The concept of the communities of practice, as developed by Jean Lave and Etienne Wenger[160], two education researchers from the USA and Switzerland who were interested in anthropology, is a social arrangement, or 'situated learning' experience[161] – to express it more clearly: organisational

---

[159] See Chapter 2.3.
[160] See Lave and Wenger 1991; Lave 1991.
[161] See also Chapter 2.3.

forms that enable learning processes which can exist and grow in ordinary, yet 'natural' situations. Communities of practice specifically should not be didactic institutions wherein teachers impart abstract knowledge to their students. It is more a matter of a living process of inspired experience, whereby *newcomers* gradually and autonomously approach the experience of the *old-timers*, and – simultaneously – not only gain knowledge and skills, but also develop their personal identities.[162]

Lave and Wenger talk about "full participants" in a community of practice and about "legitimate peripheral participants."[163] This differentiation is interesting, because even the newcomers, who do not have the knowledge and experience that the old-timers do, play a legitimate part. They are legitimate participators. The feeling of 'belonging' is a foundation of trust that is essential for any learning process. Life itself is not an exchange from 'top' to 'bottom', it is not a teacher-learner relationship. It is – as in the case of the newcomers – a continuous awareness of what the experienced members of the community actually do, to try something out by themselves; a piece of advice that is sought to answer a specific question of interest. It is, in the best sense, a relationship between master and apprentice, as an effective master is not a typical teacher. Masters rather "usually do not have a direct, didactic impact on apprentices' learning activity, although they are often crucial in providing newcomers to a community with legitimate access to its practices."[164]

An example that is often referred to by Jean Lave is interesting because it comes from a pre-modern culture: the education of the midwives in the Yucatec Maya in Mexico.[165] The 'period of apprenticeship' is incorporated in normal daily routine. This would never be understood as a process that is explicitly 'taught'. As a general rule, a Mayan girl who will eventually become a midwife in later life, has a mother and a grandmother who are also midwives, as midwifery is passed along the generations of the family line.[166] Here, the community of practice is the intergenerational cohesion of the female members in the family tradition of midwifery. There is learning *en passant*, as it were. As time passes, the newcomers eventually become the old-timers, but they are legitimate peripheral *participants* from the very start.

There are also modern examples, such as *Alcoholics Anonymous*, whereby similar participatory learning processes may be observed.[167] Additionally, our own research material also has very interesting evidence, which leads us to

---

[162] See Lave 1991: 68.
[163] See Lave and Wenger 1991: 35ff.
[164] Lave 1991: p. 68.
[165] See Lave 1991: 70ff.
[166] See also Jordan 1989: 932f.
[167] See Lave 1991: 72f.

consider a community of practice. An insightful conversation in the team illustrates this:

Matthew: *"I think what you said about filtering down is key. I remember you talking about the organisation as being a community of learning and I figure that's absolutely right. That people are drawn closer and closer and that the knowledge that we have is tacit, and it's not bullet point. You cannot kind of break it down in bullet points (...) it is an internalised and an experiential learning that you can't explain! That comes up again and again!"*
Anneliese: *"That's the next one, isn't it, how do you... I still find it sort of hard to describe the work if people ask me what I do. You can say something quite quickly, but that doesn't mean that people really understand what you're doing. And that says sort of something about it in a way, doesn't it?"*
Matthew: *"Yeah, very much so."*
Anneliese: *"And sort of how you teach it or learn it."*
Matthew: *"And it only can be through, almost apprenticeship. Isn't it? That's sort of the system that we found works the best. Yeah. As you were talking then I was just thinking about how I, I think that's the thing that binds the team together as well, because you've shared these experiences which you can't explain to anybody else. So you feel understood by each other."*
Fiona: *"Respect is the word I had in my head, again and again."*
Matthew: *"Yeah, absolutely. We have this shared experience which can't be articulated and shared with other people. Which is common with other sort of shared experiences, maybe religious experiences or family experiences. You know, a family culture where things can't be explained or shared. Friends that you shared a lot with sometimes, that's a bit a similar thing."*

Many statements in this conversation are instantly evocative of Lave and Wenger's *community of practice*: the explicit mention of a "*community of learning*", Matthew's association of the "*apprenticeship*" status, and the several references to "*shared experiences*". The most impressive aspect is perhaps the simple consensus on the difficulty of describing what one actually does: "*I still find it sort of hard to describe the work if people ask me what I do*", as Anneliese puts it. The fact that, so to speak, only he or she who shares the experience directly can know exactly what it is about, shows the implicit character of the learning process that takes place, thus gaining the competences, that one inherently possesses. "*The knowledge that we have is tacit*", Matthew appropriately comments.

The British-Hungarian natural scientist and philosopher Michael Polanyi[168] describes this 'tacit dimension' as something that we do not consciously control, but which gives us the *ability* to accomplish certain things. Polanyi

---

[168] See Polanyi 1966; 1969.

speaks about *tacit knowing,* in order to clarify the process in which this implicit knowledge – an existing disposition, not a conscious ability – is created. 'Ability' is – according to Polanyi – therefore always more than 'knowledge'.

Not only do Matthew, Fiona and Anneliese express themselves intuitively when they refer to the almost indescribable notion of 'surplus knowing', but they also refer to a dimension that they all share. Matthew quite rightly parallels this with a religious or intimate experience. The *tacit dimension,* therefore, does not only express an individual ability, but to some extent it also refers to a community of practice. Matthew elaborates on another aspect: *"There's a very strong bond between the musicians. Very strong. And it's a tricky thing with bringing new people in. It takes a while for that to develop (...) It's not just about being accepted into the wider group, but there needs to be a kind of an opening up from the new musicians as well, it's a two-way process (...) We need to be open to new people bringing new things as well to the work. And people of themselves can be very protective of the work as well. I think there needs to be some agreement about, what are the things about the work that are at the core of it that are unchangeable. Things that I don't fight what it is. That there needs to be openness as well for new musicians to bring fresh thoughts and fresh insights. I think the new musicians need to work a lot with people who have been working for a long time. They need to work alongside them a lot and build, I mean, they need to build those friendships in the same way that we want to develop with the staff."*

Matthew describes the dimension that Lave and Wenger call *legitimate peripheral participation*[169] and which constitutes the origins of the learning processes of the communities of practice. He is concerned with the question of openness for new members of the 'musical community': *"That there needs to be openness as well for new musicians..."* and the way that they may be integrated. He suggests a shared experience with the 'old-timers': *"I think the new musicians need to work a lot with people who have been working for a long time."*

Matthew's wording, that the new members should work *"alongside"* those members who have more experience, that is 'side by side' and not in a subordinate way or as a 'student', subject to instruction, is interesting. This *en passant* method of learning, on an equal footing, is precisely how Lave and Wenger's envisaged the growth into a community of practice.[170] This results in participation, cohesion and 'friendship'.

We see that Matthew connects the integration of the musical newcomers with the incorporation of the care staff here as well: *"I mean, they need to*

[169] See also Chapter 2.3.
[170] See again Lave and Wenger 1991: 35ff.

build those friendships in the same way that we want to develop with the staff." This means that he is not only concerned with a 'community of musicians', but a community that embraces the entire Music for Life project experience. Matthew continues:

"In that, for the musicians to have a sense of well-being and that they're doing a good job, they need to feel that they're playing well together, that they're expressing themselves musically, that they see the residents participating. So they're dependent on that for their sense of well-being. Dependent on the residents having a good time and that they're participating. They're dependent on the staff as well, the staff feeling relaxed and taking initiatives, expressing themselves. So the musicians kind of feed off all of that. And for the staff, for them to feel that they are finding their place within the projects. We were asking these questions before, you know, what can we do, and today there was a sense that they knew what to do. They felt comfortable about taking initiatives, they felt comfortable about expressing themselves, both musically and verbally and in a way that they're supporting the residents. There was a lightness to it as well. They have an innate knowing of what to do. But then that's uncovered, or they've been given permission to do that by the team of musicians."

Matthew makes it convincingly clear that the prerequisite to perform well in the project not only requires the feeling that the musicians are *"playing well together, that they're expressing themselves musically"*, but that the residents and staff members become involved: *"they're dependent on that for their sense of well-being. Dependent on the residents having a good time and that they're participating. They're dependent on the staff as well (...)."* This does not mean that the successful interaction of the musicians is not a central source of accomplishment when it comes to communication, but rather that there is something more: the inclusion of the residents and the care staff. The community in question therefore also encompasses musical aesthetics and communicative socialisation. This is not limited to the three musicians, but also applies to the residents and the staff.

That the care staff members open themselves, feel good – *"they felt comfortable"* – and seem to know intuitively what to do – *"They have an innate knowing of what to do"* – during the project's progress yet again points to Polanyi's *tacit knowing*[171], which is so typical for the learning process present in the communities of practice. The idea that there is an opportunity to build communities of practice from the Music for Life project, which involves all participants: the musicians, the care staff and the residents, is, without question, fascinating.

Matthew later extracts some compassionate self-criticism from this perspective in an interview: *"It's something that I would certainly consider on*

[171] See above.

all projects. Thinking about how much of the leadership can be shared with the intention of leading in that way, of allowing as much as possible for everybody to input and to feel they are leading the work. And as an idea it goes beyond the musician team. You want everybody in the group to feel that, the care staff, everybody. I forgot Brian one week. We'd talked about wanting this more direct communication with the staff and so I had this very quick conversation with Brian, and the minute I said what I'd said, I could see that I'd forgotten he's part of the team too. So it's an interesting thing, leadership is, as I'm really becoming more and more aware of, it's not about telling people what to do. Really not. If you really are truly leading it's about everybody fulfilling what is possible for them to do and almost, the ultimate achievement would be for you to disappear, for you not to be there anymore. That the group is completely able to support itself without you. That's what would be the ultimate, really. I can't remember who I was listening to the other day who said you should plan for your own extinction."

'Leadership' is, as we have seen throughout this chapter, obviously part of Matthew's identity. In the light of his experience in the project, he has grown fundamentally as a leader, recognising and understanding the principle of a community of practice, tacitly, as it were: "*If you really are truly leading it's about everybody fulfilling what is possible for them to do and almost, the ultimate achievement would be for you to disappear, for you not to be there anymore. That the group is completely able to support itself without you.*"

It becomes clear from this remarkable statement, that the Music for Life project not only represents a simple community of practice, but also more of a radical variation of it: where music and dementia encounter each other and are connected by care, all participants are *apprentices* in an equal way. No single person is the 'master'. Those who have experience at one level are 'newcomers' at another. Those who are 'newcomers' here could be 'old-timers' there. The integration of musicians and care staff members into a community is exemplary. The condition of dementia remains a challenge that can only be met with completely new and creative processes and models of practice. Music for Life is an outstanding example.

Conceptual summary

The notion of 'development' is a dichotomous one. The standard association is that certain things progress – mostly in a continuous way, occasionally in qualitative leaps. The great modern philosophers have differing opinions on this subject. We have quoted Leibniz's belief that nature cannot make leaps, and it is Hegel who tells us to envisage developmental progress as a new quality. There are, of course, many different and well-justified theories that lie somewhere between these two positions and plausibly prove a differentiation between the two. But does that help us?

Our research material proves the previously mentioned dichotomy in a rather drastic way. On the one hand, when interacting with people living with dementia, completely new qualifications and learning processes seem to be required. We can prove that such developmental processes take place. On the other hand however, the modern idea that the potential for any development is fundamentally possible must be abandoned outright: dementia blocks progress; dementia renders 'planning in advance' as absurd. Brian's somewhat aggrieved statement at the end of the project shows that what remains is a realistic experience: *"However, for the primary protagonists of Music for Life, this reliving of the experience through memory seems to be denied to them through the condition of dementia."*

This challenge is inherently applicable to modern society: Is continuous progress really possible? Or more accurately: Is indefinite progress actually useful? As we well know, dementia is, due to demographic changes, increasing. It cannot be ignored, even within the scope of an average family's daily routine, and it requires different solutions. Therefore we need time to quietly contemplate the notion of 'deceleration'. We also need new forms of cooperation, civilian and humane conditions that are needed for a meaningful life, *for* and particularly *with* those living with dementia.

The Music for Life project sets a milestone in this respect. The connection between music, care and dementia makes all of the aspects of cooperation visible. The impressive reflections provided by all participants in the researched project have revealed the inherent difficulties but have also shown the enormous possibilities, which can inspire projects elsewhere.

There are alternatives in understanding dementia. The idea that dementia seems to be an irreversible stop to human development can teach us something: it forces us to think about the modern world with its absurdly accelerating sense of urgency.[172] This questioning leads to the modest conclusion that there is no such thing as a patent remedy when 'dealing' with dementia, but rather that we need solidarity, creativity, and also new working processes, perhaps even a new *set of ethics*, to approach this problem as a community, a problem which could affect each and every one of us at some stage. Music for Life has broken new ground in this respect. The project's courage serves as an inspiration to all.

[172] See Rosa 2004.

5

…you are the music

While the music lasts

Conclusions and Discussion

It is not heard at all,
But you are the music
While the music lasts

T.S. Eliot[173]

5   Conclusions and discussion

The splendid research material which we had at our disposal, the interviews with the many participants, the group discussions, the field notes, but, above all, the reflective journals of the musicians and the staff development practitioner constitute an exceptionally detailed and highly differentiated source of data about a cooperative learning process. While this process spanned eight weeks, it also opened much wider horizons as it incorporated long-term professional experiences. It also established links and contrasted between very different perspectives on the undertaken process, for example, by comparing the perspectives of the musicians with those of the care staff, or those of both of these groups with that of the residents.

Reflections on chosen qualitative approach

Bringing together these complex experiences, processed by us as qualitatively working researchers in previous chapters into *thick descriptions* (Clifford Geertz), illustrates a further perspective. It is of course beneficial that two of us are also professional musicians, nevertheless it remains a fact that as scientists we have an alternative view on the events compared to those of the musicians or the care staff, and that our results need to be weighed up against those of all other participants. Research in the framework of *Grounded Theory*, as outlined in Chapter 3, was not done for the sake of itself, but was done in the interests of those with whom and about whom the research was undertaken.

Therefore, as we have already established, we consciously chose a qualitative approach. This again should be clarified. It means that the classic quality criteria of quantitative research need to be adapted for qualitative processes. Objectivity, then, cannot be the goal, as it is especially the subjective perspectives of the participants that form the basis of the research, be they personal views of the world or personal world-coping mechanisms. Genuine *reliability* is not attainable because the collected qualitative data gathered during 'real-life situations' is not repeatable, as it is a process of concrete interaction, observation or reflection in itself. Moreover, *validity* in the sense of the desired knowledge that what could be 'measured' should actually be measured seemed problematic as in general

---

[173] From: The Dry Salvages, 1941.

at the start of the research, it is not yet wholly clear what might be 'measurable'. Fundamentally, the question remains if 'measuring' should not be seen as an inappropriate approach to this research process.[174]

That is not to suggest that the qualitative process we selected is not justifiable, unreliable or even arbitrary. It is just that the processes of legitimation for justifiability and generalisation, for dependability and validity, are systematically different in the qualitative process of research: instead of 'objectivity', the qualitative process of research emphasises the *adequacy of the subject*. The 'process-nature' of processes, as well as 'routines', need to be observed, reconstructed and understood in their very own structure. The uniqueness of a particular process of development only comes to produce results through a lifetime of reflection. This is why the choice of this method is so important. The narrative interview is, for example, a 'best choice' option in order to reconstruct individual phases of development. Nonetheless, it is not suitable for every topic of research or, moreover, every target group. Studies in South Korea have for instance shown that, in the elderly generation of a society based on Confucian values, a biographical narrative interview is seen as a 'loss of face'.[175] Group discussions are meaningful for the collective formation of opinions, but they can also suppress the dispositions of the individual. The basic method of every ethnographical analysis is one of participatory observation. This may however run the risk of *going native*, i.e. of losing methodological distance. The research process has to be methodologically appropriate to the object of study; otherwise, persuasive results cannot be expected. It is not by coincidence that we chose a *mixture of methods* as our medium. This was necessitated by the great differences in situations as well as groups with which we worked.[176]

The 'reliability' of qualitative research cannot be based on being able to repeat identical research settings. Such arrangements may be useful in a laboratory, but these are not the goals of qualitative social research where 'natural situations' and everyday social settings are at the core. Such situations are, of course, artificial in a true sense when we look at them qualitatively. Researchers become 'co-actors' when they moderate an interview, when they openly observe a situation, or when they initiate a group discussion. This artificiality, however, is reflexively accessible as it is readily identifiable in the data and in the evaluation process. The reliability of qualitative research is therefore based on the *careful documentation and reconstruction of the research data gathered during comparatively 'natural situations'*. And it is exactly this that was achieved in the Music for Life project.

---

[174] See Alheit 2012.
[175] See Lee 2002.
[176] See again Chapter 3.3.

The 'validation' of the qualitative process is not dependent on the conclusion that 'what we wanted to measure has been measured'. Exact measurements are not the goal of qualitative analyses. More fundamentally it is a question of *understanding* complex, often fuzzy and diffuse social connections. For this, processes of construction and of interpretation are required. *Validation is only possible 'communicatively'* by balancing individual readings and proposals of interpretations with the ideas and suggestions of others. Therefore, we placed an especially high value on the reflections of the participants as we valued their interpretations and did not want to put our interpretations 'above theirs'.

In our research findings below we will focus on the musicians. There is a great need for research that can underpin the development of new practices for musicians, where they engage with audiences other than those in the concert hall.[177] It is undeniable that the care staff will also benefit from our results. This is convincingly shown by our outcomes. The available results can be of great use and provide hope, even in families where a member lives with dementia. However, the core topic is *Music and Dementia*.

Research findings

So what are the results of our research according to these criteria? What does it mean to identify the 'core categories' of our data as *Identity, Communication, Participation* and *Development*? What perceptions and associations do we have with these four categories and how can they be broadened and deepened? How are they connected, and which perspectives emerge by their connectedness?

Identity, as we have established[178] "exists on a personal level as well as on a group level. The musicians' learning process and, in the end, their development towards 'acceptance' lead to an identity that is a constructed version of 'becoming' through learning."[179] Identity develops according to George Herbert Mead's classical interpretation:

> It is not initially there at birth, but arises in the process of social experience and activity, that is, develops in the given individual as a result of his relations to the process as a whole, and to other individuals within that process.[180]

Musicians appear to be particularly sensitive in terms of this construction. Their performances are in a specific sense 'public', even if they take place privately. Part of the professional identity of the musician is also to always have in mind their own music 'teacher', the perspective of the (fictitious) audience, and even the immediate reaction of that with which 'I', as a

---

[177] See also Preface.
[178] See Chapter 4.1, conceptual summary.
[179] See Chapter 2.3.
[180] Mead 1967: 168.

musician, am currently working. This connects musical identity to the context and makes it into a social phenomenon. However, this also confirms the fragility of identity and threatens it yet again. The stage fright that every musician knows, the difficult experiment with successful improvisation,[181] even the insecurity of how to deal with an audience with dementia, show that identity must always be re-established. Musical identity is a struggle with *self-assurance* and *personal development*. And this struggle is a very personal and intimate process, regardless of the concrete context.

If *identity* is therefore a key to our data then it primarily addresses the fact that in an encounter between music and dementia a great many 'obvious expectations' get out of balance. This realisation is an individual challenge for each of the participating musicians. This, of course, applies equally to the care staff, and all participants have to be willing to engage in a *learning process*. 'Identity work' is therefore in a sense a prerequisite for the shared activity in the Music for Life project. This is not some sort of routine arrangement, but instead, it is an open process of learning that guides the whole project.

Nonetheless, this process of learning is dependent on *communication*, being the second core category that our data presents. Just as we view ourselves through the eyes of another when we try to build our own identity, so we also need to communicate with others to still further develop our identity. This is especially true when we, as musicians, are confronted with people who at first sight seem to have lost their identity and whose reaction to our performance is unpredictable.

The desire to communicate with others, to interpret and understand difficult situations, to create solutions, and to establish contact with people with dementia, and to do so with musical sensitivity, is essential and self-evident. The complexity which communication exemplifies in the Music for Life project has been presented in detail in the analysis.[182] It deals with the various forms of language: verbal and non-verbal, in essence also the language(s) of music. It is about interaction and interpretation, about places of communication and means of communication. Occasionally, it is also about overcoming misunderstandings. Communication is a social activity that relies on *self-assurance* and *social sensitivity*. As such, it moves between the extremes of 'personality' and 'sociality'.

The dimension of communication we analysed has little to do with conventional definitions of signal theory such as 'transmitters', 'receivers' and 'filters'. This is equally true of classic action-theoretical concepts that assume clear goals and obvious purposes of communication. It is easiest to comprehend the concept of communication used here by examining what

---

[181] See Smilde 2009: 146 ff.
[182] See Chapter 4.2.

George Herbert Mead wanted to express in his *game*-metaphor[183]: an intuitive rule-governed anticipation of 'players' in relation to the behaviour of other 'players'. When musicians, through improvisation and with great sensitivity, respond to people with dementia and the latter become involved in the 'playing', then what results is really a *game* in which each participant reacts sensitively to the other, and where the co-players are 'brought into the game' through their efforts. Musical communication is complex and varied, but has little to do with rational planning. It is a means of communication that is based on rule-governed intuitions that connect tensions that are intimately personal with those that are empathically social.

Our third core category *participation* is already inherent in this concept of communication. The connection of the individual with the social has a concrete focus: the *living group* in which all are participating. Belonging to the group is not, of course, a 'status', it is not a legal title that has always existed. *Belonging* is a process that has to be actively introduced. Participation, therefore, does not only mean *social sensitivity*, as is a characteristic of communication, but also implies *social activity* such as the willingness to integrate and to apply one's abilities in the group, the desire for tolerance, and to be able to respect and embrace the conceptual ideas of everyone else.

Participation in the Music for Life project has many forms: creativity and intuition, respect and empathy, and responsibility of care. It also has a great variety of participants: the musicians who create a new atmosphere through their participation, the care staff members who can make use of this ambience in their daily care work, the group members with leadership duties who observe and develop innovative real-life perspectives, and the people with dementia who are motivated to contribute their own potential to the group.

This process is however not linear; it is disrupted by conflict and problems. Plans and conceptual ideas have to be reflected upon and, if necessary, amended. Nevertheless it is not uncommon that such reflections often form the basis of greater opportunities for participation that had not been considered before. A symptomatic example is the 'exposing' scene where Rosamund is lifted from her wheelchair into an armchair by means of a mechanical hoist. The technical process 'brutally' disrupts a social communication scene. The musicians are shocked. In hindsight, however, they realise that it is exactly this which is Rosamund's reality and by recognising this they return in an even deeper way her dignity which, in their initial perspectives, seemed to have been destroyed by the event. It is a dignity that strengthens her participation in the group henceforth.

---

[183] See Mead 1967: 152ff.

This example creates a relevant bridge to the notion of *development*, the fourth and last core category. The Music for Life project, in actual fact, is not only a group in which a variety of members participate: it deals with a *community of practice* as we have learnt from Lave and Wenger, which is in itself characterised through participation, i.e. through a development of 'legitimate peripheral participation' into 'full participation'.[184]

We should envisage this process once again in real terms, and appreciate the humane idea of 'development' hidden within it. A single participant – symbolically – stands on the edge of a group. She is *permitted* to do so and is, as such, accepted as a peripheral member. Through the interaction with other group members, there is a gradual sense of development whereby she finally becomes a full member of the group. The prerequisite of full membership is not a 'status', but instead it is the learning process in which she enters and which changes her personally.

Music for Life does not evolve in a 'group' in the conventional sense, it is actually a community of practice and the transition from group to community is a *transitional learning process*. The single participant, be it a musician, a care staff member, the staff development practitioner, or a person with dementia, becomes a part of the experience that can only be created by everyone – in harmony with one another. In a sense, through this process, the individual turns into 'another', one who develops further and becomes aware of herself in a new way. Our core criteria of development lie, as it were, between the extremes of *social activity* and *personal development*. Moreover, this category encompasses collective and individual development.

This means that the four explored core categories relate to each other and they interconnect. They describe a unique process of learning whereupon the individual actors and the developing community are equally affected. The dimension of identity already shows the developmental process. Identity is not a static condition, but rather a process. This process requires contact with others. It needs communication and reflection and this connection is active and participatory. The development, which therefore becomes noticeable, also leads to a new level of identity for the participants. It is not a circle that is closed here, but a *spiral of learning* is completed, and a new process of learning begins, perhaps one on a higher level.

The space of social learning

This spiral of learning undoubtedly liberates imagination that might be encouraging to find a more general representation of the described process of learning, without claiming to reveal a pedagogical or psychological 'theory of learning' that is relevant to every imaginable process of learning. *Grounded Theory* means a theory on a particular content, a theory that

---

[184] See again Lave and Wenger 1991: 35ff.

relates to the investigated field of work and that has to be accepted by those who are active in that field.

We can therefore place the process of learning, associated with the four core categories of *Identity, Communication, Participation* and *Development*, in a symbolic space that stretches from individual to social experiences, from *self-assurance* to *social activity*, from *personal development* to *social sensitivity*. The first point of contrast relates to the polarity between the extrovert and the introvert. The second is one of inner and outer dimensions of reflexivity. In this way, a surprising *space of social learning* is created which is typical for the Music for Life project.

Fig. 4: The space of social learning within the Music for Life project

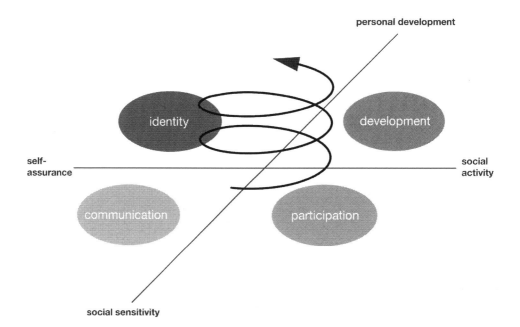

The interesting aspect is obviously that the implied arrow does not describe a simple 'development', but instead describes a spiral of development and learning that continuously leads to new 'identities', 'communications' and 'participations'. It encourages the participants *to repeat and disseminate* the described process because it is rewarding for all members, yet does not lead to a simple conclusion. Nonetheless, it appears – practically – to be so inspiring that it makes sense to apply it to processes of learning for professional musicians.

246

The space of professional learning as a musician

Development is feasible for all musical performers, not just for soloists in large concert halls. Fiona writes at some point: ..."*I think there can be a lot of cynicism in the musicians' world, sometimes in the professional world, and I feel really lucky to have these experiences [of Music for Life] sometimes. I just don't view it as my next pay cheque, it's something I can believe in and love. And so I suppose it fuels my love of music and my love of working with people and my belief in the chamber music aspect of it, the playing together, feeding off other musicians and the creativity of that.*"
This is an important given. Music can, in community settings, contribute to dealing with social problems which cannot anymore be addressed through 'classical' methods of social work. Music is a communicative, social activity. It develops into a 'language' that does not only require listeners, but also partners in order to communicate. Such a musical community becomes the more important when obviously and consistently it has to be relied upon, for instance when musicians engage with audiences in various social contexts.[185]

Music can play an empowering role for many more 'audiences' than we tend to envision. We can make this case by returning once more to Brian, when he reflects: "*Perhaps it is because the creative arts world has a different culture that it can be of benefit and enriching to the care world.*" Key behind Brian's words is the validation of both the artistic identity of the musician and the context to which she responds. Genuine artistic engagement excludes the useless debates about whether an artistic practice needs to be considered *l'Art pour l'Art* or 'social work'. Collaborative creative practice in a context like the project of Music for Life is "by definition artistically driven and shows a close interconnection between the creative passion of the artist and what the artist creates in the community."[186] Or, to put it once more in Brian's wording: "*generated by the musicians but from the residents.*" And this is, as we have seen in many examples, an artistic and social learning process on an equal and mutual basis. It is, as the musicians at some point discuss amongst themselves, a cyclical action. It has to do with others as much as with oneself. That is an important insight for musicians relevant for engaging with all sorts of audiences.

[185] If evidence would be required for this, other than this project's analysis, then a possible example could be the dance project *Rhythm is it*. This was an initiative of Sir Simon Rattle, conductor of the Berlin Philharmonic Orchestra, who enabled East Berlin working class youth to engage in quality dance performances of an exceptional and artistically high level.
[186] Rineke Smilde in Renshaw 2010: iii.

Fig. 5: The space of professional learning as a musician

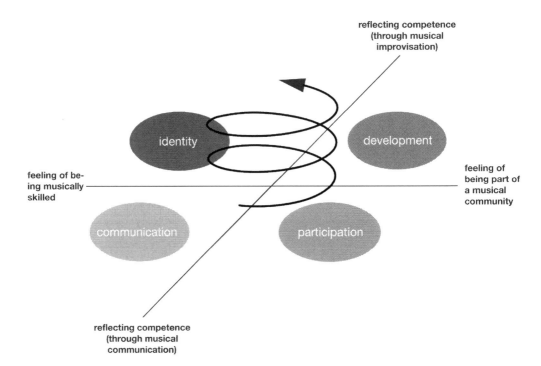

reflecting competence
(through musical
improvisation)

identity

development

feeling of be-
ing musically
skilled

feeling of
being part of
a musical
community

communication

participation

reflecting competence
(through musical
communication)

If this makes sense, then it would be important to transfer experiences like those of the Music for Life project to institutions of Higher Music Education. Moreover, training in conservatoires and music academies of musicians that engage with audiences in various social contexts should no longer be marginalised – if even offered – but be much more at the heart of the curricula, both in the interest of the professional prospects of today's music students, and in the interest of society as a whole. Here 'head and heart' can truly come together.

The space of a basic curriculum of Higher Music Education

This would drastically change the training of future musicians. *Musical skills* would of course remain the focus. However, training in improvisation should not be restricted to jazz classes, but instead be offered to all music students. The importance of the competence to improvise is not only crucial to artistic work in community contexts, like for instance this project, but also enhances musicians' possibilities for expression and can have a positive influence on overcoming performance anxiety.[187]

[187] See also Smilde 2009.

In addition, *personal skills* such as recognising potential for new venues, a willingness to approach others, as well as instilling a sense of inquisitiveness and friendliness would be required. It could be learnt in practical projects that are defined by intensive phases of reflexivity. The same can be said of *social skills* i.e., the familiarisation with collaborative skills, learning to be able to 'read' a situation or to change a point of view. Moreover, a very important social skill in this context is the ability for making observations through the eyes of another. Fiona's question: *"How can I reflect who you are and how you are in the music I play for you? How can I play music that you can own? What is your sound?"* is fundamental in this respect.

Key components are the (reflective) *learning skills*, i.e., being able to question one's own assumptions, based on new experiences, by being able to rethink one's own biographical experiences as a musician. We can for instance listen to music students, who in 2005 engaged in a community music project[188] for the first time in their lives. Their report on what they learnt was quite impressive, including:

Renewing personal motivation;

Strengthening courage, confidence, and self-esteem;

Understanding the importance of teamwork and cooperation;

Becoming more aware of roles and responsibilities in a team;

Grasping the challenges of leadership and shared leadership;

Building up trust in oneself and in the group;

Thinking on one's feet and acting in the moment;

Becoming aware of the need of quality;

Seeing the need to create new forms of music making.

These observations are well known to us after having investigated musicians' requirements for collaborating in the Music for Life project.

Such conclusions are implied by the investigated core categories of *Identity, Communication, Participation* and *Development*. These investigations collectively mean that the personal and, moreover, professional horizons should be extended, and that new challenges should be taken seriously.

---

[188] See Smilde 2006: 79.

Fig. 6: The space of a basic curriculum of higher education in music

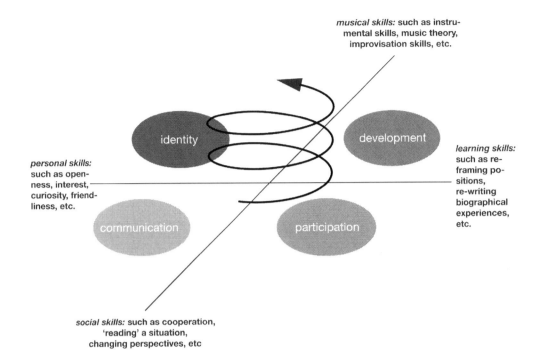

musical skills: such as instrumental skills, music theory, improvisation skills, etc.

personal skills: such as openness, interest, curiosity, friendliness, etc.

learning skills: such as re-framing positions, re-writing biographical experiences, etc.

identity

development

communication

participation

social skills: such as cooperation, 'reading' a situation, changing perspectives, etc

Final note

To reiterate: Music for Life has set a milestone. A *good practice model* was constructed from this research project despite the limited time available. It can be replicated or adapted, however it deserves critical consideration in other countries. Music for Life has shown that there are alternatives to engaging with people living with dementia. Dementia does not have to mean a 'static state' or 'infantile regression'. It means something 'in itself' and it challenges us to think critically about ourselves, and about the 'postmodern' society in which we live. Will the approach with how we deal with the current generation of the elderly, where we develop imagination, provide care, and assume responsibility, change our society? Will the capacity of music have a broader influence in this context? We will have to wait and see. Nonetheless, this documented project takes an important if modest step towards a new horizon; while the music lasts.

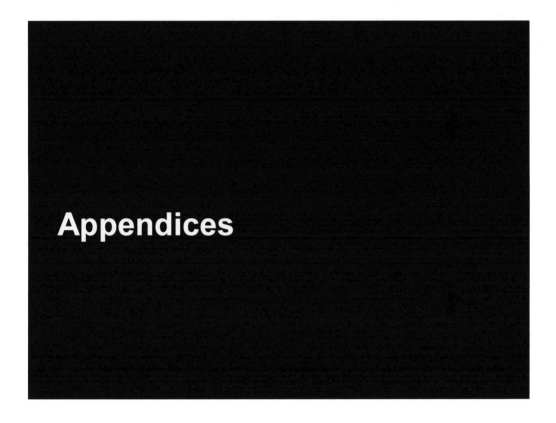

Appendices

I   The Practice of Music for Life

The following appendix details a description of a typical Music for Life project (as explored in this research), the development of the practice and aspects of management. Each of these parts entails a number of key focus areas, including:

> Project description: *duration; workshop space; resources; musical elements; delivery team; participants: people living with dementia; participants: staff; staff development; staff development practitioners; project planning; evaluation; aims and outcomes; monitoring.*

> Practice development: *impact of leadership; early practice hallmarks; contextual development; practitioner recruitment; training models; practitioner profiles; ongoing practitioner development; practice development forums.*

> Management and partnerships: *early management; collaboration and transfer of management; transition management; partnership categories (primary partnerships, associate partnerships, collaborative partnerships); context of the project within lead partner organisation; programme description; general management; dissemination; fundraising; diversification.*

I.1   The Music for Life project

Music for Life projects aim both to enhance the quality of life of its participants and to demonstrate to staff the emotional, social and physical potential of people in their care. Projects take place in residential care homes, hospitals, extra care housing and specialist day centres in association with a series of strategic and delivery partners. As the majority of projects are delivered in residential care homes, they often involve people experiencing isolation and a sense of disempowerment as a result of the advanced stage of their dementia and physical frailty.

Duration

A Music for Life project consists of eight weekly sessions lasting three hours, which usually take place in the morning. Each session involves an hour of preparation including physical set-up of the workshop area (project delivery team only), an hour of creative music workshop (involving three musicians, eight participants living with dementia and three to five participating care staff), and an hour of reflective practice (project delivery team and participating care staff).

Workshop space

The workshop takes place in a circle, usually in a shared lounge area, which is booked for exclusive use during the project period. Seating arrangements are often discussed in the preparation hour, taking into account issues of access, visibility, comfort, proximity and personal preferences of participants, with the key aim of enhancing the engagement of the group.

Resources

A selection of tuned and untuned percussion is available for each project.[189] Instruments have been carefully chosen for their size, quality, safety, visual attractiveness and appropriateness for the age group, and usually include percussion such as djembes (with timpani beaters or similar), hand drums, small gato drums, bass metallophones, alto chime bars, chime bar trees, temple blocks, maracas, a variety of ethnic instruments such as afuches, caxixi, seed shakers, etc. The instruments are laid out in the centre of the circle, on one to two small, low height tables so that they do not restrict sight lines to others in the circle. Great care is taken to ensure that the display is not cluttered with too many instruments and that it looks visually appealing.

Musical elements

Music is primarily improvised during the workshops, with an emphasis on drawing on the creativity of the group; participants engage in the music making using percussion, their voice, or through directing the music making. Consistent musical elements include a framing composition with a short, repetitive, simple theme, which commences and concludes the session and a welcome song in which participants names are sung. These elements and other recurrent approaches diverge in their manifestations dependent on the musicians involved, albeit with a shared ethical vision underlying the approaches. Some interactions may directly and actively involve the whole group, whilst other interactions appear to actively involve a smaller combination of individuals.

Delivery team

The project delivery team consists of a minimum of 3 specially trained professional musicians who deliver the creative music workshop, a project manager who manages the overall project logistics and overarching relationships as well as acting as a sounding board for the musicians, and a staff development practitioner who engages with participating care staff in a reflective format.

---

[189] See for an overview of these instruments Appendix V.

Participants: people living with dementia

The project involves a regular group of eight people living with dementia and three to five members of care staff, recruited in advance of the project. About three weeks before a project starts, the project manager, staff development practitioner and workshopleader visit the participating setting for a selection meeting. Prior to the selection meeting, a long-list of up to 15 nominated participants is prepared by settings as a starting point for discussion. During this selection meeting, care staff are briefed about the project and the project team, and undertake a process whereby 10 participants living with dementia are selected. This short-list includes two reserves, in case a situation arises in the first few weeks whereby an identified participant needs to be replaced, e.g. decline in health, or choice of person with dementia not to participate. During the selection meeting, information about hearing loss, impaired sight, physical difficulties or mental health problems is usually conveyed.

Ideally, the final selected group will be well-balanced, including a range of emotional and physical needs, personalities and gender. This nomination and selection process includes a wide consultation with setting staff, and may include staff that will not be directly involved in the project. Criteria for inclusion into the project involve selecting participants living with dementia who may be experiencing poor communication, or may be socially isolated or disengaged. Many of those selected may be recognised as needing a high level of support from care staff to draw them out to interact with other people, or those whose behaviour has often led to them being isolated within the setting.

Participants: staff

The same three to five care staff are involved consistently throughout the eight-week project. For some staff, working arrangements (i.e. rota, leave) may need to be adapted so they can be fully involved in the workshop sessions and debriefs over the eight weeks. Usually staff become aware of the project and its potential through briefings in staff meetings, usually conveyed by the setting manager (sometimes in collaboration with Music for Life), and through discussions with their team leaders. Involvement in the project can be through nomination by care management or self-selection. A range of staff have been involved in projects, including care assistants, team leaders, social care/activity coordinators, management staff and general staff (e.g. catering, handyman).

Staff development

Projects include a staff development practitioner who supports care staff to engage in reflection and discussion of their experiences and observations directly after each workshop. This reflective practice is followed up through additional visits by the staff development practitioner to the setting, engaging with both setting management and participating care staff, and focusing on developing practical ways to sustain and extend experiences and discoveries gained during the project. Activities may include creating personalized care plans, interactive training in specific areas identified by staff, or further reflection and discussion around key concepts.

Staff development practitioners

The team of staff development practitioners is made up of the Jewish Care Disability and Dementia team and freelance dementia specialists from Dementia UK. Each practitioner brings a different style in their approach within the role, drawing on their own professional experiences, expertise and personal strengths. A Dementia Facilitator forum, comprising of the above members, was established in 2010 in order to share insights and develop a united vision for this aspect of the practice.

Project planning

Each project is planned over a few months and includes a process of fixing the personnel of the delivery team, scheduling all project dates, a set-up meeting with the setting management where confirmation of project logistics occurs, a participant selection meeting, and a project preparation session for musicians. This process is reified through the creation of a pro-forma agreement, utilized by both the delivery team and the participating setting.

Evaluation

Evaluation in the project occurs on a local and global scale, on an informal and formal basis, and is targeted towards a variety of stakeholders. Evaluation occurs on an ongoing, informal basis throughout each Music for Life project, and feeds organically into the planning and delivery of subsequent sessions. At each project planning and workshop session, observers from the management team and staff development workers make observational notes that can be used as stimulus for discussion during the debrief session. Evaluation at this level generally involves those directly involved in the project, though further informal evaluation may occur more widely through other forums and modes (e.g. mentoring meetings, musician development activities, reflective journals).

After each project, a report is completed by the project manager or staff development practitioner involved, highlighting outcomes for participants and care staff during the project, and including recommendations for building upon the work of the project. The audience for this report is internal, and includes the participating care setting and the delivery team directly involved in the projects. This report is often used within the participating setting as a tool for stimulating further reflective practice, developing more personalized care plans for individuals and reporting to setting stakeholders.

At the end of each financial year, a comprehensive overview report is compiled that reflects the activities of the full programme, and draws on all of the projects undertaken. This report includes evidence of key achievements and outcomes for people living with dementia, care staff and musicians (as per an established evaluation framework), details of musician development and training opportunities, challenges and learning points faced at a practical and strategic level and strategic achievements and ambitions for the year ahead. The audience for this report is diverse and includes internal and external stakeholders, and is made publically available through the Wigmore Hall website.

Aims and outcomes

Each project has a number of conditional variables (e.g. setting type/location/culture, participant profiles, delivery team etc.), however there are a number of areas where positive outcomes have been known to consistently occur; outcomes which reflect the principles of a person-centred care approach and highlight some of the potential benefits of the project.

The primary stated aim of Music for Life projects is to improve the quality of life and potential to communicate for people living with dementia. On the basis of this, key aims for each participating group have been identified in a formal project evaluation framework, and detailed via outcomes evidenced in project reports.

For the person living with dementia, the aim of the project is to create a safe space to explore, enjoy, discover, reminisce and communicate in new ways, expressing their feelings/thoughts/emotions, and to support them to take decisions and make choices. Potential outcomes include:

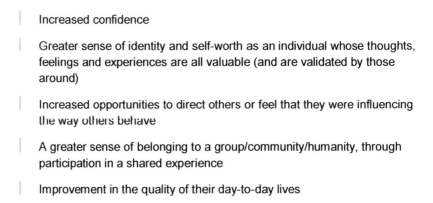

Increased confidence

Greater sense of identity and self-worth as an individual whose thoughts, feelings and experiences are all valuable (and are validated by those around)

Increased opportunities to direct others or feel that they were influencing the way others behave

A greater sense of belonging to a group/community/humanity, through participation in a shared experience

Improvement in the quality of their day-to-day lives

For staff working in the settings, the aim of the project is to create a non-hierarchical safe space to explore innovative ways to identify and acknowledge the unique qualities of those in their care (acknowledging the personhood needs of the residents) through participation and reflection.

Potential outcomes include:

- Increased confidence

- Increased competence

- Increased job satisfaction

- Greater sense of team working

- Development of emotional vocabulary

- Interactions with people living with dementia that are person-centred and meaningful to each individual

- Broader understanding of the needs of people living with dementia through discovery of their histories, interests and strengths

- Greater interest in people living with dementia, through getting to know them and through thinking creatively about providing meaningful occupation

- Developing an approach that is 'enabling' rather than 'doing for'

For all musicians involved, the aim of the project is to develop communication and musical skills and knowledge relevant to the needs of the programme. Potential outcomes include:

- Increased understanding of the communication potential and unique personality of each person living with dementia in the group

- Development of a range of strategies for engaging each person in the group

- Greater awareness of personal response in verbal and non verbal communication

- Increased confidence in musical leadership, including increased flexibility and spontaneity when improvising

- Awareness of the social, mental and physical impact of dementia on the individual, and of the broader challenges faced in dementia care environments

Monitoring

Monitoring information is required principally by funders and commissioners, and focuses on aspects of the recipient participant profile (age, gender, ethnicity) and attendance figures.

I.2   **Practice development**

Impact of leadership

At its core, Music for Life is a practice based in reflection that strongly reflects and resonates with the ethical viewpoints and learning of those deeply involved in its development and delivery. This seed from which this distinctive, ethically-driven approach germinated was firmly planted by Linda Rose, the project's founder, whose biographical history, including her formative years as an educationalist, stimulated a significant impact on the character and subsequent development of the practice (see also Appendix III). Together with a growing team of musicians, and an ongoing association with Jewish Care, the practice developed from an exploratory beginning into a cohesive approach.

Early practice hallmarks

The initial pilot of Music for Life was developed as a 12-week project, with students from the Guildhall School of Music & Drama in London, working with a small, consistent group of regular day centre service users. At this time, the project activities were not exclusive to people living with dementia, and there was no dedicated work with care staff, although they were actively involved. Activities focused on reminiscence as the key element, from which the performance of musical repertoire, sharing of stories, creation and performance of new work were explored and developed. Many of these elements were retained during further explorations, though there was a large degree of variance as each project was bespoke according to resources and delivery context.

Contextual development

Development of key aspects, approaches and scope within the work emerged organically over time, and reflect responsiveness towards internal and external contexts. For instance, the impact of changes in the National Health Service community care policy in the 1990's, which focused on maintaining independent living for older people in their own homes. This resulted in a growing number of frailer people with a spectrum of care needs being cared for in residential care homes. This had ramifications for the project, with practitioners needing to become more skilled in adapting to and engaging with a changing participant profile. Engagement with research in 1997 enabled the existing practice to be evaluated, leading to significant changes in the approach, format and scope of the project. The research firmly established many principles that are currently employed in the practice, articulating a need for: incorporating dedicated planning and debrief time, cultivating and maintaining a focused workshop environment, reassessing methodology in selection of participants and participant profile (including group size) and the use of musical elements (e.g. texture, structure). It also highlighted challenges in maintaining the well-being of the delivery team within this context; with an emphasis on building collaborative skills, self-esteem, and coping with transference of emotion. Developmental work with care staff, and a greater emphasis on participation opportunities for staff was also explored as a potential future direction.

Practitioner recruitment

Entry into the project has comprised of two distinct models: formal, structured training programmes with a group of trainees, and individual apprenticeship. As mentioned, Music for Life started as a pilot project in 1993, with a small team of students drawn from the Guildhall School of Music & Drama in London. These students were drawn from a specialist postgraduate course for musicians, which focused on widening perspectives of performance contexts and developing communication and collaborative skills. In the early stages of the project, the musician team expanded slowly, and occurred in a very fluid, organic way. In the first few years, three of the original students from the Guildhall pilot became the central forces in developing the practice, alongside a diversity of trainees who often interacted with the practice in a short-term, voluntary, casual capacity. Over time, the nature of recruitment into the project began to change with an increasing focus on professional musicians with specific qualities that would enable them to integrate into the ethos and requirements of the developing practice. Musicians were often drawn from professional music organisations and ensembles, through recommendations from members of the existing musician team, participants in associated training schemes (e.g. Wigmore Hall Trainee Animateur), and through audition-interviews. Rapid growth of the team occurred when a new influx of professional musicians joined the team around 1998 via a training programme involving the (now defunct) ensemble, Sinfonia 21. The initial collaboration with Wigmore Hall, between 2005-2008, 'Dementia Awareness' led to another rapid expansion taking the team to its present day size of 25 musicians.

Training models

The training format in these collaborations share similar traits, although recent training has been influenced by a significant body of shared experience developed by the existing team over time. Training agendas involved developing an understanding of the context and nature of dementia, and sharing practical insights and approaches regarding the performance and communication skills required of a musician in this area of work. Usually a team of four to six trainees would be involved in a project, alongside two experienced members of the existing team, with equal opportunity for each trainee to observe and participate in sessions. This initial foundation was followed, where possible, by practical experience in one to two projects.

Some trainees have been involved in projects via an individual apprenticeship model, participating fully in an eight-week project alongside an existing team of three musicians in the project. This model is generally less structurally formalized and can be more personalised.

Practitioner profiles

A sense of continuity or regularity of project experiences, and a supportive team is important in building relevant skills and a cohesive approach to the work. The development of musicians enacting a leadership role has happened gradually. Within the team there is a variety of experience; some individuals have a number of years of experience and are able to enact a leadership role, whilst some are still relatively new to the work. A general guiding principle for fixing teams recommends that two highly experienced musicians from the project should support an individual less experienced in the work.

Most of the professional musicians involved in the project specialize in acoustic instruments, although they also interact during the workshops through using their voices and percussion. The majority have a background or formal training and qualifications in a western classical music tradition, though work in a diverse range of music performance and educational contexts. The balance of a team is important in several respects; experience, relationship dynamics, personality, gender and instrumentation all play a part in influencing the flavour of a project. Within the trio of musicians, there is an experienced workshopleader, who is responsible for facilitating the overall shape of each workshop session and the project as a whole, in terms of musical direction and workshop approach.

Ongoing practitioner development

Initial training and early experiences only form one part of the ongoing learning experiences of musicians involved in the project. Engagement in reflective practice, personal approaches to reflection and professional development, learning styles and motivation, participation in informal support networks internal and external to the project (e.g. consulting a colleague for advice), formal mentoring and development forums all interact in the ongoing development of the team.

As musicians have gained more experience on the project, their development has been supported through participation in two annual development forum days with a broad range of agendas driven and delivered by the team, and smaller focus group seminars. As the team grows, issues of consistency of delivery and a sense of shared ethos have emerged, and a new forum and dedicated consultant role has been established, drawing on the expertise of the workshopleaders, aimed at developing mainstreamed, relevant and personalized avenues for musician development within the project.

Practice development forums

Practice development is influenced both through formal and informal mechanisms. Formal modes include a stakeholder advisory group and a management group (described elsewhere); and separate focused forums for project managers, staff development practitioners and musicians. These may be enhanced through participation in occasional focus activities (e.g. recent work undertaken to assess perspectives around delivery roles and responsibilities; involvement in research). The groups and forums interact at a casual level through mixed membership, with reification of advisory group and management group discussions.

I.3   **Management and partnerships**

Early management

From the inception of the practice in 1993, until takeover of management of the project by Wigmore Hall (in partnership with Dementia UK, in 2008), the overall management and leadership of the project and organisation was driven by one individual, Linda Rose, on a semi-voluntary basis.

Collaboration; transfer of management

Between 2005-2008, a pilot collaborative project between Linda Rose and Wigmore Hall Community & Education was delivered. This centred on expanding the delivery team (musicians) and developing a network of new delivery partnerships. Two years into the Dementia Awareness collaboration, discussions between primary stakeholders took place in order to establish the potential for developing and extending it into a sustained collaboration. The Dementia Awareness collaboration had highlighted great potential for the growth of Music for Life, in terms of extending delivery scope and enabling sustainability of resources (human and financial). However, it emerged that there could be potential benefit for the long-term future of the project in incorporating it within the Wigmore Hall Community & Education programme, with transfer of overall management and leadership to Wigmore Hall. In February 2007, a feasibility study was produced, and was presented to, and approved by the Wigmore Hall Board of Trustees. The study examined potential benefits and risks of the proposal to Wigmore Hall and Music for Life through SWOT analysis, acknowledged areas of shared interests and ethos, established the relevance and effectiveness of the practice in relation to the contextual environment and proposed a shared vision for future management, transition mitigation and strategic development of the project.

Transition of management

The continuing involvement and development of the musician team and continuing input of Linda Rose as project consultant were identified as critical factors in ensuring the success of the transition. A management structure was proposed, including the addition of a part-time project manager based at Wigmore Hall, and the establishment of a steering committee. Transfer of the management of the project to Wigmore Hall was launched officially in May 2009. A strategic partnership between Wigmore Hall (lead partner) and Dementia UK was established, and an additional part-time position developed, based at Dementia UK. An advisory group comprising of key strategic and delivery stakeholders was created to develop strategic vision and focus on the ongoing commitment to the ethos of the practice, particularly through this period of immense transition. A management group was created that took responsibility for strategic and practical decisions and delivery of the overall programme.

Partnership categories

There are a number of overlapping partnerships, some with an ongoing strategic role, which have been reflected here, and others of a peripheral, short-term nature, focused on delivery outputs. These partnerships fall into distinct categories, although the scope, dynamics and activities of each partnership may bridge some, or all, of these elements. Partnerships can be divided into three main categories: primary, associate and collaborative and include elements of collaboration, purchasing and commissioning.

Primary partnerships

The principal strategic partnership in Music for Life is a formalized collaboration between Wigmore Hall and Dementia UK, who together have primarily initiated and enacted the strategic direction and delivery model for all aspects of the programme of activities since 2009. Both partners contribute dedicated human and financial resources to the programme as part of the formal partnership agreement, with Wigmore Hall holding the ultimate responsibility for the delivery of the programme and formal agreements with the strategic partners detailed below.

Associate partnerships

The strategic partnership with Jewish Care is a long-term, ongoing relationship beginning in 1993, which includes elements of purchasing and collaboration. The relationship with Jewish Care was initially one of collaboration, where the practice was developed and delivered in a voluntary capacity. Later changes in structure and policy within the organisation enabled Jewish Care to purchase three projects annually – i.e. full project delivery expenditure covered by Jewish Care via a renewable service contract. This model of purchasing has recently been adopted in new and emerging delivery partnerships with other care organisations. Jewish Care is a key stakeholder in developing the strategic outlook of the programme, acting in an advisory capacity.

The strategic partnership with NHS Westminster is a long-term, ongoing relationship, which includes elements of commissioning and collaboration. The relationship with NHS Westminster was initially one of fixed-term collaboration, during the Dementia Awareness musician training pilot (2005-2008). This evolved into a longer-term partnership, in which 4 projects are currently commissioned and part-funded annually, through a formal service agreement, thus resonating with wider community incentives, and responding to local and national government priorities and policies. NHS Westminster is a key stakeholder in developing the strategic outlook of the programme, acting in an advisory capacity.

Collaborative partnerships

Other programme activities have involved the development of delivery partnerships with other organisations; either on a one-off or ongoing collaborative basis. These have usually entailed a joint-funding approach. Content of the collaborations has engaged with delivering core activities of the programme (i.e. Music for Life projects) and diversified opportunities (i.e. training events, projects, community projects with altered format, scope and audience).

Context of the project within lead partner organisation

Wigmore Hall is widely regarded as one of the world's finest venues for chamber music and song, presenting over 400 concerts per year as well as broadcasting to a wide audience on BBC Radio 3, running an award winning record label, Wigmore Hall Live and promoting two international competitions – Wigmore Hall International Song Competition and Wigmore Hall London International String Quartet Competition. Music for Life sits within the activities of Wigmore Hall Learning which is focused on providing access to chamber music and song through a range of creative programmes, online resources and events. The programme has five main areas of activity – as well as Music for Life these include: early years music making; schools; music in community settings; and events at Wigmore Hall which are open for anyone to attend and include events for families and for young people and an extensive programme of talks, masterclasses and study events for adults.

Programme description

Currently nine Music for Life projects are delivered annually, in partnership with Jewish Care, NHS Westminster and other partners. In addition the overall programme includes musician training, professional development, dissemination and diversification opportunities.

Dissemination

Dissemination of the project ethos and activities forms a core area within the management of the over-arching programme. Dissemination has traditionally occurred on both a national and local scope, primarily through: commissioned articles in printed/digital press; industry (health, music, arts) publications; commissioned appearances at conferences and seminars; membership of industry forums; Wigmore Hall- and Dementia UK-promoted events (e.g. project launch, training events, fundraising events, diversification activities), digital media, press releases and stakeholder reports; informal mechanisms (e.g. word of mouth).

Fundraising

Wigmore Hall and Dementia UK administer project and programme income and expenditure. Income is only partially sourced through purchasing and commissioning arrangements (which focus on project expenditure rather than contributions to programme costs like general administration, dissemination, professional development etc.). Both Wigmore Hall and Dementia UK are registered charities, which enables the development of a diverse range of potential relationships with donors. Income is generated through ongoing relationships or one-off grants from a range of trusts, foundations and individual donors.

Diversification

The networks, expertise and dissemination activities of the various strategic and delivery partners and individuals involved in the programme enable a host of potential opportunities for diversification outside of the practice described in this research publication. Some small-scale events and projects have been delivered or are under consideration, drawing on resources and principles from the practice, whilst extending the scope (e.g. location, duration, type of activity) and the participant profile of the activity.

II   Project management

II.1   Roles and responsibilities of a project manager

by Linda Rose

The concept of management

Beyond any formal identification of roles and responsibilities, the manager's practice needs to evolve as his or her perceptions of the work develop, deepen and broaden. The role involves knowledge and judgement, insight and risk taking. It is a role which sets a secure framework for the project and contains it, overseeing and ensuring the retention of its values whilst encouraging the work to grow through exploration.

The ways in which the manager carries out the roles are as important as the roles and responsibilities themselves. The manager is a role model for the project. The way he or she works reflect principles that are integral to the project. These include authenticity in relationships, equality, respect for individuals and their individuality, connecting to individuals and their contexts, belief in creative potential and the central place of learning through reflection.

The skills and experience of the Music for Life project manager complement those of other partners who influence the work – including musicians, residential home managers and team leaders, dementia care trainers. The manager must also recognise, acknowledge and value equally people living with dementia for whom and with whom the project has been developed. They are entitled to share an equal standing with all other partners and will have skills, careers and life experiences which have shaped them but which they are no longer able to articulate.

Conceptual framework for the management of Music for Life

Values underpinning the project	Need to be reflected in the management of the project.
Learning through the project	Giving status to feelings and personal experience in the music. Ongoing personal and group reflection, mentoring and co-mentoring.
'Being' in the project	In the moment, relating to, role modelling.
Contextualising the work	Understanding the cultures, the world of the person with dementia and need for life enhancement, the musicians' world and musician development, residential care settings and person-centred care, practice development, political perspectives on social care of older people, current thinking and practice in dementia care.
Organising the work	Planning strategies – the musicians, the home and its management and staffing issues, organisational framework of the project within a series of projects, the organisation within a home, the organisation of a session, of the music workshop environment, scheduling.

Partnerships	Identifying the need for partnerships. Identifying potential partnerships (shared values and attitudes). Building partnerships. Devolving identified responsibilities to partners. Monitoring progress and effectiveness. Learning through partnerships.
Dealing with expectations	Ensuring expectations are realistic – for home, for musicians, for trainer, for funders etc. Articulating potential outcomes for people with dementia. Identifying and specifying levels and nature of support and co-operation needed from residential homes to deliver best outcomes. Identifying musicians able to cope with and learn from and lead work with people with dementia. Partnering trainers to promote reflective practice and so build legacy.
Affecting communities	Exploring ways of broadening the impact in the home beyond the project team. Recognising and valuing the impact on musicians' work beyond the project.
Motivation	Drawing on experience of past projects to encourage, motivate.
Focussing on music	Observing, facilitating reflection on quality, appropriateness, awareness of context.
Supporting the musicians	Nurturing workshopleader qualities. Encouraging progression, ensuring pastoral care, contextual understanding, ensuring they are equipped with appropriate skills and knowledge from which to explore.
Exposure	Managing visitor interest. Protecting from over-exposure or inappropriate exposure. Finding the language to present the work in different contexts.
Legal issues	Awareness of vulnerable adult policies, Insurance issues and liabilities, police checks. Need to transmit information to teams as appropriate.
Outcomes	Recognising outcomes of the work session by session, project by project, becoming aware of patterns and trends to inform subsequent

	practice, ways of recording and purposes of recording, tracing chronology of session, facilitating debriefings.
Ownership	Creating an understanding of 'equality' in and beyond the context of the project. Promoting sense of group ownership of the project through inclusive activities, meeting structures and discussions etc. Transferring responsibility to the home manager for continued learning and integration and dissemination of project values and attitudes after the project leaves a setting.

The roles and responsibilities that follow are not intended as a job description or a checklist. They represent a detailed reflection on 17 years of developing Music for Life, with the wide range of opportunities and challenges that the role of director and manager of the project have presented. It is unrealistic to embark on the management of Music for Life with the aim or expectation of fulfilling all these roles. Rather what follows may provide reference points and perhaps some reassurance to any future managers of the project as he or she encounters the many and varied aspects of the work. It identifies the key aims of the work and the practicalities involved in setting up and running the project. It also gives an indication of the complexities and paradoxes of the work and a guide to interpreting what is observed and experienced in the process of guiding the project.

The list, although long, is not definitive. The management of the project is an ongoing learning process. There will be some responsibilities which cannot be compromised upon and form the essential framework of the project, based on the philosophy underpinning the work. Beyond that, the role unfolds continuously in response to the people and the contexts in which it operates. It is an exciting and creative role with responsibility for maintaining the values, overseeing the quality of the work and with the potential to take it in new directions as the learning continues.

Aims

To initiate a project that is likely to resonate with the residents and care staff of the home

To identify and prepare musicians to deliver the project

To ensure that the needs of people with dementia remain at the heart of the project and guide its direction

To steer and monitor the project, maintaining a secure framework for its development

To create a healthy working environment in which all participants (residents, staff and musicians) have a voice and are heard

To promote the empowerment of all participants, fostering an awareness of individual choice, decision-making, sense of identity and self-esteem

To facilitate ownership of learning by musicians and staff

To promote reflective practice of staff and musicians

To strengthen the quality of engagement of staff and musicians

To ensure the staff and musicians are able to place their work in a wider context

Principles

Ensuring that the principle of 'respect for persons' underpins all aspects of the project (e.g. ways of responding to all participants, understanding where staff, musicians and residents are coming from, appropriate use of spoken and body language, sensitivity to physical and psychological space, selection of instruments).

Encouraging authenticity and integrity (e.g. the need for everyone to strive to be honest about themselves, otherwise the project finds you out. It is in the learning who we are that we learn who the residents are).

Connecting to the particular context of the staff, home, audience and potential partners, ensuring meaningful communication is established.

Understanding of the specific dementia context (e.g. the possibilities for change as well as the limitations of the project which are defined by its context; the condition and progression of dementia itself and the nature of the institutions in which people with dementia are cared for).

Maintaining a project overview whilst keeping a grasp of detail (e.g. analysing the source of a difficulty – is it in the music, the musician, the team, the staff as individuals, the home and its management or whatever? – how do all these elements interplay?) Working out strategies from which to learn and move forward.

Raising questions that help to shape the project (e.g. the place of questions, patience and support as the picture of each resident and member of staff emerges and pathways present themselves).

Identifying and analysing ongoing issues in the wider context of the project and the home.

Managing possible paradoxes within the project (e.g. the need to build confidence in order to face insecurity and questioning, leading to growth).

Managing the confusion that dementia can throw up (e.g. what is different and distinctive about working with people with dementia? How may working in a setting with people with dementia impact on musicians and staff personally?).

Understanding the complexities and challenges of cultural change in institutions (e.g. what inhibits and promotes institutional change and development?).

Accessing and processing information about the care sector, local and national government initiatives and policies. Understanding how individual homes might respond to these different factors.

Expectations

Acknowledging and dealing with the varying expectations of partners and participants (e.g. regarding the kind of music making, improvisation rather than repertoire, music that staff may prefer rather than music derived from relationships with residents).

Briefing visitors to ensure an understanding of what they will see; protecting the project from over exposure (e.g. media interest, many who catch the excitement of team members and want to observe).

Reassuring others that pace of change and relationship building is slow whilst maintaining strong belief in possibility of change and development.

Engaging in discussion about the ways music is used in this project and the ways this differs from entertainment/ listening to recorded music.

Values and Attitudes

Ensuring that pastoral care of team reflects the values of the project.

Transmitting values and attitudes through role modeling.

Dealing with issues in the spirit of the project (e.g. being patient and taking time to work out why staff may resistant to change and how to reassure and build confidence through both music making and reflection).

Supporting reflection as tool for exploring and acknowledging values.

Valuing and acknowledging feeling experiences.

Motivating – capacity to describe and discuss the project in ways that reflect its ethos and excite interest and passion in others.

Quality Assurance

Encouraging the highest quality music-making at all times – the improvisations are as important as any concert performance.

Setting the project in wider context of local and national government initiatives and staying aware of dementia-specific issues and recent developments (e.g. keeping up to date in the 'field' and with related policies; awareness of individual home's responses to current issues).

Networking and keeping musicians and relevant staff informed of progress and new directions.

Using the skill of critical reflection to strengthen the quality of work in any project.

Staying firm about the needs of each particular project to ensure it delivers to its fullest potential (e.g. appropriate space/time/ storage/staff release etc.).

Recognising the subtlety of what counts as quality in this work; striving to describe it in clear and accessible ways.

Keeping an overview of the quality and appropriateness of the music in each particular context.

Practical procedures

Identifying, negotiating and managing context-specific agendas.

Planning – pre-meetings, identifying homes to work in, liaising with managers and trainers to secure best support for project combined with relevant client need (e.g. discussing with manager appropriate staff to participate in and gain from project, engaging with manager and staff in selection of residents).

Relating to various levels of management and understanding their issues and constraints.

Overseeing organisation of time, space, environment and logistics.

Creating physical environment and ambience that supports best possible playing from musicians with the least possible disruption to the residents.

'Fixing' the team – booking musicians, liaising at the appropriate level of management to ensure the project is to be understood and supported.

Organising – ensuring rehearsals are booked, instruments are available and transported and correctly stored.

Time management – e.g. moving out of multi-purpose rooms on time; in debriefings, giving staff and musicians time to explore their own experiences of a session balanced with tight task-orientated schedules of the home.

Protecting the physical space of the project from disruption and protecting the time from other 'imperatives' in a home such as doctor's visits and personal care, whilst acknowledging importance of these and potential conflicts of time.

Forward planning – keeping people informed of future arrangements, ensuring proformas with written agreements are completed and circulated to relevant staff managers and musicians.

Dealing with formal matters (e.g. vulnerable adult policies; police checks on musicians; permissions sought for participation of residents, visitors attending; coverage of any kind and information given).

Keeping musicians safe and within their role – ensuring musicians do not carry out tasks in a residential home that are beyond their remit (e.g. any form of lifting or moving residents, ensuring a member of staff is present at all times while musicians are with residents).

Nurturing the 'team' – approach towards musicians, care staff, managers and trainers

Team building – bringing together the musicians and staff; taking account of them as individuals and the way their work culture may define how they are and how they relate to others.

Facilitating discussion and reflection between musicians and staff.

Managing in a way that is not formulaic but relies on both judgment and insight.

Being responsive and flexible to individual situations and how they impact on the project (e.g. musicians' concerns, residential home environment, tensions, staffing issues etc.).

Understanding the parameters of project management from breadth to minutiae (e.g. looking from the wider perspective to the micro-management of individual projects, to the detail of relationships within each project, each session, each moment).

Being flexible – as each project is different, there is a need to be open and responsive to the characteristics of each project and to understand that procedures only provide a rough framework.

271

Dealing with confidential information which can inform the project but may not always be shared – and possible tensions behind the scenes which can affect the project but cannot be exposed (e.g. a project will often expose team conflict, management deficiencies, expose staff shortages or individual weaknesses). Need to be non-judgmental and work with what is there.

Musicians' learning and development

Understanding nature of learning for musicians – building foundations for learning through confidence building, self-esteem, recognising and valuing small steps forward.

Developing and maintaining a learning culture (trust, confidence, encouraging questioning, coping with vulnerability) within the team of musicians.

Recognising when issues need to be exposed and explored (e.g. recognising when a musician may have difficulties because of personal experiences of dementia, which may impact on capacity to respond openly in workshop setting).

Risk taking – personal (e.g. touching on subjects and feelings that we try to hide); musical (e.g. crossing new boundaries through improvising within particular context, managing and embracing unfamiliar combinations of instruments and voice); team work (e.g. exposing oneself musically to colleagues and finding new relationships with fellow musicians through the music created together); facing the challenges of the dementia context, both individually and as a team.

Prioritising learning – distinguishing guiding principles of project from deeper levels of learning and recognising stages each musician might be at.

Encouraging learning from each other and the place and value of observation and mentoring in mentor's own learning.

Musical and creative skills

Providing opportunities for musicians to improvise together to build up a sense of each others' musical presence (e.g. ensuring time and space to make music together before each workshop session, providing professional development days to share and explore new musical ideas both within and separate from the context of the project).

Watching the nature of the improvisations prior to each session (e.g. not only working on material specific to the project but 'freeing up' musically to re-connect with team members through music; generating musical possibilities that can then be prompted and drawn on spontaneously in the workshop).

Reminding musicians of basic musical principles of work with people with dementia (e.g. keeping musical textures uncluttered, simplicity of music lines, use of repetition to encourage processing of musical themes, clarity in music developed, verbal communication and body language, importance of silence as safe place from which new connections can be made).

Observing and note-taking and reflecting back on musical content, meeting musicians requests for feedback (e.g. tracing the musical chronology of a session, looking at how clarity is achieved, noting missed opportunities to pick up on residents responses, noticing flow or disjointedness of music).

Encouraging musical risk-taking – departing from the familiar in order to connect to individual people and their context and reflecting on this afterwards.

Developing leadership skills, e.g. team building, encouraging initiatives from team members, recognising the support needs of less experienced musicians.

Promoting an understanding of the transferability of learning on this project to other work outside the project.

Communication and social skills

Promoting understanding of ways of connecting with and relating to people with dementia, e.g. through use of appropriate language, supporting verbal connections with appropriate body language, eye contact, awareness of different sensitivities relating to personal space.

Relating ways of communicating to wider contexts and community settings outside work with people with dementia.

Understanding the ways in which residents and staff may perceive musician's expectations of them (e.g. fear of being expected to sing or play an instrument, fear of appearing inadequate in front of musicians).

Drawing attention to the reciprocal nature of relationships developed in the project.

Supporting social development – helping musicians to understand and build relationships with those working in different settings – developing awareness and tolerance of different work environments and their different priorities.

Encouraging flexibility – scheduling musicians with different team members and combinations of instruments for different projects.

Importance of inclusiveness, sustainability and legacy

Learning the language of the respective cultures – entering the world of both the musician and care staff and understanding where they are coming from.

Talking with managers and staff about their roles on the project – non-hierarchical, understanding that processes are universal, and include and affect all of us.

Developing a sense of shared ownership between Music for Life musicians and the staff of each care home.

Identifying what can remain (e.g. a pattern of meeting together to discuss experiences of being with residents; shifting from task-orientated discussion to person-centred).

Drawing attention to musicians as role models in their person-centred way of relating and not just in the music they create.

Working with staff development trainers or designated development managers to develop strategies to sustain the thinking and reflection and to affect the ways of caring for residents after the project ends.

Acknowledging the learning during the project and planning for the departure of the musicians – creating an understanding that the legacy is mostly in the capacity of and interest of staff to reflect on those in their care and see them and treat them as individuals.

Responsibilities to oneself as manager / personal care

Maintaining personal confidence and vision – carrying responsibility to take care of one's own issues (possible supervision and support required).

Maintaining a strong sense of personal identity and an informed self-awareness.

Taking care of oneself – to recognise and be resilient to projections from others, including residents, musicians and staff.

Allowing the connections made in the workshops to be a source of inspiration in guiding the project.

Monitoring and evaluation

Clarifying what is being monitored and evaluated for each of the three strands of the project (e.g. improved quality of life for people with dementia, improvement in staff capacity to deliver person-centred care, development of range of personal and professional skills for musicians, and reflective skills and self-motivated learning for all three).

Knowing what to look for in reviewing an individual project session with staff and musicians, in particular a growing capacity for staff and musicians to go beyond discussing 'what' they have seen and to start to consider 'why' (e.g. why a resident no longer shouts the same words throughout the sessions, why music is improvised in the sessions, why a musician gives a resident choice rather than imposing on them, why a resident is allowed to leave the group rather than being coerced to stay, why several people were close to tears when a resident and a musician made music together).

Recognising that the success of a project has to do not just with the increasing depth in which musicians and staff are able to reflect on their experiences of the work, but also the extent to which that may start to change their professional practice.

Understanding signs that a project has 'worked' for a resident (e.g. growing confidence to direct musicians and so own the music, interest in others in the group, tolerance of attention being on others, allowing someone into their personal space, staying rather than walking out of a session, making eye contact, celebrating others' musical achievements).

Ensuring monitoring and evaluation remain an intrinsic part of the process of the Music for Life project, and are on-going throughout the workshop series and that this is understood by managers, staff trainers and musicians.

Dealing with practical issues to support monitoring and evaluation e.g. setting up shared debriefing sessions for musicians, staff and trainers, meetings with the staff trainer to monitor staff changes, meeting with the workshopleader to feedback to musicians information on residents, meeting with musicians for feedback.

Understanding the dynamics and complexities of each project and each session and appreciating the complex interactions between musical, social, psychological, emotional, logistical factors in evaluating an individual session or a workshop series.

Practical issues relating to monitoring and evaluation

Using relevant expertise to evaluate, e.g. drawing on experts in the field of dementia and identifying recognised evaluation tools and literature in the dementia care field to learn what represents quality experience for people at different stages of dementia and with different kinds of dementia.

Encouraging staff and residents' key workers to look for and record in care plans any changes that may have occurred outside the sessions in the days between sessions that may be to do with the project.

Handing back responsibility to staff and managers for taking forward the principles of the work when the project ends and so too to evaluating its effectiveness in their own way.

Recognising that outcomes of the work will need to be described and reported on in ways that are appropriate to the audiences e.g. funders of arts programmes, funders of healthcare programmes, home managers, directors of care organizations.

What does management look like in practice? Three scenarios

Music for Life is a complex project to manage with many dimensions and many roles for the manager. In order to try to bring to life the preceding pages, there follows three scenarios, examples of the kinds of experiences which are typical of the project and which focus on and combine different elements of the management role.

Setting 1. Focus on staff

We are in the lounge of a residential home, working with eight residents from a unit for people with advanced dementia. The residents have been brought in from the unit where they live and have settled in the new space. The workshop session is well underway and at last it is quiet. Each of the three Tuesdays that we have been here, the gardeners seem to have been scheduled to mow the lawn outside the room. I have finally managed to locate the manager who, understanding our need for quiet, has authorised the rescheduling of this grass cutting so the motors have stopped and we have now achieved the calm we need for the session.

The staff trainer and I are seated outside the circle together with the two staff who are observing with us this week. Following feedback from the trainer after our debriefing session last week, the musicians are going to look out for an opportunity to involve the three staff in the circle in making a piece with the team. Building their confidence towards this has not been easy. This is a disparate group of staff who although skilled at the tasks they carry out, are not a cohesive team. We have seen that the divisions in the staff group are affecting the well-being of the residents. This is something I was alerted to in the initial meeting with the home manager and we are working on together with the trainer.

During the opening piece of music, the workshopleader moves to the centre of the circle to where the percussion instruments are carefully arranged, and draws out a djembe. He returns to his seat and introduces a new rhythm to the piece whilst the other two musicians hold the tune. As the piece takes a new direction, he passes the drum to one of the staff and then encourages her to keep the beat going to support the piece. One by one he then introduces instruments to the other two staff, still supported by the musicians. As they finally withdraw from the piece the staff hold their own for a moment and then the piece becomes fragmented and quickly falls apart. The session moves on but there is a clearly a problem amongst the staff in the group.

After the session, we all help to pack away the instruments and the staff return residents to their unit. I then begin the debriefing, knowing that the staff issue needs to be raised if the group is to grow together to strengthen the confidence of the residents. I suggest the group takes a few moments to relax. The staff sit stiffly and silently. The musicians jot down thoughts in their notebooks, or sit back in their seats with closed eyes. I then invite them to feed back initial reactions to the session. Immediately one member of staff verbally attacks another, blaming her for deliberately ruining their music. It is clear that the scenario described earlier by the manager has been played out in the workshop and the staff tensions have shown themselves in this setting. The staff training agenda is now clear. I decide that the joint debriefing should break early and that the trainer should work with the staff whilst I stay with the musicians to look at the issues they want to address in relation to the music.

Over the next few weeks there is a strong focus on strategies to bring coherence to the group. The trainer works one to one with the staff member who sabotaged the piece. She discovers that this person feels isolated from her team, passed over for promotion and is in the process of seeking other work outside the care sector. As the story unfolds the trainer also finds she is good at her work with residents. The trainer shares the unfolding story with me and, whilst not divulging the whole story of this staff member, I highlight the sensitivities and encourage the musicians to look for appropriate ways of building staff relationships through the music. As the project progresses in this home, the staff and musicians become a team and it is possible gradually to talk about teamwork within the group in later debriefings and to congratulate them all on working together. The residents thrive in this warmer, supportive environment and the trainer continues to work with the staff after we have left. I stay in touch with the manager and the trainer and hear some time later that the team is now working well together, nobody has left and the member of staff who had felt so isolated was able not only to stay and work in the team, but had gained the self-esteem to talk about her journey and her growth to others beyond the home.

Setting 2. Focus on the Home management

I arrive at the home early and pass the manager's office. She calls me in and invites me to have a coffee with her. Time is tight and I am due to check that the room is clear and ready for us to set up the workshop. I also see that for some reason, I am needed here. I decide that, as it is session 7 of eight sessions, the musicians are able to get started themselves. The instrument cupboard door is unlocked and I have met the staff on the project on the way in and know that they are all on duty and the residents are all well and able to attend, so I can afford to take a few minutes away. The workshopleader has arrived now so I meet her in the corridor, tell her where I am and join the manager.

We have had several meetings and she has been very interested and supportive of the project. Now she looks very tired. There are piles of forms on her desk and the room looks a mess. She begins to tell me about how much the project is raising morale in the home. Staff are smiling more, some residents in the group are starting to becoming more tolerant of others and wandering around less as they seem to feel more secure and family members have commented to staff on small changes they have noticed in residents. It's good to hear all this, but as I listen, I sense that this is not the reason I have been called in. Soon it becomes clear that this person is overwhelmed by her work and is under huge stress outside her job. I am aware that I need to be with the team now and gently draw our conversation to a close, suggesting that if she has time, she might come and observe the session for a few minutes. I know from a previous visit that being in the session seems to replenish some energy for her. This is often the case – managers seem to be overwhelmed with paperwork and meetings and coming into a session seems to put them back in touch with the purpose of their work. We set out the room and I leave a chair by the door in case she appears but also to minimise disruption if she enters. We usually discourage observers appearing during a workshop but feel an exception can be made here, and seat myself by the door in case she arrives.

The session begins well, the manager appears, sits quietly for a few minutes, smiles and then leaves. The session progresses, the debriefing goes well and we leave. In the week between this and the final session, the workshopleader calls and we discuss strategies for the session and debriefing. She is a new leader who is learning her new role. She has been a regular and outstanding team member for a number of years and is well accustomed to the project. However, she finds the change of responsibility a real challenge and more complex than she had anticipated, balancing the need to lead and be seen to be leading whilst also remembering to invite initiatives from her fellow musicians. We have established a pattern of speaking between sessions each week. We anticipate a good final session although we are both aware of the dangers of expecting development and progression from one week to the next. We remind ourselves of this and acknowledge the need for flexibility and caution in expectations.

Arriving the following week before the musicians, there is a sense that something has happened in the home. The manager's office is empty and locked. I can find no senior staff, and residents are not being prepared for the workshop. Searching the building for staff who may be able to help, I discover the manager has left and a sense of confusion pervades the home. The staff cannot identify for me anyone who is in charge. The musicians are already setting up and playing together and I decide that if we are to be able to get through this, the musicians should be left alone while I try and sort it out. Our workshopleader needs to focus on the set up and rehearsal as we discussed.

The written agreement which is completed with the manager before any project begins, now comes into its own. Finally discovering a senior team leader, I show him the agreement and work with him to assemble the staff and residents who need to be with us. I know that this will put pressure on an already insecure staff team and am not sure that this is the right thing to do under the circumstances, but the project is so far advanced that it is a risk to be taken. By the time the session is due to start, the musicians are ready, the staff have appeared and the residents are being brought in to the room. Despite the confusion and uncertainty outside the room, the atmosphere in the workshop is calm and the session starts in a structured and predictable way. It has been possible to keep this confusion away from the musicians and to provide some sense of continuity for residents and staff in what is clearly an unstable situation.

Setting 3. Focus on the musicians

"You told us we could only have a group of eight people and now look what's happened!" The trainer and I are meeting with the manager and laughing together at the way the day centre members have taken ownership of the group. This project has seemed to need endless flexibility. After week one, four of the eight people with dementia were absent from the group – in hospital, ill at home or in one case on a family holiday with no prior warning to the centre manager. In the succeeding weeks some have returned unexpectedly and having been replaced, insist on rejoining the group, and so the group has become fluid and flexible. As we accept this, it turns from a problem into source of interest and fun. This spirit of fun has pervaded the sessions and spirits and energy are high at the start of each session.

During the preparation hour before the workshop we discuss this particularly unusual energy amongst the group members, and as we look at this more deeply, we acknowledge that it originates from one man in particular. He like, others in the group, has mild dementia and short term memory loss. His long term memory is intact and he is fixated on his army days. In the presence of his male friends in the group, and stimulated by the presence of one of our musicians who plays trumpet, he is frequently imitating bugle calls during the session and in particular the reveille, the morning wakeup call in the army. This arouses memories in the other two men who were also in the army during the last war. They banter together, generating much laugher – but they also relate army experiences in which women are clearly objects to be used by the soldiers. We talk about this and realise that this has impacted, particularly, on our one female musician. She has come to the centre this week feeling uncomfortable and upset and not understanding why this is. As we talk, we begin to see that in her position in the group beside the bugler for the past couple of sessions, she has been turned into one of his women. She has not understood what has happened and how she has been treated but simply knows that she has been unable to be herself in the sessions and playing her cello with him has caused great discomfort. Addressing this involves thinking about both the practical seating arrangements and ways of using music to move him from his default position to a more present and real position in the group. We consider the way the trumpet is played in the session, using a mute, avoiding military style sounds and moving towards more lyricism in the music.

It is a complex session to lead, and the challenge of this workshop tells on the workshopleader. As the workshop ends, the members leave to have their lunch, and the buzz of conversation dies down. The staff and two musicians are packing away the instruments and talking with great excitement about the session and the responses they noticed. It is then that I spot the workshopleader, sitting down quietly on his own, away from his colleagues and staff. I go over to him and open up conversation. He feels the session was really unsuccessful and that his leadership was questionable. I now hold two entirely different views of the past hour and have the agenda for the debriefing. As we sit together I suggest to the group of staff and musicians that we go around the circle describing our feeling about the session. I decide to start with the workshopleader. As he describes his experience of the session, there is a stunned silence. As we progress around the circle, he begins to see that this is not the picture seen by anyone else. They describe the changed behaviour of the men in the group. They comment on the music played by the cellist, now freed up to be herself in the group. They talk about the effectiveness of the new approach of the musician playing trumpet. They compliment the workshopleader on prompting and guiding these changes. He is relieved and grateful for their feedback and now appreciates that the emotional energy it has taken to change the dynamic in the session had caused him to misread his contribution. We talk further about this, reinforcing the value of reflecting as a group and, together with the trainer, opening up wider conversation about how to take forward the learning from the session.

II.2   **Reflections on project management**

by Peter Renshaw[190]

Background

The aim of this research report is to offer further reflections on the management of projects like Music for Life, drawing on the perspectives of four members of the Music for Life project with complementary functions: that of staff development practitioner, project manager, musician and Head of Learning, Wigmore Hall. None of these interviewees have been involved in the wider research project 'Music and Dementia', but their contributions have helped to provide a broader view of the roles and responsibilities of a project manager in a Music for Life project. The following questions formed the basis of four semi-structured interviews:

From your experience of working for Music for Life, how do you perceive the roles and responsibilities of the project manager? In relation to:

     the people with dementia in a residential home

     the residential home manager

     the care staff in the home

     the staff development practitioner

     the musicians in the group

What principles, values and attitudes do you think should underpin the role of project manager?
What skills do you think are essential for effective project management? For example:

     management and organisation skills

     communication and social skills

     musical and creative skills

     monitoring and evaluation skills

     mentoring and support skills

Are there any other factors that you feel ought to be taken into account in project management?

---

[190] Peter Renshaw is a writer and researcher who lives and works in London. His special interests are in institutional change and lifelong learning. Renshaw's recent research has been in connection with the Barbican and Guildhall School of Music & Drama.

Values and qualities underpinning Music for Life projects

The success of any Music for Life project is dependent in part on developing and sustaining effective partnerships. Like any good relationship, these partnerships must be allowed to grow organically over time. Within Music for Life there is a strong feeling that if the ultimate aim of a project is to engage meaningfully with the people with dementia, all participants – project manager, residential home manager, care staff, staff development practitioner and musicians – need to be working together towards shared priorities, a shared vision and an integrity of purpose. Ideally all partners should be aiming to build up a sense of shared engagement and shared ownership in which each other's agendas are understood and supported, and possible differences and common ground are respected.

From the interviews it was clear that all successful Music for Life projects are underpinned by a cluster of values and qualities which help to characterise the humanistic nature of Music for Life. The principle of respect for persons lies at the heart of a programme that aims to enhance the quality of people's lives. It is not surprising then that the core values and qualities are seen to include: mutual respect; trust; honesty; integrity; authenticity; tolerance; openness; generosity; empathy; patience; equity of status and spirit of inclusion.

Ensuring that these values and qualities are embodied in the life of each project represents a challenge for all participants. In fact, people speak about their engagement more in terms of a 'way of life' rather than as a 'job'. Responding to different contexts, connecting to people, caring for residents, listening to different voices, supporting each other in the team, making music together in a responsive way – basically, learning from each other to make each partnership work – all these elements are fundamental to the philosophy and practice of Music for Life.

Relationships within each project

The sensitivity and intimacy of each Music for Life project necessitate that the dynamics and complexity of working relationships are understood by all team members. This is especially the case for the project manager who, in many ways, is at the hub of any one project – initiating, connecting, planning, organising, communicating, facilitating, enabling, nurturing, supporting, monitoring, evaluating and sustaining at all stages of the journey. This multifaceted role requires an insight into how residents, carers, staff development practitioners, home managers and musicians might respond in different circumstances. Responsiveness to events and people lies at its core. A few examples drawn from the interviews might help to illustrate this complexity.

Relationship between project manager and residential home manager

As the home manager is the first point of contact in any project, it is crucial to gain their support and understanding right from the beginning. The project manager must be able to explain clearly the aims and objectives of the project and the nature of the processes used to the home manager, at all times focusing on the benefits of the project for the residents: for example, helping them to make connections through reminiscence, strengthening their sense of identity and feeling of belonging, unlocking their voice and self-awareness, building up a feeling of security within a group.

The project manager has to be constantly alert to building up and sustaining a good working relationship with the home manager, who is frequently under pressure from practical, bureaucratic and human demands. Adopting an empathetic listening and supportive role is likely to be much valued by a home manager feeling stressed by the constant accumulation of circumstances, many of which are unforeseen. In many ways the smooth running of a project hangs on decisions made by the home manager – e.g. choice of residents and care staff for the project, question of space and logistics. It is therefore important for the project manager to adopt a diplomatic role vis á vis the home manager so that an appropriate environment can be created for the music making.

Relationship between project manager, staff development practitioner and care staff

For each project the staff development practitioner is the crucial link between the project manager and the care staff. He or she engages the staff to be involved in the project and together with the home manager, selects the residents likely to respond to the whole experience. The project manager, supported by the musicians, then has the responsibility to draw the care staff into the shared process of each session.

Ideally there should be a synergy between the project manager and the staff development practitioner. They should be working together from a shared vision of the project, underpinned by a shared sense of commitment, enthusiasm and imagination. They should have a mutual understanding of dementia and of the possible impact of the project on both the residents and care staff. Together, the project manager and the staff development practitioner must provide a strong structure that will enable the creative and social process to work. Basically they need to create an open climate within a clear structure from which all participants will benefit.

Relationship between musicians and project manager, staff development practitioner and care staff

First and foremost the musicians in each project team are dependent on the project manager creating a framework that will work for them. Practical matters such as space, time and logistics are a *sine qua non*, but the musicians also function best in a psychological climate that is supportive and trusting. The project manager is pivotal in making this happen.

From all accounts the care staff see the benefits of the Music for Life sessions not only for the residents but also for themselves. In his interview the staff development practitioner observed that in addition to their creative and performance skills, the musicians have important non-musical qualities that would be seen as exemplary for the care staff: for example, excellent teamwork, open and flexible attitudes, good communication (both verbal and non-verbal), sensitivity to the well-being of the residents, responsiveness to the emotional climate of the group and an awareness of the nuances within the care staff.

What stands out from the interviews is that although the project manager plays a significant role in making the project work, the responsibility for the relationships within a project is very much shared throughout the whole team. The project manager is responsible for creating a supportive environment, putting into place partnership building, helping to establish the ethos of the work and being an integral part of the reflective and evaluative process. But it is important to recognise that the musicians and staff development practitioner also have a key role in developing the relationships with the care home. The success of a project is very much dependent on the strength of the collective responsibility of the whole team.

Emergent issues

Monitoring and evaluation

Throughout its history Music for Life has generated a culture of critical reflection. This has enabled it to keep developing, connecting and adapting to changing circumstances. In practice this means that each 8-week project is viewed through a critical lens, whilst at the end of each weekly session all the professionals involved devote an hour to feedback and reflection. This is seen as an opportunity for personal and professional development.

During the interviews one key question kept recurring – should a Music for Life project manager be a musician? Most of the musicians involved in projects have a history of working closely with Linda Rose, who is a musician and an educationalist with a strong commitment to reflective forms of learning and development. All have valued her style of leadership and management over the years. As Linda would be the first to acknowledge, no leader can be replicated. On the other hand, the principles and procedures implicit in her approach are understandably still considered significant to the work and life of the project.

The wide-ranging skills required by a project manager become especially evident in the process of monitoring and evaluation. Although the creative processes used in any Music for Life project are musical, it would seem that any good project manager should be effective at facilitating a reflective conversation drawing out *non-musical* issues that have arisen in the course of a session. In many ways, a project manager can be seen as a detached observer who pays special attention to the responses of the residents with dementia, as well as focusing on shifts in behaviour that might inform the perspective of the care staff. In fact, the combined voice of the project manager and the staff development practitioner can help to highlight such key issues as:

- the success of the session in connecting to the particular context

- the quality of engagement with the residents

- the impact of the process on the residents

- responsiveness to the felt needs of the residents

- recognition of signs of well-being

- the quality of interaction and relationship building

- the effectiveness of communication with the residents and within the team of professionals (including verbal and body language)

- the openness, adaptability and flexibility of the team to the rhythm and flow of the session.

In the interviews some people considered that this non-musical role of the project manager, working in tandem with the staff development practitioner, needs to be made explicit, especially as it includes many key aspects of any Music for Life project. This would help to delineate the role of the project manager in the monitoring and evaluation process.

Similarly, it was felt that during this reflective process the voice of the care staff should be heard towards the beginning of each feedback session. Their observations are critical as they are in the frontline of daily care of the residents. They are in the position of supporting and sustaining any development in the longer term. The project manager can help to choreograph this conversation and bring observations back into the planning and development of future Music for Life projects.

Monitoring and evaluation of musical processes

As was intimated above, many of the musicians currently working in Music for Life feel that the project manager should ideally have some inside knowledge of the musical, creative and improvisatory processes that are central to each project. Anyone monitoring and evaluating such challenging processes within equally challenging contexts should have some understanding of the motivation, emotional drive and possible vulnerability of the team of musicians – basically, understanding what makes the creative musician 'tick' in a dementia care setting. This could not be more different from performing in a conventional concert hall. Judgements regarding the quality of the musical process have to be made in relation to the subtle nuances of a residential care environment.

Therefore it would seem critical that any discussion about musical processes should be led by a musician who understands the nature of such creative processes from the inside. It is suggested that an additional musician to the team could sit outside the workshop circle with the project manager observing the process from a detached perspective. Events move so quickly within a workshop that it is difficult for the musicians involved to be objective and clear about the complexity of what is happening within the creative process. For example, the following kind of issues might well arise when tracking the flow of the musical process:

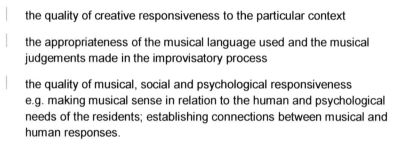

- the quality of creative responsiveness to the particular context

- the appropriateness of the musical language used and the musical judgements made in the improvisatory process

- the quality of musical, social and psychological responsiveness e.g. making musical sense in relation to the human and psychological needs of the residents; establishing connections between musical and human responses.

From these brief observations it is clear that a project manager without musical knowledge cannot be expected to facilitate a reflective conversation about the quality and appropriateness of the musical process. This role has to be taken by a musician who has experience of engaging in creative processes, preferably in dementia care settings.

In no way does this denigrate the role of the project manager whose responsibilities remain far-reaching and critical to the whole monitoring and evaluation process. Perhaps one way of choreographing the de-briefing session is to have the evaluation of the musical process led by the observer-musician, whilst the other elements are facilitated by the project manager and the staff development practitioner – another good example of collaborative teamwork.

It was suggested that for this monitoring and evaluation process to work effectively it would be good to provide opportunities for Music for Life musicians to engage in professional development programmes designed:

- to deepen their self-evaluation skills

- to strengthen their monitoring and evaluation skills as observer-musicians

- to develop their facilitation skills in leading evaluation discussions to enable them to work collaboratively with project managers and care trainers.

Providing a support structure for all staff and musicians

Different forms of staff development are seen as one necessary way of strengthening the quality of Music for Life projects. But the interviewees also felt that all staff and musicians would benefit from an effective support structure that would include reflective forms of mentoring and co-mentoring. This is hardly surprising because at one level, questions concerning identity constitute the DNA of practices like the Music for Life project. The sensitive, multi-layered process unlocks different emotional energies, capacities and feelings through both the music and the human interaction within the professional team and between the team and the residents. These responses are relevant to the musicians, project manager, home manager, staff development practitioner and care staff alike. Therefore it is suggested that appropriate support is available for those individuals and groups seeking it.

The personal and group challenges arising from the flow of creative collaborative learning embodied in a Music for Life project might be energising and inspiring, but they can also be quite daunting. Living 'on the edge', constantly taking risks, responding to the unpredictable, drawing on ones creative resources yet always listening to the voice of others – these finely tuned skills and states of being lie at the heart of any creative conversational process. But if they are to be allowed to flow and to flower, this can only take place in an emotionally supportive and understanding environment. Certain conditions, for example, can help to make this happen:

creating and sustaining a safe, receptive conversational space that is non-judgemental, trusting, empathetic and accepting

listening reflectively to the voice of others

remaining engaged with and learning from different perspectives

understanding differences and conflict as resources for learning.

The staff and musicians involved in Music for Life acknowledge the complex emotional dynamics of collaboration. If creative conversation is to flow, this process necessarily has to draw on both cognitive and affective support from within the group. The emotional connectedness that can help bind a group together can be characterised by feelings of shared motivation, shared purpose, solidarity based on shared values and a reassurance knowing that feelings of fear, vulnerability, self-doubt and marginality can also be shared. Mutual support is further strengthened when temperaments complement each other in a group. This inevitably affects the chemistry of a group and the ways in which people work together.

287

The language of reflection

Reflection lies at the heart of the processes of monitoring, evaluation, mentoring and co-mentoring. But the process of critical reflection comes with its own language that can seem threatening and alienating to those people whose normal mode of language is more descriptive and less analytical. Some musicians, for example, see themselves as pragmatic people who can feel alienated by too much reflection focusing on 'why' questions. Their identity is embedded in practical music-making, not on reflection that might raise unsettling personal and professional issues. Nevertheless, one of the significant aspects of Music for Life is that it has created a culture that has encouraged its musicians to engage in critical reflection. By and large they feel at home using more reflective forms of language, so their sense of psychological ease enables them to participate fully in any of the evaluation sessions.

On the other hand, this might not be the case with care staff who, in general, have to function in a very busy, tightly scheduled working environment. The language of reflection hardly resonates within this mechanistic, target-driven world. Therefore, in the evaluation sessions it is very much the responsibility of the project manager and the staff development practitioner to draw the care staff into the conversation in a way that makes sense to them. They need to feel that their observations and points of view are valued within the whole reflective process. The nature of the language used and the way it is expressed is critical to fostering a sense of shared ownership within the whole group.

Organisation and communication

In her profile of project management Linda Rose is very thorough in her analysis of the organisational and communication skills necessary for the effectiveness of Music for Life projects or any other comparable project. The interviews raised one important observation that is not unique to Music for Life – the danger of information overload. In this world of instant e-mail communication it is only too easy for managers to send out information indiscriminately to all members of a project. The musicians acknowledge that they need to be kept informed about those matters that are essential for the effective running of any project, but they feel that a sense of proportion needs to be maintained regarding the content and quantity of information.

Epilogue

In conclusion, I would like to thank the interviewees for their perceptive observations about project management in Music for Life. They ranged very widely in their comments and demonstrated the complexities of what is entailed in any Music for Life project. I hope this brief paper does full justice to the issues raised in our conversations.

With its commitment to fostering quality of experience and integrity of engagement, the work of Music for Life continues to demonstrate the need for thorough preparation, understanding the context of residential homes in the UK, grounded practice, effective communication and collaboration, and quality of shared reflection and evaluation. This developmental approach can only help to strengthen the sustainability and legacy of Music for Life.

II.3   Transferring the project

by Linda Rose

She surveys the room with warm authority – perhaps we are the young, nervous students in her tutorial group or perhaps we are with her on the university board, making strategic decisions under her guidance. However she casts us, we are present for her, in silence, breathing in the wisdom she so clearly imparts to us in her eyes...

A former academic, no longer able to convey her story in words, tells us so eloquently that she is once again empowered and that she has, if only for a moment, become who she was... The heart of the work you are about to engage in lies in the unwavering commitment to the person with dementia.

What needs to be in place in managing the transfer of this work to another country must be a reflection and assertion of this commitment, just as it has always been the guiding light of the work in the UK. It will be present and demonstrated in the quality of smallest interaction or connection that is made between any of the participants on this project. The ways in which those very small and sensitive connections are made, whether spoken or through music, are the models for everything else about this project. Each person recruited or involved must be willing to get close to the 'lived experience', as Padraic Garrett has described to me as we talked about this. This means there needs to be a willingness for exposure to everything from the joy and spontaneity that this can bring to the pain and suffering that is a part of the life of a person living with dementia. The work begins and ends within that framework.

Any manager must spend time in the company of people living with dementia and in the community in which they live. Decisions about the work and its growth require this firsthand knowledge. Keeping alive this experience within oneself will help guide thoughts about the development of musicians, about the building of relationships with care homes and their staff, about funding and evaluation and all the myriad of issues that are integral to the growth of the work. This may at times lead to hard decisions about where to work, who to work with, how to secure funding, how to develop criteria for assessing the progress of the work. If a manager senses that commitment seems to be lacking in any possible partnerships, if there is a shying away from the very real difficulties of this challenging area of work then it will not achieve its aims – and lives will not be affected in the very deepest way that this work is capable of achieving.

Peter Renshaw raises the complex question of whether the manager needs to be a musician. Given that other personal qualities and managerial skills and experience are in place, this question is perhaps less about whether a manager should have a music background but rather, are there points in the growth of the work when this becomes less of an issue. Tracing the growth of Music for Life in the UK, the development of the musicians could not have been achieved without knowledge of music. The musicians had much to learn about working in this new context of dementia care and it was crucial to be able both to enter their world whilst also understanding the agendas of the care settings in which the work was being piloted. The manager needed to be able to straddle both.

The growth and support of the musician is always crucial and will be particularly so at the inception of this work in the Netherlands. At this stage it will be important for the manager to understand from the inside, the thinking, the driving forces and the vulnerabilities of a professional musician. As the musicians gain in experience and in understanding of the context which defines their work, their need for this direct musical support from the project manager may lessen. However as Peter identifies it may diminish, but the external observer, mentor, colleague will always be needed and perhaps this is not a role exclusive to the manager. Realistically, the manager cannot humanly meet every need of the project, connecting cultures is complex and challenging. He or she must be able to see and feel when and how expertise needs to be drawn in and to act on this. With such a high level of responsibility and such close contact with the sensibilities of all involved, the needs of the manager must not be forgotten. It will be essential to ensure that appropriate support is in place for the manager from the outset.

Try to see the project involving a tapestry of responsibilities and try to avoid hierarchies. All involved will have a part to play in all their different functions, with one aim in mind – to keep the focus on who the project is about and be consistent and uncompromising in this. So much of the work is responsive but the framework has to be secure. This will guide decisions about the very practical aspects of setting it up, the training, the location the time and space allocated for workshops and for reflection. Recognise that the 'community' includes all those who support behind the scenes and value them equally and in the same spirit of respect and equality. The values of the work will ripple beyond the workshops and affect others so maintaining the essential focus and deepening the impact on the person with dementia.

Stay small and focussed and supported. The work will be new and could arouse great interest. It is crucial to ensure that it is not overexposed, so that participants are able to develop their relationships in a contained way. They must be free to explore, to make mistakes, to reflect and to celebrate the changes they may make as individuals, benefitting from support and encouragement from those who understand the significance of what is happening.

In the end, there are no blueprints for this work. It always raises more questions than it answers. There is no defining moment when the talking stops and we all know what to do and how to do it. And so this concludes with the most important question that must be constantly in the heart and mind of any new manager: "Am I doing everything I possibly can to take forward the core values that I know are important?"

...She no longer addresses us, but moves slowly back within herself to the person we first saw. Small, frail and enclosed... But she and her message are conveyed, and must remain with us as a constant reminder of what is important and is the inspiration for all of our future work.

III   Passionate about connection – founder Linda Rose

"And the thing that struck me is this quote by T.S. Eliot...'you are the music While the music lasts'. To me what happens is terribly subtle. But if you get it right as a musician, if you match something in your music, about the person you are working with, whose identity is lost, who very often doesn't know who they are, where they are, what's going on... if that match is right, then somewhere between you and that other person, somewhere in that space where the music is happening, is that person's identity. It's in that music. And they see themselves, they feel themselves, they notice, they know that somewhere in there, is them. And that is the essence of that connection."

Linda Rose has felt herself an educator throughout her life. Born in Cheltenham, Gloucestershire, into a Jewish family, she spent a short time in the United States as a child before the family moved to London. There at the age of seven she started learning the violin. Her father was her inspiration in music, "he was very musical in an untrained way. He used to play banjo and the ukulele in dance bands. He was a very strong influence on me as a youngster." Linda was not happy in her violin lessons: "I had a teacher who terrified me. I loved music, but I hated my lessons (...) I loved everything about music, but I didn't enjoy playing the violin. I loved to sing, I knew it was possible to make music without the fear I had experienced." She was later to discover that she wanted to be a music educator and became passionate about it.

The choice to train as a teacher was more or less coincidental. Linda started off in teacher training at the Wall Hall College in Hertfordshire where sculpture was her main study. She was shortly to change to music. Here she met the first of a few important people guiding her professional life, her education tutor Peter Renshaw. The discussions with him were a major influence: "As an eighteen year old just out of school, everything inside was melting down and starting again, and what emerged was someone who was passionate about changing things in education. Peter drove that passion, constantly challenging ideas and constantly questioning."

Linda's first teaching post was in 1970 at a primary school in Harrow, in North London, where after one year, she became Head of Music. Soon she started networking, bringing people together in the borough who, like herself, were reflecting on necessary change in music education for children: "....how to make it relevant to children, how to begin to draw on children's own ideas, instead of imposing ideas on them." An important other person she met in this period was Peter Slade, a leader in drama therapy in the UK, who became her mentor. Slade had written a book on drama education for children, finding the starting point with the child. Here she found parallels with her thoughts on music education. She was to discover Slade was quite a controversial figure in the UK, but became a strong influence on Linda's work. She describes him as "a pioneer in his field", promoting for the first time in drama education the equivalent to improvisation in music education. Through this contact Linda became more and more aware that it was not the just children who needed to undergo change, but first and foremost it was their teachers.

In order to further her education she then took a course at the London University Institute of Education, where she became excited by new approaches to action research, and together with colleagues, started a project on curriculum reform for music education in her borough.

At the beginning of the eighties a third influential person came on her path. This was John Stephens, at that time Staff Inspector for Music in the Inner London Education Authority (ILEA). Stephens appointed Linda to his newly formed team of Music Coordinators, responsible for supporting teachers in the classroom and developing music education practice across two London boroughs.

> ...my first job, was to go into a boys' secondary school in Acton, next to Wormwood Scrubs, a high security prison. Many of the boys' families had moved to that area because their fathers were in prison. The music department had wire around the windows, the boys were locked in, they had to have a pass to go out of the classroom, to be allowed to go to any other part of the school. And my job was to go in there and to change the practice of a teacher who was near to retirement. I had never taught in secondary school. I was completely and utterly terrified to do this. This was typical of the kind of work it was. I remember going in on the first day, the teacher was hugely sceptical: 'this young woman, who is this young upstart?'
> I remember turning up outside this classroom having talked to him about what I wanted to do. 'I don't want the boys in rows, I want a circle and well, leave it to me.' So the boys lined up outside the classroom, throwing their bags everywhere, like crazy fourteen-year-olds. They piled into the classroom, threw the chairs everywhere, so I sent them out of the classroom and made them line up again. Put the chairs right again. They came in again, same thing again, lolling all over the place, and I threw them out again, brought them in again, told them to take their blazers off. Take their jackets off! Well, for these boys, this was their security. But, they put their jackets behind their chairs. I'd prepared a warm–up drama game. And I remember standing in the middle of the circle thinking, 'I have one chance here. I've got about thirty seconds to capture their interest, or I've had it.' I don't know what, I did some silly clapping game or clicking, something, something fast around the circle and they did it. And I'd reached them. Every lesson was terrifying, but we built a connection... and I worked with the teacher and he came on board and he got excited. There was a steel band teacher who used to work with us too and she caught the energy and by the end it was fantastic, absolutely fantastic. So that was the nature of the job. And each one I went into, whether it was a nursery school or a secondary school or a primary school, the kids generally were a real challenge to work with. Throughout all of this time, John Stephens was a constant support and inspiration, always believing in the potential of his team to change individuals and improve lives for young people through music.

Linda reflects on the three 'significant others' she met in her professional life: "They came one after the other. And each of them believed in the parts of me that, I guess, my family perhaps did not understand (...) there was something that drove me, something that excited me, which other people hadn't seen. And that was so empowering, so supportive and exciting. It just meant that, I could actually begin to believe in and act on my hunches."

Making connections between people was increasingly recognised as her skill, a key skill in the Music for Life project which she would at a later stage start to develop: "...encouraging it. Listening to people who felt threatened by change, and trying to come in from where they were. I suppose create a relationship myself with them and help them to create a relationship with other people so there was a feeling of everybody learning and moving on together."

From 1983 till 1990 Linda worked in Birmingham as a general inspector and advisor for music in the City of Birmingham Education Department. There she was responsible for policy development for music education for the city's schools and colleges, curriculum development and teacher recruitment and development. It was not an easy time; she met initial resistance to change and difficult local politics. Nevertheless the situation changed gradually and she succeeded in developing interesting initiatives both in schools and on the wider arts and music scene, for example with the City of Birmingham Symphony Orchestra which was at that time led by a forward looking conductor, Simon Rattle.

Linda went back to London in 1990 and was then asked by Peter Renshaw to teach on a course at the Guildhall School of Music & Drama, where he had set up a postgraduate course on Performance and Communication Skills. Like pioneers will always encounter, this was also tough, having to deal with music students who had to gain 'community experience' and often not seeing the relevance of it.

The development of the Music for Life project started from 1993, as often happens, more or less coincidentally. Linda was contacted by her mother who asked her to care for a cousin who was old, very depressed and had tried to commit suicide. As Linda did not know anything about supporting older people she therefore contacted the organisation Jewish Care. This led to her starting to work as a volunteer. It was an empowering period for her: "I discovered, first of all, that I knew far more than I thought I knew. Because my experience of working with people was transferable." Linda then initiated a new idea: "I started thinking, well, we're doing all this work at the Guildhall, to introduce the students to working in schools with children, I wonder if it's possible to do any of this work with older people. And so I spoke to Peter Renshaw about it. And I spoke to a colleague in Jewish Care and said, 'might you be interested in piloting an idea?' By this time I had drawn up a draft proposal to make a link between Jewish Care and the Guildhall, a module of work to explore what the possibilities were. So we set up this project in a day centre for older people in the East End of London. This was not with people with dementia at this point; the members were in their eighties, probably most of them. And the project involved drawing on their memories. The students built relationships with the individuals, they drew out their stories and they created music with them based on their stories." Jewish Care became more and more interested and slowly the project Music for Life evolved and became embedded in Jewish Care. A few of the Guildhall students remained in the work and continued to work along with Linda. The emphasis moved to people with dementia, as more and more elderly people entered into care homes at a later age, when they were physically and mentally more frail, and had often developed dementia.

Linda developed the programme of Music for Life workshops for people with dementia and their carers, supported by research which she carried out with her colleague Stephanie Schlingensiepen, a nurse-researcher. This was also the starting point of the serious thinking about staff development. The research model, based on critical reflection, became central to the project: "So the project is now, and always will be, I hope, ongoing action research." Initially Linda worked with a few musicians, amongst them amateur volunteers but later on she was able to develop and implement a training programme for professional musicians.

Much energy has since then gone into explaining the project, e.g. that it was not aiming at cognitive improvement, nor could be measured in a quantitative way: "The long-term effects have much to do with the impact on the staff. But equally you can't deny the value of the immediate responses of the people during those sessions. You know, it is just like when you go to a concert, you can be overwhelmed by the music, but no one asks you in two weeks time, 'has your life improved because of that?' It doesn't take away the impact of that piece of music at *that* moment." A telling example is recounted by Linda:

> Alan was working with a man. He was 104, he was asleep and Alan sang to him. Alan is a singer. The whole group was just riveted, watching this little, frail man asleep, and as Alan is singing, he wakes up with a start, and Alan gently carries on singing 'good morning Mr. Rosenberg', singing that to him all the time, and then, as the sun comes into the room: 'it's a lovely morning Mr. Rosenberg.' He holds his hand and gently strokes his hand and this man very gradually refocuses, looks at Alan, smiles at him and then smiles at the carer and then beams as he notices that everyone in the circle is looking at him. It's just so moving. And, in a way *he* is leading even though he was asleep, he dictated what Alan did by the way he was sleeping. Alan had to match something about Mr. Rosenberg because he knew it was possible Mr. Rosenberg would wake up. He had to do something that was appropriate and would bring him gently into the group. He had to be real, or authentic, a word that is used a lot in dementia care, to be the real person in order to meet the real person.

Building relationships is at the core of the practice, Linda feels: "bringing together the world of a professional musician and the world of health and social care seemed to me to be one of the biggest challenges to face, and I just loved trying to find a way to do it. That was the drive during those years. I would just love to try and bring together people from different worlds. And that's the theme that probably goes through my life in different ways. It's almost like a need, it's not just a passion."

> When we started talking with individual staff you discovered that maybe somebody had travelled for hours and hours across London at six o'clock in the morning, with huge childcare problems. A member of the care staff, who would come into a home in North London and travel for hours, with very little qualifications and very little pay, to do some very hard work, all day. Possibly not understanding the language or the culture of the people they were working with, working in Jewish Care, sometimes working with Holocaust survivors, working with older people who had been brought up, if not as religious Jews, at least with the Jewish culture behind them, and they would come in and these two groups of people would not understand each other, and the stress level of the job of the carer was huge, and the status of the carer is so low. And I found that it made such a difference if you could just come in and meet them where they were, even by simply saying, 'did you have a rough journey here today', or, 'it's three in the afternoon, you must be dying for a cup of tea, you must be exhausted.' The tiniest things, I found, were ways into gaining their trust. And so each time we came into a home we were trusted more and more. And as the trust grew so the potential for learning grew. I could see this happening, and the musicians intuitively did this. They were drawn to the work because they were certain kinds of people. So they did this themselves without realising what they were doing. And I began to think, there have to be ways of using this project, the project is a tool for change, it's not just a project. It's a means, it is a medium for learning. Whoever wants to learn from it can learn from it (...) I had to be so careful not to use the language, the educational language I was so familiar with, I had to learn the language of the care setting, of health and social care. I had to learn the kind of questions to ask about what was going on in the place, so that if you met a manager, you'd know that she had spent the morning at the computer, you'd know she had problems with staff rota's and absence and cover staff. And if you could just come in and acknowledge that, then you would find she'd give you the staff you needed for the project and would support your work in so many ways.

In 2009 Wigmore Hall took over the management of the project and since then Linda has been involved as a consultant for Music for Life Wigmore Hall and Dementia UK as it is at present officially entitled. Years of careful preparation have preceded this step. Linda is happy with the development, as it is a valuable opportunity for sustainability of the project. However, she remains alert: "I do think it is important if the work is going to be replicated elsewhere, that the whole spirit, the learning, the values, the relationships, all of these things, this whole tapestry of different things that make this project, can't be compromised on. One of my team once said, 'you don't compromise, do you?' I had to think hard about this: 'No I don't compromise, not where I think it matters.'"

IV   Protagonists

Residential home

Emanuel Zeffert House

Residents

Rosamund

Rebecca

Esther

Jessica

Gabriella

Sarah

Hannah

Abigail

Musicians

Matthew, workshopleader

Fiona

Anneliese

Harry

Staff development practitioner

Brian

Staff

Anne

Diallo

Helena

Rachel

Samantha

Project manager

Deborah

Director of the residential home

Carrie

V   List of musical instruments

A note about pitches:

Using a standard 88-key concert piano, Helmholtz ascribed the following system for naming notes of the Western chromatic scale. These have been used in the analysis and descriptions:

Keys 1-3: A,, A#/Bb,, B,,

Keys 4 to 12: C, to B,

Keys 13 to 27: C to B

Keys 28 to 39: c to b

Keys 40 to 51: c' to b'

Keys 52 to 63: c" to b"

Keys 64 to 75: c''' to b'''

Keys 76 to 88: c'''' to c'''''

Tuned instruments:

Aluminum Chime Tree: Twenty narrow, hollow aluminum tubes, affixed to and hanging loosely from a tabletop stand. The lengths of the tubes range from 1.75 inches (4,5 cm) up to 6.5 inches (16,5 cm), and are arranged so that they progressively change in pitch. When stroked by hand or with a stick, the tubes produce a high tinkling sound through hitting each other, akin to wind chimes.

Chime Bars: A chime bar is a tuned metal bar mounted onto a wooden resonator box. The sound is produced by striking the metal part of the chime bar with a beater, most often a beater with a soft rubber head, or a wooden head. The set used in this project incorporated a chromatic pitch range between the notes g' to g'''. Soprano chime bars are generally in the range c" to a''', and alto chime bars in the range of c' to a'.

Bass Chime Bar, Metallophone, or Bass Bar: A chime bar metallophone is a tuned metal bar mounted onto a wooden resonator box, in the pitch range of G to a. The sound is produced by striking the metal part of the chime bar with a mallet or beater, most often soft mallets with a wool-wrapped head or hard rubber. An alternative version of the Bass Chime Bar Metallophone is the Bass Chime Bar Xylophone, where a tuned wooden bar is affixed to a wooden resonator box.

Hand chime, or Tone Chime: Tuned square tubes with an external clapper system, rung by hand, and similar to handbells. The hand chimes used in this project were pitched at c', e' and g'.

Kalimba: Also known as mbira, thumb piano, the kalimba is an African instrument. It consists of a hollow wooden board upon which varying lengths of metal 'tongues' or lamellae are affixed. The varying lengths produce a series of pitches; the wooden board acts as a resonator when the thumb and fingers are used pluck the tongues.

Spirit chime, similar to a tubaphone: Narrow, solid aluminium tubes, mounted onto a wooden resonated box. It can consist of a single pitch or a series of pitches arranged into a major scale, commonly a'' to a'''. The sound is produced through striking or stroking the tubes.

Un-tuned instruments:

African Ankle Rattle: An African instrument, traditionally worn on the ankles, consisting of a band strung with small seedpod shells. Shaking the instrument produces a raspy, rattle sound.

Agogô Bell, Wooden Agogô, Wooden Double Agogô: Originating from the West African Yoruba and used in samba music, this instrument consists of two metal conical 'bells', struck by a drumstick. The bells are both high pitched, and produce two discrete pitches. The Wooden Agogô imitates the design of the Agogô Bell, and it consists of either one or two bells. Each wooden 'bell' has grooves on it, so that the instrument can either be struck by a wooden beater, producing a semi-pitched sound much like the wood block, or scraped, producing a sound like a guiro.

Bodhran: A frame drum (see Frame Drum) with a goatskin head originating from Ireland, usually around 35 cm to 45 cm in diameter. A sound is traditionally made by using a special wooden beater (called a cipin or tipper) or by hand. The drum is struck with the dominant hand, and the non-dominant hand is used against the underside of the drum to control the pitch and tension of the drum.

Caxixi: A woven basket shaker, with a flat bottom usually made from cocoa shell, and filled with seeds or other particles. It is associated with West African and Brazilian music.

Cabasa, Afuche: A cylinder with a handle upon which loops of steel-ball chain are wrapped, adapted from the African Shekere. The Shekere is a hollowed out gourd covered with a net of beads. Both the Cabasa and the Shekere are played through holding the instrument with one hand, whilst the other hand scrapes the beads back and forth over the cylinder or gourd.

299

Castanets: Widely used in traditional dance music in Southern Europe, the castanet consists of a pair of concave shells, attached at one end by string. The loop of the string is hung over the thumb, and the pair of shells produce a loud, clicking sound when struck together, using the fingers of the hand, predominantly the middle and ring fingers. They can be made of hardwood, fiberglass and hard plastic.

Claves: Widely used in Latin American music, claves consist of a pair of thick wooden dowel, which produce a bright clicking noise when struck together. One stick is cupped in the non-dominant hand, with the space between the hand and the stick acting as a resonating chamber, and the other stick acts as the striker, and is held in the dominant hand. They can be made out a variety of wood types, most often maple, granadilla and rosewood, as well as fiberglass.

Djembe: Also known as djembé, jembe, jenbe, djimbe, jimbe, or dyinbe. Originating from West Africa, the djembe is a goblet drum with a skin head, often made of hardwood and untreated goat hide. The skin head is attached to the drum with rope, and the drum is 'rope-tuned' through a weaving process. A variety of sounds can be produced using hand strokes, a rich bass tone through striking the centre of the drum, and drier tones near the rim. In the project, a large, soft wool-headed mallet was used to produce a sound.

Gato drum: A type of hollow slit drum, crafted from wood into a rectangular shape. Varying widths and lengths of the multiple slits or 'tongues' on the top of the drum produce different pitches when struck by a mallet, wooden beater or heavy rubber beater, with the body of the drum acting as a resonating chamber.

Ghungharus: Also known as Payal, Paayal, Ghungaru, Ghungroo, Ghungur, Nupur, Ghangaroo. An Indian instrument, traditionally worn on the ankles, consisting of a band with two rows of small bells sewn into it. Shaking the instrument produces a high, light sound.

Guiro: Originating from Latin America, the guiro consists of a long hollow gourd, with a serrated surface. Scraping a stick across the serrated surface produces a ratchet-like sound.

Frame Drum: The diameter of a frame drum's head is greater than its depth. The shell is made from thin wood curved into a circle upon which a skin head is stretched. It can be played using a hand, or with a beater.

Maracas, Chikitas, Egg Shakers: The Maraca is a native instrument of South America, traditionally made of gourd or coconut shells, but also commercially out of wood, plastic and leather, occasionally clay; the shell is usually attached to a handle for ease of playing. The sound is produced when beads or small particles inside the maraca hit the inside of the shell.

Chikitas are small plastic versions of the maraca. Egg Shakers work on the same acoustic principles as the Maraca, are handle-less, and have the same size and shape as a chicken egg.

Ocean drum: A cylindrical drum that emulates the sound of the ocean. Metal beads are contained within the cylinder; rolling the drum slowly back and forth produces the sound.

Rainstick: When upturned vertically, the Rainstick produces a musical effect that sounds like rainfall. The Rainstick consists of a long, hollow tube with closed ends, often derived from a cactus plant. Cactus spikes are driven into the inside of the tube in the shape of a helix; small beans or other particles trapped inside produce a sound as they fall through the spikes.

Tambourine: A ring in which small, thin 'cymbals' are attached to, akin to the frame drum, with or without a skin head. When shaken or struck, the cymbals strike each other to produce a high, rattling sound. Tambourines can often come in an oval or half moon shape, and the ring is commonly made of a light wood or plastic.

Wood Block: A small rectangular slit drum made from a single piece of wood, most commonly maple, teak or rosewood. A slit drum is a hollow percussion instrument with slits carved into it to make tongue-like shapes; the shell acts as a resonator, and the size and shape of the tongue creates a pitch. Wood Blocks are struck using a wooden headed beater.

Seed shell shaker or seed shaker: A collection of natural seed pods connected together by thin rope, and with a loop for holding it in the hand. The sound is produced through shaking the instrument, or using the hand to stroke the pods.

Tingshas or Tibetan Bell: Small heavy cymbals connected by a leather strap, traditionally used in prayer by Tibetan Buddhist monks. When struck together, the cymbals make a high pitched, resonant sound and are typically made from a bronze alloy.

References

Alheit, Peter (1993). The Narrative Interview. An Introduction. *Voksenpaedagogisk Teoriudvikling. Arbejdstekster nr. 11*. Roskilde: Roskilde Universitetscenter.

Alheit, Peter (1994). The "biographical question" as a challenge to adult education. *International Review of Education* 40 (3-5): 283-298.

Alheit, Peter (2009). Biographical learning – within the new lifelong learning discourse. In K. Illeris (ed.), *Contemporary Theories of Learning*. London: Routledge.

Alheit, Peter (2010). Die Bedeutung qualitativer Ansätze in der Sozialforschung. In C. Barthel and C. Lorei (eds.), *Empirische Forschungsmethoden. Eine praxisorientierte Einführung für Bachelor- und Masterstudiengänge der Polizei*. Frankfurt am Main: Verlag für Polizeiwissenschaften: 39-66.

Alheit, Peter (2012). Komparatistische Ansätze im Kontext qualitativer Forschung. In B. Schäffer and O. Dömer (eds.), *Handbuch Qualitative Erwachsenen- und Weiterbildungsforschung*: 626-640. Opladen: Barbara Budrich.

Alheit, Peter and Dausien, Bettina (2002). The 'double face' of lifelong learning: Two analytical perspectives on a 'silent revolution'. *Studies in the Education of Adults*, Vol. 34, Issue I: 1-20.

Alheit, Peter and Dausien, Bettina (2007). Lifelong Learning and Biography: A Competitive Dynamic Between the Macro- and the Micro Level of Education. In L. West, P. Alheit, A. S. Andersen, B. Merrill (eds.), *Using Biographical and Life History Approaches in the Study of Adult and Lifelong Learning: European Perspectives*. Frankfurt am Main: Peter Lang.

Antikainen, Ari, Houtsonen, Jarmo, Huotelin, Hannu and Kauppila, Juha (1996). *Living in a Learning Society: Life-Histories, Identities and Education*. London: Falmer Press.

Antikainen, Ari (1998). Between Structure and Subjectivity: Life Histories and Lifelong Learning. *International Review of Education* 44 (2-3): 215-234.

Azzarra, Christopher D. (1999). An aural approach to improvisation. *Music Educators Journal* 86 (3): 21-25.

Bailey, Derek (1992). *Improvisation, Its Nature and Practice in Music*. Ashbourne: Da Capo Press.

Bauman, Zygmunt (2005). *Liquid Life*. Cambridge: Polity Press.

Ballard, Clive. *Factsheet 417: The later stages of dementia*, Alzheimer's Society UK. July 2011, http://alzheimers.org.uk/site/scripts/documents_info.php?documentID=101. Accessed 1 February 2012.

Benson, Bruce Ellis (2003). *The improvisation of musical dialogue - a phenomenology of music*. Cambridge: Cambridge University Press.

Borgo, David (2005). *Sync or Swarm: Improvising Music in a Complex Age*. London: Continuum.

Bourdieu, Pierre (1987). *Die feinen Unterschiede. Kritik der gesellschaftlichen Urteilskraft*. Frankfurt am Main: Suhrkamp.

Brodsky, Warren (1995). *Career Stress and Performance Anxiety in Professional Orchestra Musicians: a Study of Individual Differences and their Impact on Therapeutic Outcomes*. Unpublished PhD Thesis, University of Keele, Staffordshire, UK.

Burgess, Robert G. 1982. *Field Research: A Source Book and Field Manual*. London: George Allen & Unwin.

Crutch, Sebastian and Rait, Greta. *Factsheet 458: The progression of Alzheimer's disease and other dementias*. Alzheimer's Society UK. December 2011. http://alzheimers.org.uk/site/scripts/documents_info.php?documentID=133. Accessed 1 February 2012.

Cobussen, Marcel (2008). *Thresholds: Rethinking Spirituality through Music*. London: Ashgate.

Davidson, Jane S. and King, Elaine C. (2004). Strategies for ensemble practice. In A. Williamon (ed.), *Musical Excellence; strategies and techniques to enhance performance*. Oxford: Oxford University Press.

Dausien, Bettina (1996). *Biographie und Geschlecht. Zur biographischen Konstruktion sozialer Wirklichkeit in Frauenlebensgeschichten*. Bremen: Donat.

Dewey, John (1986/1972). The Reflex Arc Concept in Psychology. In *John Dewey. The Early Work*, Vol. 5, Carbondale: 96ff.

Dewey, John (1938). *Experience and Education*. New York: The Macmillan Company.

Dewey, John (1917). *Creative Intelligence. Essays in the Pragmatic Attitude*. New York: Henry Holt and Company.

Flick, Uwe (2009). *An Introduction to Qualitative Research*. London: Sage.

Garrett, Padraic (2009). *Can Music for Life enhance the well-being of people with dementia and develop the person-centred care skills of care workers?* Unpublished MSc Dissertation, University of Bradford.

Geertz, Clifford (1973). Thick Descriptions: Toward an Interpretative Theory of Culture. In *The Interpretation of Cultures: Selected Essays*. New York: Basic Books.

Geiger, Arno (2011). *Der alte König in seinem Exil*. München: Hanser Verlag.

Giddens, Anthony (1991). *Modernity & Self-Identity*. Stanford: Stanford University Press.

Glaser, Barney G. and Strauss, Anselm L. (1967). *The Discovery of Grounded Theory. Strategies for Qualitative Research*. Mill Valley: The Sociology Press.

Gregory, Sean (2004). *Quality and Effectiveness in Creative Music Workshop Practice: an evaluation of language, meaning and collaborative process*. Unpublished MPhil Thesis, Royal College of Art, London.

Gregory, Sean (2005). The creative music workshop: a contextual study of its origin and practice. In G. Odam and N. Bannan (eds.), *The Reflective Conservatoire*. London: Guildhall School of Music & Drama / Aldershot: Ashgate.

Hegel, Georg Wilhelm Friedrich (1955). *Ästhetik*, Vol. 1 and 2. Berlin: Aufbau Verlag.

Illeris, Knud (2004). *The three dimensions of learning*. Frederiksberg: Roskilde University Press / Leicester: Niace.

Joas, Hans (1988). Symbolischer Interaktionismus. Von der Philosophie des Pragmatismus zu einer soziologischen Forschungstradition. *Kölner Zeitschrift für Soziologie und Sozialpsychologie*, 40, nr. 2: 417ff.

Jordan, Brigitte (1989). Cosmopolitical obstetrics; some insights from the training of traditional midwives. *Social Science and Medicine*, 28 (9): 925-944.

Kegan, Robert (2009). What "form" transforms? A constructive-developmental approach to transformative learning. In K. Illeris (ed.), *Contemporary Theories of Learning*. London: Routledge.

Kelle, Udo (1994). *Empirisch begründete Theoriebildung. Zur Logik und Methodologie interpretativer Sozialforschung*. Weinheim: Deutscher Studien Verlag.

Kitwood, Tom (1997). *Dementia reconsidered: the person comes first*. Maidenhead, Berkshire: Open University Press.

Kors, Ninja and Mak, Peter (2007). Vocal Students as Animateurs, a Case Study of Non-Formal Learning. In: P. Mak, N. Kors and P. Renshaw, *Formal, Non-Formal and Informal Learning in Music*. Groningen / The Hague: Research group Lifelong Learning in Music. ISBN 978-90-811273-3-2.

Lave, Jean and Wenger, Etienne (1991). *Situated Learning: legitimate peripheral participation.* Cambridge: Cambridge University Press.

Lave, Jean (1991). Situating learning in communities of practice. In L. Resnick, J. Levine, and S. Teasley (eds.), *Perspectives on socially shared cognition* (p. 63-82). Washington DC: APA.

Lee, Seong-Hie (2002). *Individuelle Modernisierungsprozesse im Alter und Generationsbeziehungen der Frauen in Südkorea.* Diss. phil. University of Goettingen.

Leibniz, Gottfried Wilhelm (1704/1765). *Nouveaux Essais sur l'entendement humain (original title and manuscript* 1704). Published in German as *Neue Abhandlungen über den menschlichen Verstand.*
http://www.zeno.org/Philosophie/M/Leibniz,+Gottfried+Wilhelm/Neue+ Abhandlungen+über+den+menschlichen+Verstand/Vorrede.
Accessed 4 January 2013.

Mead, George Herbert (1903). The Definition of the Psychical. In *Decennial Publications of the University of Chicago,* first series, Vol. III: 77ff.

Mead, George Herbert (1934). *Mind, Self, & Society from the Standpoint of a Social Behaviorist.* Chicago: The University of Chicago Press.

Mead, George Herbert (1967). *Mind, Self and Society. From the Standpoint of a Social Behaviorist.* Edited and with an Introduction by Charles W. Morris. Works, Vol. 1. Chicago and London: The University of Chicago Press.

Mezirow, Jack (1990). How Critical Reflection Triggers Transformative Learning. In J. Mezirov and associates, *Fostering Critical Reflection in Adulthood.* San Francisco: Jossey Bass.

Mezirow, Jack (2009). An overview on transformative learning. In K. Illeris (ed.), *Contemporary Theories of Learning.* London: Routledge.

Nachmanovitch, Stephen (1990). *Freeplay: Improvisation in Life and Art.* New York: Penguin Putnam.

Peirce, Charles Sanders (1991). *Schriften zum Pragmatismus und Pragmatizismus,* hg. von Karl-Otto Apel. Frankfurt am Main: Suhrkamp.

Parsons, Talcott (1951). *The Social System.* New York: Free Press.

Peters, Gary (2009). *The Philosophy of Improvisation.* Chicago: University of Chicago Press.

Platon (1988). *Sämtliche Dialoge.* Vol. 5. Hamburg: Meiner.

Polanyi, Michael (1966). *The tacit dimension.* New York: Doubleday.

Polanyi, Michael (1969). *Knowing and Being.* Edited with an introduction by Marjorie Grene. Chicago: The University of Chicago Press.

Renshaw, Peter (2001). *Globalisation, Music and Identity*. Unpublished keynote address presented to the International Music Council in Tokyo, September 2001.

Renshaw, Peter (2006/2009). *Lifelong Learning for Musicians: The Place of Mentoring*. Groningen / The Hague: Research group Lifelong Learning in Music. ISBN 90-811273-2-2.

Renshaw, Peter (2007). Lifelong Learning for Musicians. Critical issues arising from a case study of *Connect*. In: P. Mak, N. Kors and P. Renshaw, *Formal, Non-Formal and Informal Learning in Music*. Groningen / The Hague: Research group Lifelong Learning in Music.
ISBN nr. 978-90-811273-3-2.

Renshaw, Peter (2010). *Engaged Passions: Searches for Quality in Community Contexts*. Delft: Eburon Academic Publishers.

Rogers, Carl R. (1961). *On Becoming a Person: A therapist's view of psychotherapy*. London: Constable & Robinson.

Rosa, Hartmut (2004). *Beschleunigung. Die Veränderung der Zeitstrukturen in der Moderne*. Frankfurt am Main: Suhrkamp.

Rose, Linda and Schlingensiepen, Stephanie (2001). Meeting in the dark: a musical journal of discovery. *Journal of Dementia Care* vol. 9, nr. 2: 20-23.

Rose, Linda and De Martino, Hilary (2008). Music for Life: a model for reflective practice. *Journal of Dementia Care* vol. 16, nr. 3: 20-23.

Sacks, Oliver (2008). *Musicophilia, Tales of Music and the Brain*. London: Picador.

Sawyer, Keith (2000). Improvisation and the Creative Process: Dewey Collingwood and the Aesthetics of Spontaneity. *The Journal of Aesthetics and Art Criticism,* 58/2: 149-161.

Schön, Donald A. (1983). *The Reflective Practitioner; How Professionals think in Action*. Aldershot: Ashgate.

Schön, Donald A. (1987). *Educating the Reflective Practitioner; Toward a new Design for Teaching and Learning in the Professions*. San Francisco: Jossey-Bass.

Schütz, Alfred and Luckmann, Thomas (1979). *Strukturen der Lebenswelt*. Vol. 1. Frankfurt am Main: Suhrkamp.

Smilde, Rineke (2006). Lifelong Learning for Musicians. *Proceedings of the 81st Annual Meeting of the National Association of Schools of Music, held in Boston, USA in 2005*. Reston: NASM.

Smilde, Rineke (2009a). *Musicians as Lifelong Learners: Discovery through Biography*. Delft: Eburon Academic Publishers.

Smilde, Rineke (2009b). *Musicians as Lifelong Learners: 32 Biographies*. Delft: Eburon Academic Publishers.

Smilde, Rineke (2011). Musicians Reaching out to People Living with Dementia: Perspectives of Learning. In H. Herzberg and E. Kammler (eds), *Biographie und Gesellschaft; Ueberlegungen zu einer Theorie des modernen Selbst*. Frankfurt/New York: Campus Verlag.

Steptoe, Andrew S. (1989). Stress, Coping and Stage Fright in Professional Musicians. *Psychology of Music* 17: 3-11.

Strauss, Anselm L. (1987). *Qualitative Analysis for Social Scientists*. Cambridge: Cambridge University Press.

Strauss, Anselm L. and Corbin, Juliet (1990). Grounded Theory Research: Procedures, Canons and Evaluative Criteria. *Zeitschrift für Soziologie*, 19: 418ff.

Strauss, Anselm L. and Corbin, Juliet (1990a). *Basics of Qualitative Research: Techniques and Procedures for Developing Grounded Theory*. London: Sage.

Weber, Max (1947). *The Theory of Social and Economic Organisation*. Edited by T. Parsons. London: William Hodge and Company Limited.

Wenger, Etienne (1998). *Communities of Practice, Learning, Meaning and Identity*. Cambridge, USA: Cambridge University Press.

Wenger, Etienne (2009). A social theory of learning. In K. Illeris (ed.), *Contemporary Theories of Learning*. Oxon: Routledge.

Wigram, Tony (2004). *Improvisation: Methods and Techniques for Music Therapy Clinicians, Educators and Student*. London: Jessica Kingsley Publishers.

List of graphics and musical transcriptions

Index

Shared leadership: see Leadership

Shared ownership: see Ownership

Situated learning: 24, 232

Social activity: 244, 245, 246

Social sensitivity: 243, 244

Social skills: 249

Socrates: 212

Sound (world): 90, 122, 164, 167, 203

Space (as a concept and physical): 26, 31, 75, 85, **100ff.**, 145, 146, 147, 153, 164, 166, 168, 171, 172, 173, 174, 196, 197, 201, 205, 206, 207, 208, 210, 214, 215, 229

Space of social learning: 245

Spirituality: 14, 15, 143, 204

Staff development practitioner: 5, 18, 46, 53, 67, 73, 76, 78, 85, 88, 217, 227, 240, 245

Stage fright: 243

Strauss, Anselm: 34

Support (as a concept): 193, 202, 203, 204, 214, 215, 216, 217, 220

Sustainability (as a concept): **222ff.**

Synchronicity (as a concept in applied improvisation): 28

Tacit knowledge, tacit dimension: 23, 28, 236

Tactile: 30, 142, 164, 167, 189

Thick description: iv, 240

Threatened identity: see Identity

Timalation: 11, 142

Transformative learning: 23, 194

Transformative processes: 23

Transition: 8, 9, 21, 22, 101, 103, 147, 152, 163, **180ff.**, 181, 182, 183, 184, 185, 231, 245

Transitional knowledge: 22

Transitional learning: 23, 85, 212, **228ff.**, 229, 230, 245

Translation (as a concept in applied improvisation): 29, 32, 72, 100, 168

About the authors

Rineke Smilde PhD is a flautist, musicologist and music educationalist. She is Professor in Lifelong Learning in Music at Hanze University of Applied Sciences (Prince Claus Conservatoire) in Groningen and Professor of Music Pedagogy at the University of Music and Performing Arts in Vienna. Rineke Smilde co-leads the international research group 'Lifelong Learning in Music', part of the Centre of Applied Research and Innovation 'Art and Society' of the Hanze University. The research group examines questions about the relationship between musicians and society, and what engaging with new audiences means for the different roles, learning and leadership of musicians. Rineke Smilde's particular research interests are the learning styles of musicians and the role of biographical learning in the context of lifelong and lifewide learning. She has published various articles and book chapters on different aspects of lifelong learning in (higher) music education. She lectures and gives presentations worldwide and has led various international research groups for the European Association of Conservatoires (AEC).

Kate Page, MMus (in Leadership; Guildhall School of Music & Drama) is a musician, specialising in the facilitation of creative music workshops, alongside her work as an oboist and multi-instrumentalist in collaborative performance projects, arts management, research and tuition. Based in Perth, Western Australia, she develops creative projects in partnership with a variety of organisations in the public and private sector, working in both formal and informal learning environments alongside a diverse range of people right from babies to older people. She was formerly the project manager for Music for Life at Wigmore Hall In London.

Dr. Dr. Peter Alheit is educationalist and sociologist, Emeritus Professor at the University of Goettingen, Germany and former holder of the Chair of General Pedagogy. He is considered a world expert on biographical research and lifelong learning. He was one of the founders of the European Society for Research on the Education of Adults (ESREA), held numerous guest professorships and has been involved in a number of European research projects. Peter Alheit is a member of the editorial board of various international research journals. His publications include more than 50 books, an abundance of articles in sociology and education with selected examples of translations into 15 languages. He serves as scientific advisor of the research group 'Lifelong Learning in Music' at Hanze University of Applied Sciences in Groningen, the Netherlands.

Printed in Great Britain
by Amazon

20994419R00189